T0339672

Minimizing the Risk of Alzheimer's Disease

MINIMIZING THE RISK OF ALZHEIMER'S DISEASE

FRANK MURRAY

Algora Publishing
New York

Library of Congress Cataloging-in-Publication Data —

Murray, Frank, 1924-
  Minimizing the risk of Alzheimer's disease / Frank Murray.
    pages cm
  Includes bibliographical references.
    ISBN 978-0-87586-934-6 (hard cover: alk. paper) — ISBN 978-0-87586-933-9 (soft
cover: alk. paper) — ISBN 978-0-87586-935-3 (ebook) (print) 1. Alzheimer's disease—
Risk factors. 2. Alzheimer's disease—Prevention. I. Title.
    RC523.M86 2012
    616.831—dc23
                                2012031384

Printed in the United States

TABLE OF CONTENTS

INTRODUCTION

As baby-boomers start to reach retirement age, government statistics predict an epidemic of Alzheimer's disease which threatens to overwhelm America's health-care system. As a nation, we have a problem, but as individuals, we each can work to minimize the risk to ourselves and our families. Throughout the book, we will be discussing vitamins, minerals, and lifestyle choices that each of us can use to protect ourselves against Alzheimers and other forms of age-related dementia.

Over half of the Alzheimer's cases in the world could be prevented if we eliminated those risk factors that we have control over, such as depression, obesity, and smoking, either with lifestyle changes or treatment of underlying conditions.

That was the conclusion of researchers participating in the Alzheimer's Association International Conference that was held in Paris, France, July 19, 2011, and reported in The Lancet Neurology/HealthDay News. Many additional points were highlighted at this conference, including these:

Just a 25% reduction in 7 common risk factors could prevent up to 3 million Alzheimer's cases around the world and up to 500,000 in the United States alone.

Some risk factors appear to have a greater impact on Alzheimer's risk than others, according to Deborah Barnes, M.D., of the University of California at San Francisco. Worldwide, she said, 19% of the AD cases are linked to low education; 14% to smoking;

13% to physical inactivity; 10% to depression; 5% to mid-life high blood pressure; 2.4% to diabetes; and 2% to obesity.

In the United States, 21% of the cases could be traced to physical inactivity; 15% to depression; 11% to smoking; 8% to mid-life hypertension; 7% to mid-life obesity; 7% to low education; and 3% to diabetes.

In 2008, the most recent tabulations, an estimated 5.2 million Americans were living with Alzheimer's disease, and that number is expected to grow to 16 million by 2050, according to the Alzheimer's Association in Chicago.

Alzheimer's disease is the 7th leading cause of death in the United States, and the 5th leading cause of death for those over the age of 65, the Association said. From 2000 to 2005, deaths attributed to Alzheimer's disease increased 45%. In contrast, during the same period, deaths from heart disease decreased by 8.6%; deaths from breast cancer went down by 8%; prostate cancer deaths dropped 4.9%; and stroke deaths dropped 14.5%.

"People with Alzheimer's disease, in general, have decreased survival in the general population," the Association said. "One study noted that those with AD survive about half as long as those of similar age who do not have Alzheimer's. Survival time is generally 4 to 6 years after diagnosis, but survival time can be as long as 20 years from the detection of the first symptoms....The direct costs to Medicare and Medicaid for care of those with Alzheimer's and other dementias, and the indirect cost to business for employees who are caring for Alzheimer's patients, amounts to over $148 billion annually," the Association added.

In fact, Medicare currently spends more than three times as much for those 65 years of age and older with Alzheimer's and other dementias than for other beneficiaries. In 2005, Medicare spent $91 billion on patients with Alzheimer's and other dementias who also have a coexisting chronic condition. This figure is considerably higher than that for patients with a chronic condition alone. The Association reported that Medicare costs for those with dementia and diabetes are more than twice that for those with diabetes alone.

Here are other grim statistics concerning Alzheimer's diseases:
- About 500,000 Americans under the age of 65 have Alzheimer's dementia. About 40% have been diagnosed with Alzheimer's.
- One in 8 Americans aged 65 has AD.

- 10 million baby-boomers in the United States will develop AD. By mid-2008, the latest tabulations, it was estimated that an American would be diagnosed with Alzheimer's every 33 seconds.
- One in 6 women and one in 10 men who reach age 55, can expect to develop AD in their lifetime. More women will be diagnosed with the disease since, on average, they live longer than men.
- 69% of nursing home residents have some degree of cognitive impairment.
- 46.4% of nursing home residents have a diagnosis of Alzheimer's disease or another form of dementia in their medical records.

As you will discover throughout this book, it is not too late to adopt lifestyle and nutritional measures to prevent or delay Alzheimer's disease and dementia. Baby-boomers, as a group, are usually financially secure, which means that they have time and money for productive things that stimulate the mind, and that is one key to avoiding dementia in old age. Activities such as traveling, writing, teaching, reading, playing crossword puzzles, lecturing, performing, competing in sports, watching "Jeopardy" and other mind-stimulating TV programs, and building toys or model airplanes are beneficial activities. As explained in the book, use your brain or lose it.

Although I suspect that many professionals may disagree with this view, I think that many Alzheimer's patients suffer from a subclinical deficiency of vitamins, minerals, and other essential nutrients and their aging brains are not getting sufficient nutrients from their impoverished diet. To compound the problem, we do not absorb nutrients as readily as we did when we were younger. As for subclinical deficiencies, you may not have, say, full-blown scurvy, but you can still have a vitamin C deficiency that prevents you from enjoying optimal health.

In addition to a deficient diet, many seniors are taking 5, 6, or more medications, and only a qualified pharmacist can tell if there are any serious consequences of this witch's brew. We do know that when two drugs interact, they can form an entirely new chemical whose profile and side-effects are unknown.

How many seniors are getting an adequate supply of brain-building nutrients each day, such as meat, fish, eggs, dairy, whole grains, fruits, vegetables, and other nutritious fare? Of special interest are fish, fruit, carrots, spinach, walnuts, and berries.

Many seniors do not have money to buy supplements or health-ful foods; they may not have an appetite for nutritious food; many older people do not absorb the nutrients they are getting from their diet due to a lack of the 'intrinsic factor'; and some may not have good enough teeth to chew meat and other fibrous foods. To add to their dilemma, many seniors are very sedentary and may not be able to shop for nutritious fare.

Family and friends can help seniors eat a more nutritious diet by encouraging them to save money by buying sale items at the supermarket; buying in bulk; using supermarket coupons; buy-ing local produce, since it is often cheaper; buying at farmer's mar-kets; and applying for food stamps if they are eligible. If the senior has a chewing problem, offer suggestions for nutritious foods and menus they can use. If they have a chewing problem, suggest they dine on meatloaf rather than meat. Oatmeal, farina, and eggs are wonderful suggestions.

The National Institutes of Health panel issued a consensus statement on Alzheimer's disease. Carl Bell, M.D., one of the panel members, said that, "We don't have any solid evidence that there is anything that will prevent either kind of decline or dementia."[1] Many people, including the scientists at the aforementioned Par-is conference, would disagree. One wonders if the panel members have read the extensive literature, some of which is reported in this book. The panel did admit that many of the studies used in-consistent definitions of cognitive decline; had too few partici-pants; did not cover a long enough timeframe; or had high drop-out rates among the participants.

They forgot to mention, as well, that studies often do not use high potencies of vitamins and other nutrients. Vitamin C and the B-Complex are water-soluble and are very sensitive to heat, light, etc. The vitamin C you had for breakfast exited your body by noon.

Another fly in the gumbo is that information about diet is usu-ally based on food questionnaires filled out by volunteers. How ac-curately do people remember what they ate yesterday, let alone last week?

Panel member Martha Daviglus, M.D., of Northwestern Univer-sity's Feinberg School of Medicine in Chicago, rightly mentioned that physical exercise, anti-depressive medications, and consump-tion of omega-3 fatty acids (fish oils) are promising interventions. These and many other options are explored in this book.

---

1 Reported in the June 23/30, 2010 issue of the Journal of the American Medical Association (JAMA).

In the same issue of JAMA, Martha Clare Morris, Sc.D., and Christine C. Tangney, Ph.D., of Rush University Medical Center in Chicago, in the article "Diet and Prevention of Alzheimer Disease," said that "the investigation of dietary risk factors in the prevention of AD is a relatively young field of research. There are a limited number of studies, and the study findings have not shown consistent evidence for any one dietary factor."

The best evidence, they added, is for antioxidant nutrients, such as vitamin E, omega-3 fatty acids, folic acid, the B vitamin, and others.

There is no valid reason why someone in their 30s, 40s, 50s, and beyond should manifest Alzheimer's disease or dementia. There is plenty of evidence that it can be warded off, and much of it is enumerated in the following pages. Perhaps this book will encourage the naysayers to look more closely. It just might lead to additional breakthroughs in understanding and fighting AD and similar debilitating diseases.

Frank Murray
New York, N. Y.

1. What Is Alzheimer's Disease?

Alzheimer's disease is the most frequent cause or form of dementia. In fact, Alzheimer's accounts for 70% of all cases of dementia in Americans 71 years of age and older. In those 90 and older, Alzheimer's disease is responsible for 80% of all dementias, compared with 47% in those 71 to 90. However, some 500,000 people in their 30s, 40s, and 50s have Alzheimer's or a related dementia, according to the Alzheimer's Association.[1] The disease is named after Alois Alzheimer (1864–1915), a German neurologist.

It is estimated that as many as 5.2 million Americans are living with Alzheimer's disease. By 2050, that number could reach 16 million. Every 71 seconds someone in the U.S. is diagnosed with Alzheimer's.

As might be expected, the number of Alzheimer's cases follows population density, except that Florida, with its large aging population, had the most cases in 2000 (360,000). That number is expected to have increased to 450,000 by 2010.

Next on the list is California with 440,000 in 2000, and this number is expected to have increased to 480,000 by 2010; New York (330,000, to decline to 320,000 by 2010; Pennsylvania (280,000, remaining the same by 2010; Texas (270,000 and 340,000); Illinois (210,000 and remaining the same); and Ohio (200,000 and 230,000).

---

1 "Alzheimer's Disease," Alzheimer's Association, Chicago, Illinois, 2008.

WARNING SIGNS

The Alzheimer's Association has identified ten warning signs to help recognize the disease:

1. Memory loss.
2. Difficulty performing familiar tasks.
3. Problems with language.
4. Disorientation to time and place.
5. Poor or decreased judgment.
6. Problems with abstract thinking.
7. Misplacing things.
8. Changes in mood and behavior.
9. Changes in personality.
10. Loss of initiative.

CAUSES

For the most part, the cause of Alzheimer's disease is unknown, "but most experts agree that the disease, like other chronic conditions, likely develops as a result of multiple factors rather than a single cause," according to the Association. "However, the greatest risk factor is increasing age." In a small percentage of cases Alzheimer's is caused by rare genetic variations; these are found in a few hundred families worldwide. In these inherited forms of Alzheimer's, the disease tends to strike younger people. When the disease is initially recognized in a person under the age of 65, it is referred to as early-onset or young-onset Alzheimer's.

Women are more likely than men to have Alzheimer's disease and dementia. The Association estimates that 14% of those aged 71 and over have dementia. This includes 16% of women and 11% of men in that age group, accounting for 1.4 million people.

Studies find that having fewer years of education can be associated with a greater likelihood of developing dementia. One study found that those with less than 12 years of education had a 15% greater risk of developing dementia than those with 12 to 15 years of education, and a 35% greater risk of developing dementia than people with more than 15 years of education.

"Scientists believe that whatever triggers Alzheimer's begins to damage the brain years before symptoms appear," the Association says. "When symptoms appear, nerve cells that process, store, and retrieve information have already begun to degenerate and die."

Experts consider two abnormal microscopic structures called "plaques" and "tangles" as the hallmarks of Alzheimer's disease. Amyloid plaques are clumps of protein fragments that accumulate between the brain's nerve cells. Tangles are twisted strands of another protein that forms inside brain cells. However, scientists have not yet determined the exact role that plaques and tangles have in the development of the disease.

Just 25 years ago, many textbooks considered Alzheimer's disease to be rare, according to Current Diagnosis and Treatment in Psychiatry. Before 1975, a computer search of the medical literature identified fewer than 50 papers that addressed Alzheimer's disease as a key word. However, a search in 2000 found 12,718 citations.[1]

Behavioral manifestations of the disease, such as temper outbursts, screaming, agitation, and severe personality changes, are more troubling than the cognitive difficulties, the publication said. No two patients are exactly alike when it comes to these behavioral manifestations. Only recently has this aspect of the disease received substantial attention.

"Alzheimer's disease represents an imbalance between neuronal injury and repair," the publication added. "Factors contributing to injury may include free-radical formation, vascular insufficiency, inflammation, head trauma, hypoglycemia (low blood sugar), and aggregated beta-amyloid protein."

Factors which contribute to ineffective repair may include the presence of Apo lipoprotein E (ApoE)-E4 gene, altered synthesis of amyloid precursor protein, hypothyroidism (diminished production of thyroid hormone), and estrogen deficit.

Plaques and tangles identify the illness at the microscopic level, and amyloid plaques occur in large numbers in severe cases, according to Current Diagnosis and Treatment in Psychiatry. These plaques were first recognized in 1892. PAS (p-aminosalicylic acid) or Congo Red stains (an acid direct cotton dye) identify these structures. PAS is an abbreviation for periodic acid-Schiff stain, which was named after Hugo Schiff (1834–1915), a German chemist who lived in Florence, Italy. The stain is used to identify proteins.

The beta-amyloid protein appears early in the brain of Alzheimer's disease, and some studies suggest it is toxic to mature neurons in the brains of AD patients.

1 Ebert, Michael H., M.D., et al., editors. Current Diagnosis and Treatment in Psychiatry. New York: McGraw-Hill/Lange Medical Books, 2000, pp. 203ff.

"Neurons in these areas begin to develop neurofibrillary tangles, and amyloid plaques and tangles gradually accumulate in the frontal, temporal, and parietal lobes," says Current Diagnosis. "The density of plaques determines postmortem diagnosis. Researchers find that the number of neurons and synapses is reduced, and this is especially true of acetylcholine-cholinergic-containing neurons in the basal nucleus of Meynert, which project to wide areas of the cerebral cortex. Theodor H. Meynert (1833–1892), a Vienna neurologist, first isolated these retroflex (bent) bundles."

PET (positron emission tomography) stains demonstrate a reduction in acetylcholinesterase and decreased binding of cholinergic ligands (groups of molecules). Hirano bodies and gramulovascular generation occur in the hippocampus and represent further degeneration.

"Neurofibrillary tangles contain an abnormally phosphorylated protein named tau, and the abnormal phosphorylation of this protein probably causes defective construction of microtubules and neurofilaments," the publication says. "Neural thread protein is found in the long axonal processes that emerge from the nerve cell body, and it is found in conjunction with neurofibrillary tangles. This protein may be involved in neural repair and regeneration." Furthermore, neurons bearing neurofibrillary tangles often project to brain regions that are rich in senile plaques containing beta-amyloid. These plaques are found in areas innervated by cholinergic neurons, and cholinergic neurons in the hippocampus and the basal nucleus of Meynert degenerate early in AD, causing impairment of cortical and hippocampal neurotransmission and cognitive difficulty.

The affected cortical areas become automatically disconnected, and one of the earliest areas to be severed is the hippocampus, which is why memory disorder is one of the earliest manifestations of AD.

In time, there is a loss of communication between other cortical zones, and the subsequent loss of higher cognitive abilities.

Chromosome 21 has been implicated in Alzheimer's disease, since it is well known that patients with Down's syndrome are very likely to develop the histological features of AD, according to the same publication. Named after John Langdon H. Down (1828–1896), an English physician, Down's syndrome is a chromosomal disturbance in chromosome 21. The incidence of leukemia is increased and Alzheimer's disease is almost inevitable by the age of 40.

Several mutations of the amyloid precursor protein gene on chromosome 21 have been described by researchers, and these mutations increase the production of an abnormal amyloid that has been associated with neurotoxicity.

"Another early form of early onset disease has been localized to a variety of defects on chromosome 14, and these mutations are associated with presenilin 1 and account for the majority of familial Alzheimer's cases. A mutation of chromosome 1 is associated with presenilin 2, and both of these mutations also cause increased production of amyloid."

The ApoE-4 gene is associated with the risk of late-onset familial and sporadic forms of AD. ApoE is a plasma protein involved in the transport of cholesterol, and it is encoded by a gene on chromosome 19. Disease risk increases in proportion to the number of these gene alleles (genes).

DIAGNOSIS

Experienced doctors can make a diagnosis with more than 90% accuracy, according to the Association. Because there is no single test for Alzheimer's, diagnosis usually involves consideration of a thorough medical history and physical examination, followed by tests to assess memory and the overall function of the mind and nervous system. Changes observed by friends and families in the patient's memory or thinking skills also contribute to a diagnosis.

It can be, however, difficult to distinguish Alzheimer's from the various types of dementia. Dementia is a general term for a group of brain disorders that affect memory, judgment, personality, and other mental functions, although Alzheimer's disease is the most common form of dementia.

"Vascular dementia, another common form, results from reduced blood flow to the brain's nerve cells," the Association said. "In some cases, Alzheimer's disease and vascular dementia can occur simultaneously in a condition called 'mixed dementia.' Other causes of dementia include front temporal dementia, dementia with Lewy bodies, Creutzfeldt-Jakob disease, and Parkinson's disease."

A diagnosis of Alzheimer's disease is usually made by a process of elimination — only an autopsy of the brain can reveal the definitive evidence — and it is important when suspecting Alzheimer's to eliminate other factors that can cause memory loss or that mimic Alzheimer's, explained Robert M. Griller, M.D.[1]

Some other factors that may mimic Alzheimer's include:

1. Drug interactions. Many people, especially older people, take various prescription and nonprescription medications that could be having an effect on their memory, either alone or due to an interaction with another drug.

2. High blood pressure. Uncontrolled blood pressure, often caused by hardening of the arteries, can cause strokes that destroy brain tissue and result in memory loss.

3. Infections. Various infections, including syphilis, can cause symptoms that result in Alzheimer's. Lyme disease has recently been recognized as a cause of symptoms that have been mistaken for Alzheimer's.

4. Poor thyroid function. A thyroid gland that is not functioning poorly can also cause Alzheimer's-like symptoms.

5. Brain tumor. The pressure from a brain tumor can disrupt the normal functioning of the brain, causing symptoms that involve memory.

He recalled a fascinating study by which simple forgetfulness can be distinguished from Alzheimer's. Patients were asked to draw the face of a clock with the time showing 2:45. Those who were able to do so, in spite of other symptoms, were found to be normal. Those with Alzheimer's could not draw the clock.

An important goal of the diagnostic workup is to determine whether symptoms may be due to a condition other than Alzheimer's. For example, depression, medication side effects, certain thyroid conditions, excess use of alcohol and nutritional imbalances are all potential factors that may sometimes impair memory or other mental functions. Even if the diagnosis is Alzheimer's disease, timely identification enables people to take an active role in their own treatment decisions and planning for the future, the Association added.

Early detection of Alzheimer's disease is beneficial in that it gives patients a chance to plan for the future and to take medications to keep symptoms from worsening, reported Shirley S. Wang.[2] "Screening proponents say the Alzheimer's tests are quick, easy to use, and can identify most people with memory problems who warrant further evaluation. Screening can involve just a few

---

1 Giller, Robert M., M.D., and Matthews, Kathy. *Natural Prescriptions*. New York: Carol Southern Books, 1994, p. 8.
2 Wang, Shirley S. "How Soon Is Too Soon to Screen People for Alzheimer's Disease?" *The Wall Street Journal*, December 18, 2007, p. D1.

tests, such as word recall. And it could be part of a routine physical for patients over 65 years of age."

This is a proposal from the Alzheimer's Disease Screening Discussion Group, a group of academic health centers, drug companies, and patient-advocacy groups that met at a drug-industry meeting in November 2007.

However, some researchers, physicians and patient advocates, including the Alzheimer's Association, suggest the current push for widespread screening is premature, since there are no data to suggest any benefit from screening people who do not have memory complaints. In addition, there are potential negative consequences, including false positives (data may suggest potential Alzheimer's when there is none) that put patients at risk for depression and anxiety. Patients may worry that if they screen positive, they might lose their driving licenses or jobs, or have trouble getting life insurance, even if their symptoms don't affect their daily functioning.

"Some doctors also note that it doesn't help to diagnose people who don't have noticeable memory problems because existing medications appear to help only those who are already suffering clear symptoms," Wang continued. "A recent study in the Journal of General Internal Medicine found that of 524 adults screened in a doctor's office, only 1 in 5 who screened positive was referred to a specialist or received a diagnosis or a prescription for medication."

Here are places to find information and support on the Web:
- Alzheimer's Foundation of America (www.alzfdn.org)
- Alzheimer's Association (www.alz.org)
- Alzheimer's Disease Education and Referral Center (www.nia.nih.gov/alzheimers).

Most older adults, including those with dementia, depend on general practitioners for their health care, reports Christopher M. Callahan, M.D., and colleagues at the University Center for Aging Research in Indianapolis.[1] Primary care physicians prescribe the majority of psychiatric medications to older patients, but the primary care setting appears to be poorly designed and undersourced to provide comprehensive management approaches for dementia."

Quality efforts for geriatric syndromes in primary care have focused on decision support, care management, and other systems-level innovations to deliver guideline-level care," the researchers added. "Although recent evidence that early recognition and

---

1 Callahan, Christopher M., M.D., et al. "Effectiveness of Collaborative Care for Older Adults with Alzheimer Disease in Primary Care," JAMA 295(18) :2148-2157, 2006.

treatment of cognitive impairment may improve patient outcomes, there is continued controversy about the cost and utility of screening and early diagnosis, and continued debate about the effectiveness of cholinesterase inhibitors. Found in cobra venom, cholinesterase is a family of enzymes capable of catalyzing (altering) the hydrolysis of acylcholines and other chemicals.

"Behavioral and psychological symptoms of dementia represent a major challenge in the care of older adults with Alzheimer's disease," the research team continued. "These symptoms, which include a broad range of distressing behaviors and psychological reactions, affect the health and quality of life of both the patient and his/her caregiver, since over 90% of patients with dementia will experience symptoms at some time during their illness."

Leaving patients' behavior and psychological symptoms of dementia untreated has been associated with caregiver burnout, nursing home placement, poor management of comorbid (an unrelated disease) conditions, and excess health care costs.

In their study, intervention patients received one year of care management by an interdisciplinary team led by an advanced practice nurse working with the patient's family, caregiver, and integrated within primary care. The team utilized standard protocol to initiate treatment and identity, monitor, and treat behavioral and psychological symptoms of dementia, stressing nonpharmacological management.

The researchers concluded that, "Collaborative care for the treatment of Alzheimer's disease resulted in significant improvement in the quality of care and in behavioral and psychological symptoms of dementia among primary care patients and their caregivers. These improvements were achieved without significantly increasing the use of antipsychotics or sedative hypnotics."

The amyloid plaques found in the brain of Alzheimer's patients may form more rapidly than previously suspected, according to Tracy Hampton, Ph.D.[1]

Using a microscopic imaging technique called longitudinal in vivo multiphoton microscopy to examine brain tissue in animals with the disease, researchers from Neurodegenerative Disease in Charlestown, Massachusetts, found that plaques form quickly every 24-hour period. They also observed that within 1 to 2 days of a new plaque's appearance, microglia (small nervous system cells) are activated and recruited to the site. "The findings may help to solve a long-standing debate regarding whether plaques precede

---

1 Hampton, Tracy, Ph.D. "Alzheimer Plaques," JAMA 299(13):1533, 2008.

and induce the neuronal abnormalities seen in dementia, or are simply a byproduct of other alterations in the brain."

Although the ApoE-4 gene is associated with an increased risk of developing Alzheimer's disease, it appears that having two ApoE-4 genes is associated with a slower clinical course, according to Archives of Neurology. The findings are consistent with hypotheses that the biological process contributing to the onset of AD are different from those determining its clinical course.[1]

At the Alzheimer's Disease Research Center in St. Louis, Missouri, researchers determined that follow-up clinical data found that brain volume reduction associated with socioeconomic status (SES) was greater in those who later developed very mild dementia, compared with those who remained nondemented.[2]

The researchers reported that privileged nondemented older adults have more preclinical brain atrophy that is consistent with their having greater reserves against Alzheimer's disease.

A research team at the Veterans Affairs Puget Sound Healthcare System in Seattle, Washington, evaluated 3,308 elderly residents of Cache County, Utah. They were aware that Apo-E is a strong genetic risk factor for AD.[3] They estimated that the 100-year lifetime incidence of AD at 72%, suggesting that 28% of the people would not develop AD over any reasonable life expectancy. They added that ApoE-4 acts as a potent risk factor for AD by accelerating its onset. However, the risk of the disease appears heterogeneous in ways independent of ApoE, and it appears that some people escape Alzheimer's, even over an extended lifespan. This suggests other genes or environmental factors that need to be investigated.

A chemical, a common class of drugs, and lifestyle factors are all implicated as a risk for cognitive decline or neurological disease, reported Bridget M. Kuehn in the May 28, 2008 issue of the Journal of the American Medical Association. This was the gist of observations from the Annual Meeting of the American Academy of Neurology, which met April 2008 in Chicago, Illinois.[4]

The meeting reported that formaldehyde exposure is linked to an increased risk of amyotrophic lateral sclerosis (ALS, Lou Geh-

---

1 Hoyt, B. D., et al. "Individual Growth Curve Analysis of ApoE-4 Associated Cognitive Decline in Alzheimer Disease," Archives of Neurology 62:454-459, 2005.

2 Fotenos, A. F., et al. "Brain Volume Decline in Aging: Evidence for a Relation Between Socioeconomic Status, Preclinical Alzheimer Disease, and Reserve," Archives of Neurology 65:113-120, 2008.

3 Khachaturian, A. S., et al. "Apolipoprotein E4 Count Affects Age at Onset of Alzheimer's Disease, But Not Lifetime Susceptibility: The Cache County Study," Archives of General Psychiatry 61:518-524, 2004.

4 Kuehn, Bridget M. "Researchers Identify Neurological Risks," JAMA 299(20):2375-2376, 2008.

rig's disease), the use of anticholinergic drugs to faster cognitive decline, and heavy smoking and drinking to an earlier onset of Alzheimer's disease.

One of the participants indicated that previous studies have linked anticholinergic medications with poor cognitive outcome in patients with Alzheimer's disease. Anticholinergic drugs (Atropine, etc.) are drugs that block the effects of acetylcholine, a chemical that is released from nerve endings in the autoimmune nervous system. They stimulate muscle contraction, slow the heart beat, etc.

However, Jack Tsao, M.D., of Uniformed Services University of Health Sciences in Bethesda, Maryland, confirmed that he and his colleagues have found patients without preexisting cognitive impairment experience rapid — and, in some cases — reversible — cognitive decline while taking an anticholinergic medication for an overactive bladder.

Tsao added that it appeared that medications with the strongest anticholinergic activity, predominantly those for overactive bladder, had greater effects on cognition, and he and his colleagues are doing further analysis of the data to determine whether there may be an additive effect on cognition when patients take multiple drugs in this class, Kuehn added.

"Many drugs with anticholinergic effects, including tolterodine, ranitidine, warfarin, hydrochlorothiazide, and furosemide, are commonly used to treat elderly patients," Kuehn continued. "Tsao recommended that physicians refer elderly patients for baseline cognitive assessment to monitor for cognitive effects."

Another speaker, Ranjan Duara, M.D., of the Wien Center for Alzheimer's Disease and Memory Disorders at Mount Sinai Medical Center in Miami Beach, Florida, and colleagues, examined the impact of having the ApoE-4 gene, smoking, and drinking and the age at the onset of AD. The research team analyzed data on 938 people from the Late Onset Alzheimer's Disease Trial, who were older than 60, and who had a possible or probable diagnosis of AD. Commenting on this, Kuehn said "Those who carried the ApoE-4 variant developed AD 3 years earlier on average than those who were not carriers. Those who had a history of smoking one or more packs of cigarettes per day developed the disorder 2.3 years earlier than these who smoked less than one pack or none at all."

In addition, those who drank more than 2 drinks/day developed AD 4.8 years sooner than those who drank two or fewer drinks a day or not at all. "The risk factors were also additive, with people who had all 3 risk factors developed the disease 8.5 years earlier than those who had none of the 3 risk factors," Kuehn continued. "The 17 people in the study who had all 3 risk factors developed Alzheimer's at an average of 68.5 years, while the 374 people with none of these risk factors developed the disease on average at 77 years of age."

Duara was quoted as saying that, since the prevalence of Alzheimer's increases with age, delaying the age of onset by 5 years could reduce the prevalence of the disease by 50%.

In another study reported at the meeting, Deniz Erten-Lyons, M.D., of the Oregon Health and Science University in Portland, and colleagues, reported that having a large hippocampus may protect against the development of dementia. The hippocampus is a carved ridge that extends over the floor of the brain, and it consists of gray matter covered on the ventricular surface with white matter.

The research team conducted postmortem exams of the brains of 12 people who exhibited healthy cognitive function a year before their death, but whose brains contained many AD-type plaques when compared with 23 people who had the same level of plaques but who were diagnosed with AD prior to their death. It was found that the hippocampus was 20% larger in the group that maintained good cognitive function, compared with those who developed dementia, Kuehn added.

Researchers at the Stockholm Gerontology Research Center in Sweden, reported that both low diastolic (resting) and high systolic pressure (beating) are associated with an increased risk of Alzheimer's disease and dementia in the elderly populations, Low diastolic pressure is thought to increase dementia risk by affecting cerebral function.[1]

A community-based dementia-free cohort of volunteers, ranging in age from 75 to 101, were examined twice within 6 years to detect dementia. During the trial period, 339 patients (out of 1,270) were diagnosed with dementia, including 256 with Alzheimer's disease.

Those with a very high systolic pressure (over 180 vs. 141-180 mmHg) had an adjusted relative risk of 1.5 for Alzheimer's disease and 1.6 for dementia. Low systolic pressure (less than 140 mmHg) was not related to dementia. In contrast, high diastolic pressure (over 90 mmHg) was not associated with dementia incidence, but

---

1 Qiu, Chenghuan, et al. "Low Blood Pressure and Risk of Dementia in the Kungsholmen Project; A 6-Year Follow-up Study," Archives of Neurology 60:223-228, 2003.

extremely low diastolic pressure (less than 65 vs. 66-90 mmHg) produced an adjusted relative risk of 1.7 for AD and 1.5 for dementia. The latter was especially pronounced in those who used antihypertensive drugs.

Researchers are predicting that it may be possible to detect the development of Alzheimer's disease and to track its progress using positron emission tomography (PET), reported the New England Journal of Medicine.[1]

Researchers have focused on 2 proteins — beta-amyloid and tau — that accumulate in various regions of the brain as mild cognitive impairment indication of AD. Unfortunately, these patterns are usually not identified except by autopsy or biopsy.

In the study, the research team injected an amyloid-binding radiotracer into patients with reported memory impairment to determine whether or not they had AD, mild cognitive impairment, or no discernible symptoms.

The study involved 83 patients, ranging in age from 49 to 84, who had undergone neurologic and psychiatric evaluation using PET. It was found that 25 had AD, 28 had mild cognitive impairment, and 30 had normal cognitive functioning.

The volunteers were then injected with FDDNP, a fluorescing constituent that binds to senile plaques and neurofibrillary tangles and subjected to PET and magnetic resonance imaging. With these procedures, researchers are able to accurately track the progression of Alzheimer's disease, the publication reported.

Disruptive behavior is rather common in Alzheimer's disease, and this predicts cognitive decline, functional decline, and institutionalization, reported Archives of Neurology. However, mortality was not affected.[2]

The study involved 497 patients with early-stage AD — having a mean Felstein Mini-Mental State Exam score 20 of 30 at the beginning of the study — who underwent semiannual follow-up as long as 14 years. Recruits came from five university-based AD centers in the United States and Europe.

Using the Columbia University Scale for Psychopathology in Alzheimer Disease — administered every 6 months — the presence of disruptive behavior (wandering, verbal outbursts, physical threats/violence, agitation/restlessness, and sundowning) was extracted and examined as a time-dependent predictor in Cox mod-

---

1 Small, G. W., et al. "PET of Brain Amyloid and Tau in Mild Cognitive Impairment," New England Journal of Medicine 355(25): 2652-2663, 2006.
2 Scarmeas, N., et al. Disruptive Behavior As a Predictor of Alzheimer Disease," Archives of Neurology 64: 1755-1761, 2007.

els. The Cox II inhibitors allow practical use of nonsteroidal anti-inflammatory agents for the prevention of AD. (Sundowning is the onset or exacerbation of delirium during the night, but usually disappears during the day. It is seen in the later stages of AD.)

When both parents have Alzheimer's disease, there is an increased risk of the disease in their children, according to Archives of Neurology. However, the role of family history and the genes involved require a better definition.[1]

In the study involving 111 couples, 297 of the children surviving to adulthood or 22.6% of the adult children have developed AD. The risk of AD in these children increases with age, being 31.0% in those older than 60, and 41.8% in those older than 70.

As is often the case, ApoE-4 gene played an important part in this development, although it did not explain all cases of AD in the children.

In the largest twin study at the time, Swedish researchers confirmed that heritability for Alzheimer's disease is high and that the same genetic factors are influential for both men and women, according to Archives of General Psychiatry. However, nongenetic factors also play an important role and might be the focus for interventions to reduce the risk or delay onset of the disease.[2]

The study involved 11,884 twin pairs, among whom there were 392 pairs in which one or both had Alzheimer's disease. The participants were 65 or older. The group included male monozygotic twins, female monozygotic twins, male dizygotic twins, female dizygotic twins, and unlike-sex twins. Monozygotic means derived from a single egg, while dizygotic refers to fraternal twins.

Heritability for Alzheimer's was estimated to be 58% in the full model, and 79% in the best-fitting model, with the remaining of variations explained by nonshared environmental influences. There were no significant differences between men and women.

A urinary tract infection is the most common cause of delirium in patients with Alzheimer's disease. Constipation is a common and lesser cause of the disease.[3] Patients tend to become confused and agitated because they do not know how to deal with their uncomfortable predicament. However, it is important for physicians or caregivers to rule out nongastrointestinal medical conditions

1 Jayadev, S., et al. "Conjugal Alzheimer Disease: Risk in Children When Both Parents Have Alzheimer Disease," Archives of Neurology 66:373-378, 2008.
2 Gatz, M., et al. "Role of Genes and Environments for Explaining Alzheimer Disease," Archives of General Psychiatry 63:168-174, 2006.
3 Jancin, B. "Urinary Tract Infections, Constipation Can Cause Alzheimer's Dysfunction," Family Practice News, December 1, 2000, p. 12.

that can affect personality before turning to antipsychotic medications, the publication added.

Benzodiazepines are not good medications to use in this instance, since they cause sedation, thus increasing confusion and falls. Therefore, these medications require close monitoring, the publication said.

In evaluating 1,283 traumatic brain injury cases, 31 developed Alzheimer's disease, which is similar to a number that would be expected, according to the American Journal of Epidemiology. The observed time from traumatic brain injury to Alzheimer's disease was less than the expected time to the onset of AD — median of 10 years versus 18 years.[1]

The data suggest that traumatic brain injury reduces the time of onset of AD among those at risk of developing the disease.

A study at Johns Hopkins University School of Medicine evaluated 68 Alzheimer's disease patients, 46 of whom were living, 22 were deceased, and 34 were nondemented controls.[2] An earlier head injury was reported in 20 of the AD patients (29%) and 1 control subject (2.9%). Twenty percent of the familial and 43.5% of the sporadic Alzheimer's cases reportedly had a head injury prior to their death.

A head injury had no effect on the age of dementia onset, but this data suggests that a head injury may be a predisposing factor in the development of Alzheimer's disease, said Zeno Rasmusson, Ph.D.

Scientists have found that near-infrared light, which cannot be seen by the human eye, can pass easily through the skull and brain to pinpoint the plaques and tangles that may indicate Alzheimer's disease, reported AARP Bulletin.[3] The procedure, which is being tested in clinical trials, could be a major advance in detecting the disease earlier and thereby better slowing the progress of the disease.

The research is spearheaded by Eugene Hanlon of the U.S. Department of Veterans Affairs, who is leading a team of experts from the Harvard Medical School and Boston University in Massachusetts.

A research team at the University of Pennsylvania in Philadelphia reported that their study implied about those with mild cog-

1 Nemetz, P. N., et al. "Traumatic Brain Injury and Time to Onset of Alzheimer's Disease: A Population-Based. Study," American Journal of Epidemiology 149(1): 32-40, 1999.
2 Rasmusson, Zeno, Ph.D., et al. "Head Injury As a Risk Factor in Alzheimer's Disease," Brain Injury 9(3):213-219, 1995.
3 Yared, Rebecca. "Shining a Light on Alzheimer's," AARP Bulletin 49(4): 20, May 2008.

nitive impairment (MCI) have increased brain oxidative damage before the onset of symptoms of dementia.[1]

The isoprostane component, a specific marker of lipid peroxidation in the body, is increased in Alzheimer's disease, the researchers said. The pathological changes associated with Alzheimer's have a long silent phase before the appearance of clinical symptoms.

A number of studies have revealed that AD is preceded by a prodromal (early symptom) phase characterized by mild cognitive impairment, the researchers added.

To investigate levels of this biomarker in patients with mild cognitive impairment, the researchers used gas chromatography — mass spectrometry analysis levels in urine, blood, and cerebrospinal fluid of those with Alzheimer's, those with MCI, and cognitively normal elderly patients. Participants were enrolled in the Memory Disorders Clinic.

The research team found higher levels of isoprostane in cerebrospinal fluid, blood, and urine in those with MCI, compared with the normal controls.

Cases of early-onset Alzheimer's disease with an autosomal dominant inheritance pattern are rare, but this condition has greatly advanced understanding of the molecular pathogenesis of AD, according to Archives of Neurology.[2]

The researchers describe a patient with very early onset familial AD (less than 40 years of age), with unusual pathological features and a novel mutation in the Presenilin 1 (PSEN-1) gene.

The patient underwent full clinical assessment and postmortem examination at the Washington University Alzheimer's Disease Research Center in St. Louis, Missouri. However, limited pathological samples and autopsy records of two affected family members were not available.

The research team reported that dementia developed in 3 family members at a mean age of 27, and the patient that was studied had myoclonus (shock-like contractions), seizures, and rigidity; that was similar to findings in previously studied patients with PSEN-1 mutations.

All 3 family members were confirmed to have AD by neurological exams, and the patient that was studied also had widespread Lewy body pathology in the brainstem, limbic areas, and neo-

---

1 Domenico, Pratico, et al. "Increase of Brain Oxidative Stress in Mild Cognitive Impairment: A Possible Predictor of Alzheimer Disease," Archives of Neurology 59:972-976, 2002.
2 Snider, B. J., et al. "Novel Presenilin 1 Mutation (5170F) Causing Alzheimer Disease with Lewy Bodies in the Third Decade of Life," Archives of Neurology 62: 1821-1830, 2005.

cortex. Lewy bodies were not performed on the other two family members. The patient also had a single mutation in Exon 6 of the PSEN-1 gene, which segregates with disease. Lewy bodies are constituents that are found in pigmented brainstem neurons, especially in Parkinson's disease patients. The researchers said that, to their knowledge, this was the earliest reported onset of pathologically confirmed familial AD and dementia with Lewy bodies.

Neurology reported on 406 spouse caregivers of AD patients who were evaluated for 17 years, with half of them given standard care, and the remaining received specialized counseling. Special counseling involved the patient's spouse caregiver, other family members, support group meetings, as well as telephone counseling.[1] Often, the caregivers are so exhausted from taking care of the patient that they opt to put him/her in an institution. The caregivers and the patients were evaluated for their physical and emotional health at the beginning of the study, and for every 4 months during the first year of evaluation, and then every 6 months.

The research team said that, in the intervention group, there was a 28.3% reduction in the rate of nursing home placement when compared with the controls, which delayed placement of the patient in a special-care facility for 557 days.

The researchers observed that 61% of the caregivers delayed placement in a home due to the caregiver's increased tolerance for the patient's behavior, less depression, as well as satisfaction with the social support.

Creutzfeldt-Jakob's disease, a rare presenile dementia, has a worldwide distribution, reported Carl C. Pfeiffer, Ph.D., M.D. It is caused by a transmissible viral agent, although the symptoms are not characteristic of an infection. There is a premature mental deterioration with lesions occurring in the gray area of the brain. It, and Alzheimer's disease, have the characteristics of senile dementia, although with an earlier onset.[2]

At the former Brain-Bio Center in Princeton, New Jersey, Pfeiffer and his colleagues found a correlation between low spermine levels in the blood and the recent memory loss displayed by presenile and senile dementia patients. Spermine, which is a simple polyamine containing four aminonitrogens, is known to occur in large quantities in semen, blood tissue, and the brain. When measured in the blood, it has been found in high concentrations in pa-

1 Mittelman, M. S., et al. "Counseling Spouse Caregivers of Patients with Alzheimer's Disease," Neurology 67(9): 1592-1599, 2006.
2 Pfeiffer, Carl C., Ph.D., M.D. Mental and Elemental Nutrients, New Canaan, CT: Keats Publishing, Inc., 1975, pp. 447ff.

tients and normals with adequate memory for recent events, and low in patients with presenile and senile dementia.

"Patients on estrogen therapy, those with low blood sugar, and patients with normal aging are found to have low blood spermine levels," Pfeiffer added. "The level is lower in senility than in hypoglycemia (low blood sugar)."

A theory holds that recent memory depends on the brain's ability to synthesize ribonucleic acid (RNA), Pfeiffer continued. "The synthesis of RNA depends on RNA polymerase, which is activated by spermine.

"The four aminonitrogen groups of spermine neutralize the acidic phosphate groups of the nucleic acids in RNA, allowing the synthesis of more RNA," Pfeiffer added. "Recent memory is encoded in the RNA, so that without adequate spermine the recent memory may be faulty. Most of the presenile and senile dementia patients seen at the clinic showed exceedingly low blood spermine levels when compared with controls."

Since spermine levels in the blood decrease with age, young patients with Tourette's syndrome (cursing and motor tics) are also especially low in spermine for their ages. The constituent can be elevated with trace mineral supplements, with manganese appearing to be the most important. The combination of zinc with manganese is most effective in mobilizing copper within the tissues.

He went on to say that copper is high in many neoplastic diseases, and it may be a factor in reversing the usual spermine to spermidine ratio to less than 1. Spermidine is a polyamine found with spermine in many organisms and tissues, such as sperm, and it is necessary for cell and tissue growth.

Emily R. Rosario, M.S., and colleagues, reported that testosterone levels in the brain are depleted as a normal consequence of male aging, and that low brain levels of the male hormone increase the risk of developing Alzheimer's disease.[1] To investigate their hypothesis, the research team analyzed testosterone and estradiol levels in postmortem brain tissue of elderly men, and compared it with their neuropathological diseases. Estradiol is the most potent naturally occurring estrogen, which is found in testes and ovaries. "Brain levels of testosterone significantly decrease with age in men who lack any evidence of neuropathology, suggesting that neural androgen depletion is a normal consequence of aging," the researchers said. "In comparison with the controls, men with Alz-

---

1 Rosario, Emily R., M.S., et. al., "Age-Related Testosterone Depletion and the Development of Alzheimer Disease," JAMA 291(12): 1431-1432, 2004.

heimer's disease exhibit significantly lower testosterone levels in the brain. However, the data suggest that estrogen levels in the male brain are affected neither by advancing age nor AD diagnosis."

While it is not known how testosterone depletion may contribute to AD, the researchers theorize that androgen depletion in male rodents increases brain levels of beta-amyloid, the protein implicated as a causal factor in AD, and decreases neuronal survival upon exposure to toxic insult. "Collectively, these findings suggest that normal, age-related testosterone depletion in the male brain may impair beneficial neural actions of androgens and thereby act as a risk factor for the development of Alzheimer's disease," the researchers added. Androgen is a generic term for hormones such as testosterone, and resterone, etc.

An experimental drug that depletes the body of a protein that helps anchor damaging deposits of amyloid protein in tissues may provide a new therapeutic approach for amyloidosis and other disorders, such as Alzheimer's disease, in which amyloid is present, reports Joan Stephenson, Ph.D.[1] Amyloidosis is an extracellular accumulation of the protein amyloid in various organs and tissues. "In amyloidosis, abnormally folded protein is deposited as insoluble fibrils that lead to tissue damage and disease," Stephenson says. "Another protein, serum amyloid P component (SAP) binds to amyloid fibrils and makes them especially resistant to degradation by the body." She cites a research team in England, Switzerland, and Japan that identified the compound — a small-molecule drug called CPHRC — that interferes with SAP binding to amyloid fibrils, which leads to rapid clearance of SAP by the liver.

In earlier studies, 19 patients with systemic amyloidosis were treated with CPHRC for 9.5 months, and it dramatically reduced plasma SAP by almost 95%. The researchers hope that the efficient surging of SAP will destabilize amyloid deposits and promote their regression, Stephenson continued.

"This new approach offers great promise for treating both peripheral amyloid disorders, and possibly Alzheimer's disease," commented Leslie Iverson, Ph.D., of King's College in London, England.

Lipofuscin (age pigment) accumulates with age in the various areas of the central nervous system (CNS) in parallel with activities of oxidative enzymes, according to Richard P. Huemer, M.D. Age pigment is formed by oxidative polymerization of lipids (probably mostly mitochondrial) and proteins. However, the ac-

---

1 Stephenson, Joan, Ph. D. "Eroding Amyloid Deposits," JAMA 287(22): 2937, 2002.

cumulation of lipofuscin can be altered with antioxidants.[1] "Relatively large amounts of lipofuscin may be associated with adverse effects in the central nervous system, including loss of neurons," Huemer said. "Large deposits of neuromelanin — essentially a melanized lipofuscin — also appears to be associated with detrimental changes. Vitamin E-deficient diets increase CNS lipofuscin and depress function," Melanin is a dark brown or black animal or plant pigment.

It is a reasonable possibility that the excessive loss of neurons in the nucleus basalis of Meynert and other areas of the brain associated with senile dementia of the Alzheimer's type is due to free-radical reactions associated with the accumulation of pigment," Huemer continued.

Free radicals are highly damaging molecules or ions that contain oxygen. Once produced, they can multiply by chain reactions, making them more dangerous to cells. Free radicals can be generated inside the body, as well as outside the body via cigarette smoke and other pollutants.

Patients with Down's syndrome, like those with Alzheimer's disease, show a tendency toward premature mental aging, which is attributable to accelerated peroxidative damage to their brain tissue. Down's syndrome is characterized by moderate to severe mental retardation, Huemer added.

Lipid peroxidation is an interaction between lipids/fats and oxygen, which can lead to the destruction of cells.

A great deal of research has indicated that high intakes of vitamin E from foods and supplements reduce the risk of developing Alzheimer's disease, according to P. P. Zandi and colleagues in Archives of Neurology. A large clinical trial, mentioned earlier, found that very high doses of vitamin E slowed the progression in late-stage Alzheimer's disease, the rationale being that the use of the vitamin and other antioxidants may reduce the free-radical damage to the brain.[2]

In the study, a research team investigated the relationship between vitamin supplementation and the risk of Alzheimer's disease among 4,740 elderly residents of Cache County, Utah.

The volunteers were studied for those who took more than 400 IU/day of vitamin E, and at least 500 mg/day of vitamin C. Over 97% of the participants had used the supplements for at least two

---

1 Huemer, Richard P., M.D., editor. "The Roots of Molecular Medicine: A Tribute to Linus Pauling. New York: W. H. Freeman and Co., 1986, pp. 79, 80, 98.
2 Zandi, P. P., et al. "Reduced Risk of Alzheimer Disease in Users of Antioxidant Vitamin Supplements," The Cache County Study," Archives of Neurology 61: 82-88, 2004.

years, multivitamin users took smaller quantities of vitamins E and C, and B-vitamin users took supplements containing all 8 of the B vitamins.

The patients were evaluated for Alzheimer's disease in the mid-1990s and again in the late 1990s. Analysis of data from the mid-1990s found that those using a combination of vitamins E and C were 78% less likely to be diagnosed with Alzheimer's disease.

During the follow-up in the late 1990s, those taking vitamins E and C had a 64% lower risk of the disease. Those taking vitamin E supplements, plus a multivitamin supplement containing vitamin C, showed a slight reduction in Alzheimer's disease risk. No benefit was found in those taking only vitamin E, only vitamin C, multivitamins with low-dose vitamins E, C and B vitamins.

The study confirms the body of existing research suggesting that moderately high-dose antioxidant supplements, especially vitamins E and C, may reduce the risk of developing Alzheimer's disease, the researchers added.

Food sources of vitamin E include wheat germ oil, sunflower oil, safflower oil, peanut oil, soft and hard margarine, wheat germ, sunflower seeds, almonds, peanuts, soybean oil, brown rice, butter, oatmeal, and peanut butter.

Vitamin C in the diet is available from citrus fruits, berries, acerola cherries, pineapple, guava, cabbage, turnip greens, broccoli, tomatoes, kale, parsley, green peppers, papaya, mustard greens, cantaloupes, and other foods.

EARLY INTERVENTION

Early intervention is essential in preventing and treating Alzheimer's disease, according to Ralph Golan, M.D. Therefore, it is essential to take antioxidants and other nutrients that have a bearing on neurotransmission synthesis and brain function. He recommends:[1]

1. Take the following brain nutrients daily: B Complex — with at least 100 mg/day of the various B vitamins: 400 to 800 mcg/day of folic acid; extra vitamin B12 (1,000 mcg sublingual or injected); niacinamide (B3) — 500 to 1,500 mg/day; glutamine (500 to 1,000 mg/day); phenylalanine (500 to 2,000 mg/day: tyrosine (500 to 2,000 mg/day); zinc (30 to 60 mg/day); essential fatty acids (1 tsp or 3 capsules of flaxseed oil) and 2 to 3 capsules of borage oil. The B vitamins are: B1 (thiamine), B2 (riboflavin), B3 (niacin, niacinamide or nicotinic acid), B6 (pyridoxine), B12 (cobalamin), fo-

---

1 Golan, Ralph, M.D. *Optimal Wellness.* New York: Ballantine Books, 1995, p. 328.

lic acid, pantothenic acid, and biotin. All are recommended in milligram dosages, except that folic acid and B12 are usually listed in micrograms. There are 3 vitamin B cousins: Inositol, PABA (para-amino-benzoic acid), and choline.

2. Antioxidant support is important to preserve brain tissue from free radical injury. This includes N-acetyl-cysteine (1,500 mg/day), beta-carotene/provitamin A (25,000 to 50,000 IU/day), vitamin E (800 IU/day), vitamin C (3,000 mg/day), and selenium (200 mcg/day).

3. Take Aminomine (2 capsules 2 to 3 times daily).

4. Injectable nutrients, intravenous or intramuscularly, may bring faster results, especially if absorption from the gastrointestinal tract is not up to par.

Vitamin B12 may be the most important nutrient when given by injection, since it is the most difficult to absorb. An intramuscular injection of 1,000 mcg (1 milliliter), with the addition of up to 5 mg of folic acid (½ milliliter), and B Complex, with 400 mg of B1, plus varying amounts of other B vitamins (1 milliliter) can bring results within a day. If a person is severely deficient, several daily injections may be needed to produce results. Weekly and then bi-monthly injections may be necessary indefinitely.

Some individuals respond better to intravenous injections of the B vitamins, magnesium and other minerals, and vitamin C.

A research team at the University of Washington Alzheimer Disease Research Center, in Seattle, evaluated 136 family members and a separate group of 29 affected parent-child pairs, in an effort to determine the genetic risk factors for late-onset Alzheimer disease (LOAD).[1]

The patients were asked: 1) does early-onset Alzheimer disease (LOAD) occur in families with predominantly LOAD; and 2) does the APO-E genotype explain the wide difference in onset age in LOAD families?

The researchers reported that about 25% of the LOAD families have at least one person with LOAD, and, in those individuals, the ratio of men to women is nearly 50%, suggesting a possible subtype of familial Alzheimer's disease. The APO-E genotype plays

1 Brickell, K. L., et al. "Early-Onset Alzheimer Disease in Families with Late-Onset Alzheimer Disease: A potential Important Subtype of Familiar Alzheimer Disease," Archives of Neurology 63:1307-1311, 2006.

an important role in these early-onset cases; however, at least one fourth of the risk must represent the influence of other genetic and/or environmental factors.

The researchers added that LOAD families with early-onset cases represent an important resource for investigation of these factors, Archives of Neurology reported. Aging with and without dementia of the Alzheimer's type is associated with weight loss, but weight loss may accelerate before the diagnosis of the disease.[1]

Specific factors contributing to weight loss are unknown: however, this study suggests that they operate before the development of dementia of the Alzheimer type. Therefore, weight loss may be a preclinical indicator of Alzheimer's disease, according to researchers at the Alzheimer's Disease Research Center at Washington University School of Medicine in Seattle.

A gene variant linked to Alzheimer's disease may play a role in the progression of HIV — which may later develop into AIDS — according to Tracy Hampton, Ph.D.[2]

A research team at the University of California at San Francisco discovered that a variant of the gene encoding APO-E is a risk factor for accelerated AIDS progression and promotes entry of HIV into cells.

The study Involved 1,257 European and black individuals with HIV, and 1,132 ethnically matched seronegative controls. It was reported that there was a much faster disease course and progression to death in patients with 2 gene copies of the APO-E variant or allele than in those with two copies of the APO-E-3 allele.

The APO-E-4 allele is also a known risk factor for Alzheimer's disease. Thus, efforts to convert APO-E-4 to a molecule resembling APO-E-3 for the treatment of Alzheimer's disease also might have clinical applications for HIV, Hampton added.

The use of estrogen replacement therapy (ERT) in women after menopause was not associated with a risk of developing Alzheimer's disease, according to researchers at the University of Massachusetts Medical Center in Worcester. Previous findings have been inconsistent.[3]

The study, from the United Kingdom-based General Practice Research Database, consisted of 112,481 women who were given ERT, and 108,925 who did not receive the drug.

---

1 . Johnson, D. K., et al. "Accelerated Weight Loss May Precede Diagnosis of Alzheimer Disease," ibid, pp. 1312-1317.

2 Hampton, Tracy, Ph.D. "Alzheimer Disease and HIV," JAMA 300(5): 496, 2008.

3 Seshadn, Sudha, et al. "Postmenopausal Estrogen Replacement Therapy and the Risk of Alzheimer Disease," Archives of Neurology 58: 435-440, 2001.

The odds ratio for developing AD were similar for estrogen recipients who received estrogens alone, and those who were given combined estrogen-progestin treatment, the researchers said.

Plasma markers of amyloid precursor protein metabolism and C-reactive protein may be associated with the rate of cognitive and functional decline in those with Alzheimer's disease, according to Archives of Neurology.[1]

Amyloid is a waxy translucent substance which consists of protein in combination with polysaccharides (carbohydrates) that are deposited in tissues under abnormal conditions, such as in Alzheimer's disease.

C-reactive protein is a beta-globulin found in the serum of those with various inflammatory, degenerative, and neoplastic diseases.

A newly identified genetic mutation increases the risk of Alzheimer's disease, the second major gene to be linked to the disease, reported Barbara Juncosa in the September 2008 issue of Scientific American.[2]

The mutation was discovered in the Calhm-1 gene, which controls calcium concentrations in nerve cells, according to Philippe Marabaud of the Feinstein Institute for Medical Research in Manhasset, New York, the lead researcher.

The research team found that mutant Calhm-1 led to increased accumulation of amyloid beta plaques, the protein clumps that are characteristic of Alzheimer's.

It is estimated that 1 in 20 Americans, ages 65 to 74, carrying the risk is 1 in 14 — and 1 in 10 with 2 defective copies, leading to an earlier onset of AD. Marabaud added that the newly discovered gene, along with APO-E, which was discovered 15 years ago, will be an important screening tool for the disease.

A research team at the Stockholm Gerontology Research Center in Sweden explored whether the risk of dementia and Alzheimer disease due to a positive family history is explained by APO-E genotypes. While both family aggregation and APO-E-4 allele are known risk factors for dementia, the relation between these two factors remains unresolved.[3]

In the study, 907 nondemented people, 75 and older, were observed for up to 6 years to detect incident dementia and Alzheimer disease cases according to the diagnostic criteria of the Diag-

1 Locascio, J. J., et al. "Plasma Amyloid Beta-Protein and C-Reactive Protein in Relation to the Rate of Progression of Alzheimer Disease," Archives of Neurology 65(6): 776-785, 2008.
2 Juncosa, Barbara. "Another Gene for Alzheimer's" Scientific American, September 2008, p. 36.
3 Huang, Wenyong, et al. "APO-E Genotype, Family History of Dementia, and Alzheimer Disease Risk," Archives of Neurology 61: 1930-1934, 2004.

nosis and Statistical Manual of Mental Disorders, Revised, Third Edition.

It was found that those who had at least two siblings with dementia were at an increased risk of Alzheimer's disease. Those with both APO-E-4 and at least two affected first-degree relatives had a higher risk of dementia and Alzheimer's disease when compared with those without these two factors.

The researchers added that similar results were obtained for history of dementia separately in parents or siblings. Among the E-4 allele carriers, those with two or more first-degree demented relatives had increased risk of dementia and Alzheimer's, whereas no increased risk was detected among non-E-4 carriers.

According to Pam Belluck, writing in the New York Times, some studies have shown that many Hispanics may have more risk factors for developing dementia than other groups, and a significant number appear to be getting Alzheimer's earlier.[1] Latinos are less likely to see doctors because of financial and language barriers, and more often mistake dementia symptoms for normal aging, thereby delaying diagnosis. It is not that Hispanics are more genetically predisposed to Alzheimer's, but, rather, experts say several factors may be linked to low income or cultural dislocation, which may put Hispanics at greater risk for dementia, including higher rates of diabetes, obesity, cardiovascular disease, stroke, and possibly high blood pressure. "This is the tip of the iceberg of a huge public challenge," said Yanira L. Cruz, president of the National Hispanic Council on Aging. "We really need to do more research in this population to really understand why it is that we're developing these conditions much earlier."

Steven E. Arnold, M.D., of the University of Pennsylvania at Philadelphia, studied 2,000 white, African-American, and Latino Alzheimer's patients, and found the Latinos, mostly from low-income, poorly educated Puerto Ricans, many with diabetes, have more depression and their scores on tests (given in Spanish) measuring dementia averaged about 15% lower than African-Americans, and about 30% lower than non-Hispanic whites.

Mary N. Haan, a University of Michigan epidemiologist heading the Sacramento Area Latino Study on Aging, studied 1,800 Mexican-Americans over 10 years, and reported a greater likelihood of Alzheimer's in those more "acculturated" to American society. Pam Belluck adds, "Dr. Haan found more acculturated peo-

---

1 Belluck, Pam. "More Alzheimer's Risk Factors for Hispanics, Studies Suggest," The New York Times, October 21, 2008, pp. A1, A20.

ple more prone to diabetes, and people with diabetes or obesity more likely to have Alzheimer's."

Researchers theorize that high insulin levels and poor cerebral blood flow can cause brain changes that accompany Alzheimer's, according to Jose A. Luchsinger, M.D., of the Columbia University Medical Center in New York.

DIETARY SUPPLEMENTS

In subsequent chapters, we will talk further about vitamins, minerals, and nutritional supplements as they relate to weight management, depression, sleep disturbances and other issues. For starters, here is a list of daily supplements recommended by Giller and Matthews[1]:

- Vitamin C: 1,000 mg/day
- Vitamin E: 400 IU/day
- Beta-Carotene: 10,000 IU/day
- Selenium: 50 mcg/day
- Vitamin B12: 1,000 mcg/day, dissolved under the tongue
- Ginkgo biloba: 40 mg 3 to 4 times daily
- Choline: 650 mg, 3 times daily
- Zinc: 50 mg/day

In one study, 30 patients with Alzheimer's took these supplements daily: 6 g of evening primrose oil, 90 mg of zinc sulfate, and 2 mg of selenium. They had significant improvements in performance tests.

In another study, patients who were given supplements of L-carnitine had less deterioration in attention span and performance of tasks. They received 2.5 g of L-carnitine daily for 3 months, followed by 3 g/day for 3 months.

Compared with men, women appear to be at increased risk of Alzheimer's disease after ages 80 to 85.[2] "Postmenopausal depletion of endogenous estrogens may contribute to this risk. Estrogens may exert several neuroprotective effects on the aging brain, including inhibition of beta-amyloid formation, stimulation of cholinergic activity, reduction of oxidative stress-related damage, and protection against vascular risks."[3]

The researchers go on to say that several studies have examined whether hormone replacement therapy (HRT) is associated with

1 Giller, Robert M., M.D., and Matthews, Kathy. *Natural Prescriptions*. New York: Carol Southern Books, 1994, pp. 11-12

2 Zandi, Peter P., Ph.D. "Hormone Replacement Therapy and Incidence of Alzheimer Disease: The Cache County Study," *JAMA* 288(17): 2123-2129, 2002.

3 Skoog, I., et al. "HET and Dementia," *Journal of Epidemiol. Biostat.* 4: 227-251, 1999.

reduced risk of AD in older women, and case-control studies have been mixed. "One such study reported no relation of AD and HRT ascertained from pharmacy records within a 10-year period of observation. Another study using prescription records showed no inverse relation of AD with lifetime HRT use."

The researchers added that two prospective studies suggesting benefit of lifetime use, but a study conducted using the U.S. General Practice Research Database found no relation of AD to HRT prescriptions within a 10-year period. Therefore, the relationship of HRT and AD remains uncertain. The researchers concluded that prior HRT use is associated with reduced risk of AD, but there is no apparent benefit, with current HRT use unless such use has exceeded 10 years.

Patients with AD have several options for drug treatment, but these agents only ameliorate cognitive symptoms for a year or two, and their effect is modest, reported M. J. Friedrich in the Journal of the American Medical Association. In fact, a recent review and guidelines by the American College of Physicians, and the American Academy of Family Physicians, found little evidence that such effects are actually clinical meaningful.[1] Friedrich added that, to date, no long-term therapies to slow or halt disease progression have proven effective in clinical trials.

In fact, some of the drugs that haven't panned out in clinical trials may not be working because they are being administered after the disease has progressed too far and is too late for them to have a beneficial effect, added Ronald Petersen, M.D., of the Mayo Clinic of Medicine in Rochester, Minnesota. He added that enrolling patients in clinical trials at an earlier stage of the disease would allow treatments to be tested before the brain deteriorates.

Early detection of Alzheimer's disease is crucial in diminishing the impact, since, by the time most people become symptomatic — even mildly so — and certainly by the time they have clinical AD, a lot of damage has already been done, explained Petersen.

"Autopsy findings from patients who died with a clinical diagnosis of mild cognitive impairment (MCI), the condition that often precedes AD, showed neuropathological features intermediate between people with normal aging and patients with AD," Friedrich said.

Identifying incipient AD is one of the primary goals of the Alzheimer Disease Neuroimaging Initiative in which Petersen and

1 Friedrich, M. J. "Alzheimer Researchers Focus Efforts on Early Development and Earlier Detection," JAMA 300(22): 2595-2597, 2008.

his colleagues are participating. This facility's study is working in developing standardized neuroimaging and chemical biomarkers for diagnosing AD, along with monitoring the disease-modifying effects of therapies.

Many biomarkers are constantly being studied, reported Virginia Lee, Ph.D., of the University of Pennsylvania School of Medicine in Philadelphia. A lab test to predict conversion from MCI to AD, using a combination of chemical biomarker changes in the cerebral spinal fluid may be available in 2 to 3 years.

At the International Conference on Alzheimer's .disease, held in Chicago, Illinois, in July 2008, Petersen said that data from this study showing that incidence rates of cognitive impairment are higher than previously thought, about 3.5% per year for those 70 to 79, and 7.2% for people 80 to 89. "One of AD's hallmarks is the deposition of plaques of the A-beta-42 peptide in the brain," Friedrich continued. "But while amyloid is believed to play a fundamental role in AD pathogenesis, a complete understanding of the mechanisms underlying the disease — especially in sporadic, late-onset AD — remains elusive."

Friedrich quoted Sam Gandy, M.D., of Mount Sinai Medical School in. New York, as saying that amyloid peptide became the primary villain in the AD story a few decades ago, when investigators found that the genetic mutations that give rise to the rare forms of early onset AD are in the gene encoding the amyloid precursor protein (APP), or one of the enzymes involved in the mechanism, such as presenilin 1 or 2 (PS1 or PS2).

According to the amyloid hypothesis of AD, Friedrich added, this peptide forms clumps in the brain that poison nearby nerve cells, which, as they die, develop intraneuronal tangles.

Gandy said that the amyloid hypothesis is clearly true in the rare forms of early onset familial AD, but whether amyloid accumulation in the brain is the final common pathway in the sporadic form of the disease, which accounts for 97% of all cases, is not clear.

"A different strategy involves aiming at another key neuropathologic feature of AD — the protein tau — which is found in the intraneuronal tangles," Friedrich said. "Tau normally regulates the stability of the cell's internal skeleton, but hollow microtubules that also transport nutrients throughout the cell. However, under pathologic conditions, tau contributes to the brain dysfunction of AD."

Recent years have seen a surge of interest in tau-based treatments for AD, said Erik Robertson, M.D., of the University of Alabama at Birmingham. Amyloid was the natural first target for drug development, but some very progressive studies in animal models looking at the role of tau in AD have supported the idea of focusing on tau as a target.

Since tau is often hyperphosphorylated in AD, another tau-based approach to treatment involves inhibiting the kinases that phosphorylate tau, added Lennart Mucke, M.D., of the Gladstone Institute of Neurological Diseases at the University of California at San Francisco. However, many kinase inhibitors of tau are promiscuous, meaning they aim at other protein within cells, which poses the challenge of designing kinase inhibitors that are more specific to tau. (A kinase is an enzyme catalyzing the conversion of a proenzyme to an active enzyme.) Phosphorylation is the addition of phosphate to an organic compound.

Gandy adds that instead of being the main instigator of AD, amyloid may be a toxic byproduct of a different primary injury, such as a problem with the regulation of calcium or oxidation, which is itself neurotoxic but also promotes amyloid formation. "In these situations, amyloid accumulation would be a contributing factor but it would be the only cause of AD, as it is in early onset cases."

The absence of a distinct genetic cause of sporadic AD implies that amyloid accumulation originates from another dysfunction in the cell, according to Ralph Nixon, M.D., of the New York University School of Medicine. "One possible culprit is an abnormality in the lysosomal system, which has been reported to contribute to the development of several neurodegenerative disorders. The lysosomal system includes two major pathways to the cell: the autophagic pathway and the endocytic (inner) pathway. Both of them are involved in processing and degrading various substances, and both are sites of amyloid-beta production." (Autophagy is segregation and disposal of damaged particles in cells.)

While the lysosomal system functions throughout the body, mutations in genes involved in the lysosomal system seem to affect the nervous system preferentially, explains Nixon. These pathways may be especially necessary in helping neurons remove waste products and keep their axons and synapses in good working order. The axon is the process of a nerve cell that conducts nervous impulses away from the cello. Synapse is the functional membrane-membrane contact of a nerve cell. Antiamyloid therapeutics may still be beneficial. While the negative results of the clinical trials of these agents don't prove that there's no merit to an amyloid-lowering strategy, it may not be sufficient. Nixon comments,

"I believe it's going to require a cocktail of strategies to effectively treat AD."

Vascular factors, such as including medical history — heart disease, stroke, diabetes, hypertension, smoking, and prediagnosis blood lipid measurements (cholesterol: total, HDL and LDL), and triglyceride concentrations, may be predictors for the development of Alzheimer's disease.[1]

In the study at Washington Heights/Inwood Columbia Aging Project, New York, researchers evaluated 156 patients with incident Alzheimer's disease for 3.5 to 10.2 years. Mean age at diagnosis was 83. The research team reported that higher prediagnosis total cholesterol and LDL-C concentrations, as well as a history of diabetes, were associated with faster cognitive decline in those with incident AD, providing further evidence for the role of vascular risk factors in the development of Alzheimer's disease.

In a prospective community-based cohort study conducted in northern Manhattan, researchers reported that a history of high blood pressure is related to a higher risk of mild cognitive impairment (MCI).[2]

The study suggests that prevention and treatment of hypertension may have an important impact in reducing the risk of cognitive impairment. The association was said to be stronger with the nonamnestic than the amnestic type of MCI. (Amnestic/amnesia refers to loss of memory due to a brain injury, shock, fatigue, repression or illness.)

The association between the pathological features of Alzheimer's disease and dementia is stronger in the younger-old patients than in the older-old patients.[3] Therefore, age must be taken into consideration when assessing the likely effects of interventions against dementia in those patients.

By the time Alzheimer's disease has reached its end stage, the brain is riddled with plaques, tangles, cavities, and fissures, and has lost a substantial percentage of its weight.[4] However, researchers believe that most people living with the disease are not yet at this stage, and still have a good portion of working neurons with which to learn, be creative, and enjoy life.

---

1 Helzner, E. P., et al. "Contribution of Vascular Risk Factors in the Progression of Alzheimer Disease," Archives of Neurology 66(3): 343-348, 2009.

2 Reitz, C., et al. "Hypertension and the Risk of Mild Cognitive Impairment," Archives of Neurology 61(12): 1734-1740, 2007.

3 Savva, George M., Ph.D., et al. "Age, Neuropathology, and Dementia," New England Journal of Medicine 360: 2302-2309, 2009.

4 Friedrich, M. J. "Therapeutic Environmental Design Aims to Help Patients with Alzheimer Disease," JAMA 301(23): 2430, 2009.

That was the conclusion of John Zeisel, Ph.D., president of Hearthstone Alzheimer Care, Ltd., of Lexington, Massachusetts, a sociologist who focuses on the therapeutic effects of residential environment design among patients with AD. Therapeutic environmental design seeks to tap into the areas of the brain that are still functioning, rather than focusing on the parts of the brain that do not work, Zeisel explained.

"A well designed environment can help compensate for damage to executive function, a deficit that makes it difficult for people with AD to meld complex sequences of events into a single process, such as brushing your teeth," Friedrich said. "However, if appropriate props for a task are at hand and the environment provides cues, those with AD are more apt to complete the task successfully."

Zeisel added that environments also can help address memory deficits in those with AD, especially when memory is still present in the brain, but access to it is not, by helping to jog access in old memories. As an example, using family photos and mementos as visual landmarks for a person's own room. Since the environment tells them where they're going and gives them memories, patients are comforted and less confused, which helps them to control impulses, such as aggression, and reduce their anxiety and agitation.

Joanne Westphal, D.O., Ph.D., professor of landscape architecture at Michigan State University, East Lansing, bridges medicine and design to create the ancient concept of "healing gardens" that provide benefits, such as relieving stress and improving the sense of well-being for patients, as well as for staff and family members. A significant aspect of the work is to build into the design process standards and criteria for evaluating the site after it is constructed, including how the garden affects the medical status of the patients.

In a study at a Michigan nursing home, Westphal compared 8 indicators of the general health and well-being of patients with dementia, fathered before and after construction of a dementia garden in the fall of 1999. "The variables included aggressive and non-aggressive behavior, medication use, pulse rate, systolic and diastolic blood pressure, and weight change." The researchers then divided the patients into 3 groups, based on how much time per day they spent in the garden — less than 5 minutes, 5-10 minutes, and more than 10 minutes — and compared with patient data collected in April and May (before the garden was open), with that gathered during July and August.

"We were excited to find that there were improvements in 7 criteria — all but the physician-ordered medications — and no deteriorating parameters in the residents who spent more than 10 min-utes daily in the garden," Westphal said. "In contrast, the other two groups experienced improvements in only 2 or 3 areas and de-teriorated in several others. I'm not saying a garden will be the an-swer to all the problems that families have, but it does place people in an environment where respite and restoration can occur."

2. Dementia Is On the Increase

What is Dementia?

Dementia is a clinical syndrome of loss or decline in memory and other cognitive abilities, according to the Alzheimer's Association in Chicago. It is due to a variety of diseases and conditions that damage brain cells. In order to be classified as dementia, the syndrome must include decline in memory and at least one of the following cognitive abilities:[1]

1. Ability to generate coherent speech and understand spoken or written language.

2. Ability to recognize or identify objects, assuming intact memory function.

3. Ability to execute motor activities, assuming intact motor abilities, sensory function, and comprehension of the required task.

4. Ability to think abstractly, make sound judgments, and plan and carry out complete tasks.

"Different types of dementia have been associated with distinct symptom patterns and distinguishing microscopic brain abnormalities," the Association said. "Increasing evidence from long-term epidemiological observations and autopsy studies suggest that many people have microscopic brain abnormalities associated

---

1 2008 Alzheimer's Disease Facts and Figures. Chicago, IL: Alzheimer's Association, 2008, pp. 4-6.

with more than one type of dementia. The symptoms of different types of dementia may overlap, further complicating the diagnosis."

Here are the common types of dementia and their typical characteristics:

1. Alzheimer's disease. The most common type of dementia, it accounts for 60 to 80% of the cases. Difficulty in remembering names and recent events is often an early clinical symptom. Later symptoms include impaired judgment, disorientation, confusion, behavioral changes, and trouble speaking, swallowing, and walking. Abnormalities are deposits of the protein fragment beta-amyloid (plaques) and twisted strands of the protein tau (tangles).

2. Vascular dementia (multi-infarct or post-stroke dementia). This is considered the second most common type of dementia. Impairment is due to decreased blood flow to parts of the brain, often due to small strokes that block arteries. Symptoms often overlap with Alzheimer's although memory may not be as seriously affected.

3. Mixed dementia. Characterized by the presence of the abnormalities seen in Alzheimer's and another type of dementia, most commonly vascular dementia, but also other types, such as dementia with Lewy bodies, frontotemporal dementia and normal pressure hydrocephalus, which is marked by an excessive accumulation of fluid. Named after Frederic H. Lewy (Lewey), a German-American neurologist (1885-1950), Lewy bodies are pigmented brainstem neurons often found in Parkinson's disease.

4. Dementia with Lewy Bodies. A pattern of decline may be similar to Alzheimer's and the severity of cognitive symptoms may fluctuate daily, and visual hallucinations, muscle rigidity, and tremors are common. Hallmarks include Lewy bodies (abnormal deposits of the protein alpha-synuclein) that form inside nerve cells in the brain.

5. Parkinson's disease. These patients may develop dementia in the later stage of the disease. Hallmark abnormality is Levy bodies (abnormal deposits of the protein alpha-synuclein) that form inside nerve cells in the brain.

6. Frontotemporal dementia. This involves damage to brain cells, especially in the front and side of the brain. Typical symptoms include changes in personality and behavior and difficulty with language. No distinguishing microscopic abnormality is linked to all cases. Pick's disease, characterized by Pick's bodies, is one type of frontotemporal dementia. Friedel Pick (1867–1926) was a German physician.

7. Creutzfeldt-Jakob disease. This is a rapidly fatal disorder that impairs memory and coordination, and it causes behavior changes. Variant Creutzfeldt-Jakob disease is Alfons, thought to be caused by consumption of products from cattle affected by mad-cow disease. It is caused by the

misfolding of prion protein throughout the brain. Hans Gerhard Creutzfeldt (1885–1964) was a German neuropsychiatrist, as was Allkons M. Jakob (1884–1931).

8. Normal pressure hydrocephalus. This is caused by a buildup of fluid in the brain. Symptoms include difficulty walking, memory loss, and inability to control urine. It can sometimes be corrected with surgical installation of a shunt (bypass) in the brain to drain excess fluid.

Dementia is a prevalent problem, ranging from 2.4 million to 4.5 million people in the United States, depending on how cases are defined, according to Tracey Holsinger, M.D., of the Durham VA Medical Center in North Carolina, and colleagues at various facilities. In addition, many older adults notice difficulty with memory and other cognitive functioning.[1] "Primary care physicians often do not recognize cognitive impairment in the brief time available for an office visit," the researchers said. "Studies have found between 29 and 76% of cases of dementia or probable dementia are not diagnosed by primary care physicians."

Dementia is a major cause of disability among the elderly, and Alzheimer's disease is responsible for around 70% of the cases, according to Elizabeth J. Johnson and Ernst J. Schaefer of the Jean Mayer-USDA Human Nutrition Research Center on Aging at Tufts University in Boston, Massachusetts.[2]

The social cost of caring for dementia is said to be $100 billion annually, with most of the direct costs attributable to inpatient services, home health care, and skilled nursing facilities. During the coming decade, the increasing number of older adults presages an abrupt increase in the burden of dementia, the researchers added.

"Without scientific advances that lower the incidence and progression of Alzheimer's disease and related dementia conditions, between 11 and 18.5 million people in the United States will likely experience some level of dementia by 2050."

The research team recommends screening for the disease when it is either clinically undetectable or in its early stages when interventions can prevent or delay the consequences of the underlying disorder. A definitive diagnosis of dementia allows patients and family members the opportunity to have important conversations

1 Holsinger, Tracey, M.D., et al. "Does This Patient Have Dementia?" JAMA 297(21): 2391-2404, 2007.
2 Johnson, Elizabeth J., and Schaefer, Ernst J. "Potential Role of Dietary Omega-3 Fatty Acids in the Prevention of Asmentia and Macular Degeneration," American Journal of Clinical Nutrition 83: 1494S-1498S, 2006.

about desired future care, and the chance to arrange financial and legal matters while decision-making capacity remains.

"Early intervention can also provide early safety monitoring in such areas as medication administration, safe use of appliances and tools, and driving," the researchers said. "These family and safety issues might justify screening even if early diagnosis affected no other outcomes."

As the population ages and the number of patients with dementia increases rapidly, primary care settings will see many more patients at various stages of dementia. Clinicians should pick one primary tool that is population appropriate, then consider adding one or two others for special situations as needed, the researchers concluded.

Ongoing studies have suggested that there is an association between depression and the risk of dementia. However, as reported by R. S. Wilson, et al., in Archives of General Psychiatry, they found no increase in depressive symptoms during the prodromal (early stage) phase of Alzheimer's disease.[1] For up to 13 years, the research team evaluated 917 older Catholic nuns, priests, and monks without dementia. Changes in depressive symptoms were reported on the Center for Epidemiologic Studies Depression Scale. It was reported that those who developed Alzheimer's disease exhibited no increase in depressive symptoms before the diagnosis was made, and this finding was not modified by age, sex, education, memory complaints, vascular burden, or personality. Also, there were no changes in depressive symptoms after the Alzheimer's diagnosis was made. However, symptoms tended to decrease in women with regard to men, with a higher premorbid level of openness and a lower premorbid level of agreeableness.

The research team also found that in the volunteers without cognitive impairment at the beginning of the study, depressive symptoms did not increase in those who later developed mild cognitive impairment.

Dementia, which is characterized by global (overall) cognitive decline sufficient to affect functioning, is a serious public health problem with an increasing prevalence because of the aging of the population, explained Constantine G. Lyketsos, M.D., and colleagues at the Johns Hopkins Hospital in Baltimore, Maryland.[2]

---

1   Wilson, R. S., et al. "Change in Depressive Symptoms During the Prodronal Phase of Alzheimer Disease," Archives of General Psychiatry 65(4): 439-446, 2008.

2   Lyketsos, Constantine G., M.D., et al. "Prevalence of Neuropsychiatric Symptoms in Dementia and Mild Cognitive impairment; Results from the Cardiovascular Health Study," JAMA 288(12):1475-1483 2002.

MILD COGNITIVE IMPAIRMENT AND NEUROPSYCHIATRIC SYMPTOMS

Mild cognitive impairment (MCI) describes cognitive impairment in elderly people not of sufficient severity for a diagnosis of full-blown dementia. Those with MCI have complaints of impairment in memory or other areas of cognitive functioning usually noticeable in those around them. "In addition," the researchers said, "their performance on memory and cognitive tests is below that experienced for their age and education. However, their day-to-day functioning is generally preserved."

Several operational definitions for MCI have been proposed, with MCI being a chronic condition and may be a precursor for Alzheimer's-type dementia. Neuropsychiatric symptoms are a common accompaniment of dementia, the researchers continued. These include agitation, depression, apathy, delusions, hallucinations, and sleep impairment. These symptoms have serious consequences for patients and caregivers, such as greater impairment in activities of daily living, more rapid cognitive decline, worse quality of life, earlier institutionalization, and greater caregiver depression.

In their study, 3,608 patients were cognitively evaluated using data collected over 10 years, and additional data collected in 1999–2000 in four U.S. counties. Dementia and mild cognitive impairment were classified using clinical criteria and adjudicated by committee review by expert neurologists and psychiatrists. Of the 682 people with dementia or MCI, 43% of those with MCI exhibited neuropsychiatric symptoms in the previous month — 29% rated as clinically significant with depression (20%); apathy (15%); and irritability (15%) being most common. Among those with dementia, 75% had exhibited a neuropsychiatric symptom in the past month. The most frequent disturbances were apathy (36%); depression (32%); and agitation/aggression (30%).

"Our findings further confirm the high prevalence of neuropsychiatric symptoms in dementia, and indicate a moderate prevalence of MCI," the researchers concluded. "Clinical evaluations of patients with suspected MCI and dementia must include specific assessment of and treatment for such symptoms. This also has significant implications for further studies of the pathophysiology and treatment of neuropsychiatric symptoms in cognitively impaired elderly people."

SLEEP DISRUPTIONS AND LIGHT THERAPY

Dementia can lead to several types of sleep disruptions, including an increased number of nighttime awakenings, less efficient sleep, increased daytime napping, altered proportions of rapid eye movement (REM) and non-REM sleep, and increased latency to the first episode of REM sleep, according to Catherine Cole, Ph.D., and Kathy Richards, Ph.D., in the May 2007 issue of the American Journal of Nursing.[1]

One study that used subjective reports from people with dementia found that 10 to 20% of sleep occurred during the daytime, and another study that used 72 continuous hours of polysomnography — the monitoring of physiologic parameters during sleep — found that those with severe dementia had more disrupted sleep than elderly patients without dementia. Unfortunately, the authors continued, in standards of care of these with dementia, sleep often is not mentioned. The American Academy of Neurology's guidelines on detecting, diagnosing, and managing dementia noted that no Class 1 evidence could be found for the pharmacologic treatment of sleep disturbances in dementia, and research on non-pharmacologic treatments is needed.

"One possible cause of sleep fragmentation in people with dementia is damage to the neuronal pathways that initiate and maintain sleep and regulate cognitive arousal and sleep-wake cycles," the authors added.

Cholinesterase inhibitors, a class of drugs used to treat the cognitive symptoms of dementia that includes donepezil (Aricept) and galantamine (Razadyne), are another cause of sleep disruption in those with dementia, the authors said.

"For many caregivers, disrupted sleep — both their own and that of the people they are caring for — is the primary reason for placement of the patient with dementia into long-term care," they added.

An exciting new approach to the sleep problem as well as behavior disorders is light therapy. Behavior disorders in the dementia group are believed to be related to a decrease in the amplitude of the sleep-wake rhythm, and a decrease in melatonin secretion.

In one 2-month trial, 14 demented inpatients with sleep and behavior disorders (average age of 75), and 10 elderly controls, were evaluated for 4 weeks. This involved each person to sit for 2 hours, 9 to 11 a.m., while exposed to morning light therapy. This consist-

---

1 Cole, Catherine, Ph.D., and Richards, Kathy, Ph.D. "Sleep Disruption in Older Adults," American Journal of Nursing 107(5): 40-49, May 2007.

ed of desk-top full-spectrum fluorescent lamps, which provided an illumination of 3,000 to 5,900 lux. (A lux is a unit of illumination equal to 1 lumen per square meter.[1]) The participants were instructed to frequently gaze into the light source. The researchers reported that morning light therapy significantly increased total and nocturnal sleep time, and significantly reduced daytime sleep time.

These results suggest that morning bright light is a powerful synchronizer that can normalize sleep patterns and reduce the frequency of behavior disorders in elderly patients, according to a research team at Akita University School of Medicine in Japan.

A double-blind study from 1999 to 2004 with 189 residents of 12 group care facilities in The Netherlands involved those with an average of 85.8. Ninety percent were women, and 87% had dementia.

Changes in the circadian pacemaker of the brain, located in the hypothalamic suprachiasmatic nucleus, may contribute to cognitive, mood, behavior, and sleep disturbances. Increasing the illumination level in group care facilities ameliorated symptoms of disturbed cognition, mood, behavior, functional activities, and sleep. While melatonin improved sleep, its long-term use by elderly people can only be recommended in combination with light to suppress adverse effects on mood. Whole-day bright light did not have adverse effects, and it could be considered for use in facilities catering to elderly people with dementia.[2]

SOME POSSIBLE INDICATORS

Blood Pressure

A research team at Karolinska Institute in Stockholm, Sweden, evaluated 1,642 patients ranging in age from 75 to 101, for the relationship between blood pressure and dementia. Those with systolic (beating) blood pressure less than 140 mmHg were more often diagnosed as demented than those with systolic blood pressure greater than 140 mmHg, reported Zhenchao Guo, M.D.[3] Similar results were observed in those with diastolic (resting) pres-

---

1 Mishima, K., et al. "Morning Bright Light Therapy for Sleep and Behavior Disorders in Elderly Patients with Dementia," Acta Psychiatrica Scandinavia 89: 1-7, 1994.

2 Riemersma-van Lek, Rixt F., M.D., et al. "Effect of Bright Light and Melatonin on Cognitive and Noncognitive Function in Elderly Residents of Group Care Facilities," JAMA. 299(22): 2642-2655, 2008.

3 Guo, Zhenchao, M.D., et al. "Low Blood Pressure and Dementia in Elderly People: The Kuugsholmen Project," British Medical Journal 312: 805-808, 1996.

sures less than 75 mmHg, when compared with those with higher diastolic blood pressure.

Both systolic and diastolic blood pressure are inversely related to the prevalence of dementia in elderly people, Guo said. Low blood pressure may predispose a subpopulation to developing dementia.

A study involving 382 volunteers who initially were nondemented at age 70, were followed for 15 years, and it was revealed, that increased blood pressure may increase the risk of dementia by inducing small-vessel disease and white-matter lesions.[1] The research team reported that the risk of developing dementia between ages 79 and 85 increased when diastolic pressure increased when the patient turned 70.

Homocysteine

A research team in Sweden evaluated 44 women and 36 men, with an average age of 77.3 years, with symptoms of organic brain disease. The controls were 20 women and 30 men, average age of 76.1 years, who were healthy.[2] Blood levels of homocysteine were increased by 45% of the psychogeriatric population, and blood levels of the amino acid correlated with the severity of dementia, the Berger scale, and the score of symptoms in the psychogeriatric population. Homocysteine is normally a benign amino acid, but it can build to toxic levels and impact on health. Blood levels of folic acid, the B vitamin, were significantly correlated with the just-named measures, but the correlations of blood levels of vitamin B12 and methylmalonic acid were not.

Total homocysteine level was the only significant predictor of the severity of dementia and symptom scores, the researchers added. Other researchers have reported that folic acid, vitamin B6, and vitamin B12 can often lower homocysteine levels.

Zinc

The possibility of a causal link between zinc and Alzheimer's is still being studied. However, the addition of zinc supplements may prevent the onset of dementia in those at risk. Zinc is important in enzymes dealing with DNA replication, repair, and tran-

---

1   Skoog, Ingmar, M.D., et al. "15-Year Longitudinal Study of Blood Pressure and Dementia," The Lancet 347: 1141-1145, 1996.

2   Niisson, K., et al. "The Plasma Homocysteine Concentration is Better Than That of Serum Methylmalonic Acid As a Marker for Sociopsychological Performance in a Psychogeriatric Population," Clinical Chemistry 46(5): 691-696, 2000.

scription, as well as in neuronal DNA polymerases.[1] (Polymerase is a general term for any enzyme catalyzing a polymerization, as of nucleotides, to polynucleotide's, such as p-alpha, p-beta, and p-gamma, etc.)

Docosahexaenoic Acid (DHA)

In an article in Lipids, a research team evaluated 20 patients, with an average age of 83, living in a home for the elderly and diagnosed with mild to moderate dementia of cerebrovascular origin. Ten of the patients were given 6 DHA capsules containing 0.72 g of docosahexaenoic acid daily for one year, while another group received a placebo.[2] In the DHA group, different mental assessment scores improved, but not in the controls. There were significant differences in the dementia scores 3 to 6 months after DHA supplementation.

In the treatment group, the content of DHA and eicosapentaenoic acid (EPA) increased without altering other fatty acid compositions, including arachidonic acid, the researchers said. Red blood cell deformability significantly improved with DHA supplementation. Also, there was a positive correlation between DHA/arachidonic acid ratios and dementia scores.

Arachidonic acid is an unsaturated fatty acid essential for proper nutrition, since it is the biological precursor of the prostaglandins, thromboxanes, and the leukotrienes, collectively referred to as eicosanoids.

Calcium

In evaluating 18 non-demented patients, 22 with Alzheimer's-type dementia, and 20 with vascular-type senile dementia, the Alzheimer's-type group showed significant decreases in blood levels of calcium, increases in blood levels of parathyroid hormone and urinary calcium, and a tendency of reduced vitamin D (1,25-dihydrcxyvitamin D), compared with the nondemented group, according to Gerontology.[3] The researchers added that calcium and calcium-regulating hormones may play a role in senile dementia.

Researchers have found that there are marked differences in cerebrospinal fluid (CSF) levels of both calcium and phosphorus

---

1 Burnet, P. M. "A Possible Role of Zinc in the Pathology of Dementia," Lancet, January 24, 1981, pp. 186-188.

2 Terano, T., et al. "Docosahexaenoic Acid Supplementation Improves the Moderately Severe dementia from Thrombotic Cerebrovascular Disease," Lipids 34: 8345-8346, 1999.

3 Ogihara, T., et al. "Possible Participation of Calcium-Regulating Factors in Senile Dementia in Elderly Female Subjects," Gerontology 36(Suppl. 1): 25-30, 1990.

in dementia patients, and aged controls when compared to adult controls, according to Neurobiology and Aging.[1]

A significant decrease in both minerals in CSF was found in Alzheimer's-type dementia. The lower calcium-phosphorus in CSF may play a role in the pathology of age-related disorders, the researchers said.

Thyroid Problems

The thyroid gland, which lies at the base of the neck, produces the hormones thyroxine and triiodothyronine, which regulate the body's metabolism. Without these hormones, a person may lapse into chronic fatigue and depression.

At the Jewish Home for the Ageing in Reseda, California, Dan Osterwell, M.D., evaluated 54 nondemented hypothyroid (deficient activity of the thyroid gland) patients, ranging in age from 31 to 99, who had documented biochemical hypothyroidism, and 30 euthyroid (normal thyroid function) controls.[2] The volunteers were evaluated for attention, orientation, memory learning, visual-special abilities, calculation, language, visual scanning, and motor speed, using standardized neuropsychological tests. The hypothyroid patients showed significantly lower scores on the Mini-Mental Status Test, and on 5 of the 14 neuropsychological tests, when compared with the controls.

Osterwell concluded that hypothyroidism in nondemented older people is associated with impairment in learning, word fluency, visual-special abilities, and some aspects of attention, scanning, and motor speed.

In evaluating 1,843 people who were 55 years of age or older, those with reduced thyroid stimulating hormone (TSH) levels at the beginning of the study had a more than 3-fold increased risk of dementia and Alzheimer's disease, after adjusting for age and sex, reported Clinical Endocrinology.[3] In addition, those with reduced TSH levels, thyroxine (T4) levels appeared to be positively related to a risk of dementia, however, none of the patients who became demented had T4 levels above the normal range of over 140 nmol/l. The researchers reported that the risk of dementia was increased in those with low TSH levels, who were positive for thyroid peroxide

1 Subhash, M. N., et al. "Calcium and Phosphorus Levels in Serum and CSF in Dementia," Neurobiology and Aging 12(4): 267-269, 1991.
2 Osterwell, Dan, M.D., et al. "Cognitive Function in Nondemented Older Adults with Hypothyroidism," Journal of the American Geriatric Society 40(4): 325-335, 1992.
3 Kalminjin, S., et al. "Subclinical Hyperthyroidism and the Risk of Dementia: The Rotterdam Study," Clinical Endocrinology 53: 733-737, 2000.

antibodies. Thyroxine T4 is an iodine-containing compound that increases metabolic rate, and it is used to treat thyroid disorders.

Omega-3 Fatty Acids

Age, family history, and the presence of an apolipoprotein gene have been found to be significant risk factors for the development of Alzheimer's disease and all-cause dementia. More recently, high blood levels of homocysteine were also shown to be risk factors for both conditions.

Docosahexaenoic acid (DHA), a fatty acid found in the diet as well as in many tissues of the body, also appears to be important in affecting the risk of dementia, the researchers said. The phospholipids in the brain membranes are enriched in DHA, and it appears to be important for central nervous system function.

Several investigators have analyzed the links between plasma DHA status and dementia, and patients with dementia due to Alzheimer's disease have been reported to have 30% less DHA in brain tissue than age-matched controls.

Low dietary intakes and blood concentrations of DHA have been reported to be associated with dementia, cognitive decline, and Alzheimer's disease risk, the researchers said. The major dietary sources of DHA are fish and fish oils, and dietary supplements are available.

"Our own unpublished observations from the Framingham Heart Study suggest that over 180 mg/day of dietary DHA — around 2.7 fish servings per week — is associated with an approximate 50% reduction in dementia risk," the research team continued. "At least this amount of DHA is generally found in 1 commercially available 1 g of fish oil capsules given daily. From the available data, the World Health Organization recommends that between 1 and 2% of calories should come from omega-3 fatty acids, and this is certainly not unreasonable."

Low-Density Lipoprotein Cholesterol Next to Alzheimer's disease, vascular dementia is the second most common form of dementia in the elderly, yet few specific risk factors have been identified.[1] In the study, 1,111 nondemented volunteers, with a mean age of 75.0, were followed for an average of 2.1 years. During that time, 280 of the people developed dementia during follow-up; 61 were classified as having dementia with stroke; and 225 as having probable Alzheimer's disease.

---

1   Moroney, Joan T., M.D., et al. "Low-Density Lipoprotein Cholesterol and the Risk of Dementia with Stroke," JAMA 282(3): 254-260, 1999.

Levels of low-density lipoprotein cholesterol (LDL, the harmful kind) were significantly associated with an increased risk of dementia with stroke, the researchers said. Compared with the lowest quartile, the highest quartile of LDL-cholesterol was associated with an approximate 3-fold increase in risk of dementia with stroke. However, lipid and lipoprotein levels were not associated with Alzheimer's disease.

"These findings may have important implications for the management of elderly patients with a history of stroke and should be a focus of future research," the researchers concluded. "Dietary modification, physical activity, and therapy with lipid-lowering drugs are among the interventions that should be evaluated to determine whether they provide protection against dementia for elderly patients with stroke and elevated LDL cholesterol levels."

Gender

While women tend to live longer than men, new research reported by Maria M. Corrada-Bravo, M.D., of the University of California at Irvine, suggests that after age 90, women are more likely to have dementia than men who live to the same age.[1]

In the study involving 911 nonagenarian Americans, it was found that 45% of the women had dementia when compared with 25% of the men. It was also reported that dementia among women in their 90s doubled for every 5 years added to their age, but men did not show increased rates of dementia as they aged. "With increasing numbers of people living to a very old age, especially women, we are seeing that there are going to be millions and millions of people with this condition," Corrada-Bravo added.

Is the current definition of dementia obsolete? Vladimir Hachinski, M.D., of the University of Western Ontario in London, Ontario, Canada, thinks so.[2] "The concept of 'dementia' for ascertaining and addressing cognitive impairment has failed," he reported in the November 12, 2008 issue of the Journal of the American Medical Association. "It is too categorical, exclusive, and arbitrary."

Creating a dichotomy between dementia and non-dementia ignores the spectrum of cognitive impairment, he said. Converting soft data into hard categories fails to capture the complexity of the common coexistence and probable interaction of cerebrovascular and Alzheimer disease on the moving background of aging. It

---

1 Venkataraman, Bina. "Women May Live Longer with Dementia," New York Times, July 29, 2008, p. F6.
2 Hachinski, Vladimir, M.D. "Shifts in Thinking About Dementia," JAMA 300(18): 2172-2173, 2008.

is time to shift the focus from thresholds to a continuum of cognitive impairment, from the late to the early stages and from effects to causes.

He goes on to say that cerebrovascular disease and Alzheimer disease share similar risk factors, most of them treatable. Treating vascular risk factors can prevent stroke and possibly may delay the onset of dementia, however, before a shift in age of onset can occur, there must be a shift in thinking. "The concept of dementia is obsolete," he continued. "It combines categorical misclassification with etiologic impression. As an example, in one study of 1,879 patients diagnosed with consensus as having dementia, the number of those so identified varied by a factor of up to 10, depending on which of 5 commonly used criteria for dementia were applied. The accuracy of the etiologic diagnosis is not much better, either for Alzheimer disease or vascular dementia."

Currant definitions of dementia imply that the cognitive impairment is so severe that it interferes with self-sufficiency, he continued. Most definitions require memory impairment plus involvement of another cognitive domain. While the memory requirement works fairly well for Alzheimer's disease, it misses most cases of vascular cognitive impairment, that is, any cognitive impairment associated with or caused by vascular causes.

"The earliest cognitive manifestations of cerebrovascular disease are changes in executive function, such as planning, organizing, and deciding," he added. "Moreover, most epidemiologic and clinical studies of cognition use the Mini-Mental State Examination, This test is sensitive to memory disorders but insensitive to executive function impairment typically associated with vascular cognitive impairment, thus systematically biasing the literature in favor of the ascertainment of Alzheimer disease and to the exclusion of vascular disorders."

He added that common standards for the description of early stages of cognitive impairment, including vascular cognitive impairment and Alzheimer disease, have been recommended, mainly for research purposes. While these standards were developed mostly for vascular cognitive impairment, they were chosen so they would also apply to Alzheimer disease, and the concurrence of cerebrovascular disease and Alzheimer disease.

As an example, he continued, the standards include a 5-minute screening battery based on the Montreal Cognitive Assessment instrument, originally developed to test for Alzheimer's disease. The identification of a vascular component can then be achieved using the Hachinski Ischemic Scale, which requires no further investigation, and it has 89%, sensitivity and 89% specificity. Hachinski said that the patient's provisional diagnosis would be vascular cognitive impairment if that patient has a vascular component, implying the existence of treatable or preventable factors. Vascular risk factors should be identified and treated aggressively, if the patient does not have a vascular component, the provisional diagnosis would be cognitive impairment, cause uncertain.

However, he continued, neither label implies anything about prognosis, which is highly variable in the early stages of cognitive impairment. These minimum standards do not preclude investigators from concluding additional tests. The intent is to have common data points, so that several provisional criteria can be applied to the same patients and tested simultaneously against commonly agreed outcomes. "This would allow the development of data-based criteria to replace the current dogma-based criteria," he said. "The minimum data points could then be built into phenotypes that make clinical sense."

Neuritic plaques and neurofibrillary tangles in the brain, notably in the hippocampus, entorhinal cortex, and isocortex, are telltale signs of Alzheimer's disease and dementia in the elderly, reported Archives of Neurology.[1]

Unfortunately, this association has not been extensively studied in the rapidly growing population of the very old, the researchers said.

The study involved 317 brains of those 60 years and older, who were selected to have either no remarkable neuropathological lesions or only neuritic plaques and neurofibrillary tangle lesions. Brains with either neuropathological conditions, alone or in addition to Alzheimer's, were excluded from the study. The researchers found that, while the density of neuritic plaques and neurofibrillary tangles rose considerably by more than 10-fold as a function of the severity of dementia in the youngest-old group, significant increases in the density of the plaques and tangles were absent in the brains of the oldest-old.

"These findings suggest that the neuropathological features of dementia in the oldest-old (90 to 107) are not the same as those of cognitively impaired younger-old people (60 to 80), and compel a vigorous search for neuropathological indices of dementia in the

---

1 Haroutunian, V., et al. "Role of the Neuropathologic Neuropathology of Alzheimer Disease in Dementia in the Older-Old," Archives of Neurology 65(9): 1211-1217, 2008.

most rapidly growing segment of the elderly population," the researchers said.

Spikes in blood sugar can take a toll on memory by affecting the dentate gyrus, an area of the brain within the hippocampus that helps form memory, reported Roni Caryn Rubin in the January 6, 2009 issue of the New York Times.[1] Researchers have found that the effects can be seen when levels of blood sugar (glucose) are only moderately elevated, a finding that could explain normal age-related cognitive decline, since glucose regulation worsens with age.

The ability to regulate glucose starts deteriorating by the third or fourth decade of life, according to Scott A. Small, M.D., of the Columbia University Medical Center in New York. He added that, since glucose regulation is improved with physical activity, physical exercise is important.

"When we think about diabetes, we think about heart disease and all the consequences for the rest of the body, but we usually don't think about the brain," added Bruce S. McEwen of Rockefeller University in New York.

Rubin went on to say that, "previous observational studies have shown that physical activity reduces the risk of cognitive decline, and studies have also found that diabetes increases the risk of dementia. Earlier studies had also hinted at a link between type 2 diabetes and dysfunction of the dentate gyrus."

A research team at Kaiser Permanente in Oakland, California, headed by Rachel A. Whitmer, Ph.D., found that those with one severe hypoglycemia (low blood sugar) episode were 45% more apt to experience dementia in their later years, compared to those who had not had blood sugar crashes.[2]

Hypoglycemia occurs when there is too low a level of sugar in the blood. This happens when a person with diabetes has injected too much insulin; eaten too little food; or exercised without extra food. Typically, the person may feel nervous, shaky, weak, or sweaty and have a headache, blurred vision, and hunger. Taking small amounts of sugar, sweet juice, cheese, nuts, etc., will usually help the person to feel better within 10 to 15 minutes. "Among older patients with type 2 diabetes, a history of severe low blood sugar episodes was associated with a greater risk of dementia," the

---

1 Rabin, Roni Caryn. "Elevated Blood Sugar Found Bad for Memory," New York Times, January 6, 2009, p. D5.
2 Whitmer, Rachel A., Ph.D., et al. "Hypoglycemia Episodes and Risk of Dementia in Older Patients with type 2 Diabetes Meilitus," JAMA 301(15): 1565-1572, 2009.

researchers said. "Whether minor hypoglycemia episodes increase the risk of dementia is not known."

Diabetes mellitus increases the risk of dementia in the elderly, although its underlying mechanisms, its connection with Alzheimer's disease and vascular cognitive impairment, and effects of therapy remain unclear, according to Archives of Neurology.[1]

The number of microvascular infarcts was greater in deep cerebral structures in those with dementia whose diabetes was treated, amyloid plaque load tended to be greater for untreated diabetic patients with dementia.

The novel characterizations of different patterns of cerebral injury in patients with dementia depending on diabetes status may have etiologic and therapeutic implications, the researchers said.

Researchers who study those who reach exceptional old age are finding that the inexorable march toward the end of life need not be a steady decline, M. J. Friedrich reported in the Journal of the American Medical Association.[2] "In the last decade, investigators have been studying the growing number of people who celebrate their 100th birthday, and have found that many centenarians remain hale and hearty well into their 90s, delaying the onset of age-related diseases and compressing the time they are ill into a short period at the end of their lives."

While a geriatrics fellow at Harvard Medical School in Boston, Massachusetts in the early 1990s, Thomas Perls, M.D., was impressed by this phenomenon. While working with patients at a rehabilitation center for the aged, he found two 100-year-olds who stood out, not because of severe illness, but because they were busy members of their community. One of the centenarians played the piano for her friends, while the other, a tailor all of his life, mended clothes for others at the center, "when he was not courting his 85-year-old girlfriend."

To better understand the health and functional status of centenarians, Perls began recruiting 100-year-olds from 8 towns in the Boston area for the New England Centenarian Study. Perls and his colleagues found that this group is much healthier cognitively and physically than had been thought. Perls later became assistant professor of medicine at Boston University School of Medicine, and with his colleagues continued to study siblings and their children

---

1 Sonnen, J. A., et al. "Different Patterns of Cerebral Injury in Dementia with or Without Diabetes," Archives of Neurology 66(3): 315-322, 2009.

2 Friedrich, M. J. "Biological Secrets for Exceptional Old Age — Centenarian Study Seeks Insight into Aging Well," JAMA 288(18): 2247-2253, 2002.

to find out the genetic and environmental factors that help people reach exceptional old age.

One of their early observations was that about 90% of the centenarians were still functioning independently until they reached an average age of 92 (Lancet 354:652, 1999).

Through neuropsychological evaluation, Margery Silver, Fd.D., of the Massachusetts University, discovered that about one third of the group of Boston centenarians did not have dementia. "Studies carried out in older populations — but not in centenarians — suggested that Alzheimer's disease prevalence increases exponentially as the population ages, leading to the possible implication that by age 100 everyone would have some degree of dementia. However, once researchers, such as Silver, began to study centenarians, this notion was dispelled," noted Perls. He added that the genetics of exceptional longevity is likely a combination of having certain protective genes, and not having certain risk-producing genes. And, of course, environmental factors also play a role.

However, he said, for those who reach exceptional old age, healthy lifestyles may be less important than genes. "We simply don't learn very much from centenarians in terms of what you should do that's right — in terms of healthy behaviors — because they have the genes to get away with it — not emphasizing healthy behavior." Researchers are trying to identify the genes that lead to insights as to why some people age slower than others, and are more resistant to disease associated with aging.

"Such information could be used to help reduce the impact of age-related diseases on the rest of the population," Perls said. "For example, the centenarians and their children demonstrate that rather than 'the older you get the sicker you get,' it is much more likely that 'the older you get the healthier you've been.'"

If this positive view of aging is accepted, perhaps people will be more willing to take better care of themselves, thereby giving them a better chance of living to a significantly older age in better health, Perls concluded.

A growing number of Americans are dying of dementia, and prior work suggests that patients with advanced dementia are under-recognized as being at high risk for death and receive suboptimal palliative care, according to Susan L. Mitchell, M.D., of Hebrew SeniorLife, Boston, Massachusetts, and colleagues.[1] The researchers followed 323 nursing home residents with advanced dementia

---

1 Mitchell. Susan L., et al. "The Clinical Course of Advanced Dementia," New England Journal of Medicine 361: 1529-1538, 2009.

and their health care providers for 18 months in 22 nursing homes. During 18 months, 54.8% of the residents died. The probability of pneumonia was 41.1%; a febrile episode (running a temperature), 52.6%; and an eating problem, 85.8%. Distressing symptoms including dyspnea (shortness of breath), 46%; and pain, 39.1%, were common.

In the last 3 months of life, 40.7% of the patients underwent at least one burdensome intervention (hospitalization), emergency room visit, or parenteral (tube) feeding.

"As the mortality rates for many leading causes of death have declined during the past decade, deaths from dementia have steadily increased," the researchers said. "Patients, families, and health care providers must understand and be prepared to confront the end stage of the disease, which is estimated to afflict more than 5 million Americans currently, and is expected to affect more than 13 million by 2050." They added, "we have shown that an understanding of the prognosis and expected complications on the part of health care proxies reduces the likelihood that nursing home residents with advanced dementia, who are nearing the end of life, will undergo potentially burdensome interventions of unclear benefit. This study underscores the need to improve the quality of palliative care in nursing homes in order to reduce the physical suffering of residents with advanced dementia who are dying."

Homocysteine, a normally benign amino acid, is an independent risk factor for both dementia and cognitive impairment without dementia (CIND), reported Mary N. Haan, et al., at the University of Michigan in Ann Arbor, in the American Journal of Clinical Nutrition in 2007.[1]

Higher blood levels of vitamin B12 may reduce the risk of homocysteine associated with dementia and CIND, they added.

Homocysteine, a sulfhydryl amino acid, is a product of the methionine cycle that is derived from dietary protein, the researchers said. The homocysteine concentration is influenced by folic acid, a B vitamin, and vitamin B12, and is modifiable through B vitamin supplementation.

SAM-e — S-adenosylmethionine or "sammy" — deficiencies are common among people with neurological problems, such as Alzheimer's disease, Parkinson's disease, and HIV (AIDs) that can lead to dementia, according to Richard Brown, M.D., et al., in

---

1 Haan, Mary N., et al. "Hococysteine, B Vitamins, and the Incidence of Dementia and Cognitive Impairment: Results from the Sacramento Area Latino Study on Aging," *American Journal of Clinical Nutrition* 85: 511-517, 2007.

"Stop Depression Now." Dr. Brown is associate professor of clinical psychology at Columbia University in New York.[1]

SAM-e is made from substances normally found in the body — methionine and adenosine triphosphate (ATP). Methionine is an essential amino acid, a building block of protein that is found in meat and fish, and it is also made in small amounts by our cells, but hardly enough to meet the body's needs.

Two B vitamins — vitamin B12 and folic acid — are required for the production of methionine, and a deficiency of either one can result in depression and problems in mental health, especially among older people. "ATP is a high-powered fuel that is produced by the cells to provide energy to run the body," the researchers continued. "It is present in almost every cell and provides the juice to run all of the body's machinery. Fortunately, there is plenty to go around."

Many researchers believe that an excess of free radicals contributes to both Alzheimer's disease and Parkinson's disease. "SAM-e enables the body to produce more of its free radical scavenger, glutathione," the researchers added. "At the same time, it boosts the levels of transmitters involved in mood, memory, and learning. In a sense, SAM-e restores the brain to a more youthful environment."

The researchers went on to say that those with Alzheimer's disease have lower-than-normal levels of SAM-e. They are not suggesting that taking SAM-e can prevent or cure Alzheimer's, but, by boosting antioxidant levels, it might help to maintain a healthier environment in the brain, which could have an effect on Alzheimer's disease.

The starting dose of SAM-e is 400 mg/day. The researchers say this dose is usually effective for those with mild to moderate depression. Since the supplement works quickly, an improvement of at least 25% will be evident within 2 weeks. "If you do not see a 25% improvement after 2 weeks, increase your dose to 800 mg/day. After increasing the dose, if there is no improvement of 25% after 2 more weeks, we recommend you seek professional evaluation."

They added that you may need a higher dose of SAM-e, or the supplement in combination with another antidepressant, or a different antidepressant. "If you have a history of extreme sensitivity to medications, start out with a lower dose of 200 mg/day for the first week," the researchers said. "If you do not experience any problems, you can increase your dose to 400 mg/day." SAM-e is

---

1 Brown, Richard, M.D., Bottiglieri, Teodoro, Ph.D., and Colman, Carol. Stop Depression Now. New York: G. P. Putnam's Sons, 1999, pp. 62-63, 122ff., 230ff.

sold in tablet form, and it is best to buy enteric-coated products. SAM-e should be taken on an empty stomach about half an hour before meals. If the tablet should cause heartburn on an empty stomach, take it with meals.

If you are taking 400 mg, you can take the full amount in the morning, or take 200 mg before breakfast and 200 mg before lunch. Larger dosages can also be taken in divided doses.

On rare occasions, people may develop a mild headache when taking SAM-e, but it usually disappears after the first week or two. At higher doses — higher than those recommended here — some people may experience diarrhea. However, the supplement does not cause weight gain, sexual dysfunction, anxiety attacks, and chronic gastrointestinal distress that are side effects of other antidepressants, the researchers said.

However, they continued, SAM-e should not be taken by patients with bipolar depression, unless they are under the supervision of a psychiatrist knowledgeable in mood disorder treatments. Like other antidepressants, SAM-e can induce a manic phase in bipolar patients. (Bipolar depression is characterized by alternating periods of depression and euphoria).

3. You Don't Have to Be Depressed

How Widespread Is Depression?

According to the World Health Organization, depression is the leading global cause of years of life lived with disability, and the fourth leading cause of disability-adjusted life-years, a measure that takes premature mortality into account, reported Thomas R. Insel, M.D., and Dennis S. Charney, M.D., of the National Institute of Mental Health in Bethesda, Maryland.[1]

"Depression is not only widespread and common, but it may be fatal," they said. "An estimated 90% of suicides are associated with mental illness, most commonly depression. There were almost 30,000 suicides in the U.S. in 1999, almost twice the number of homicides, the third leading cause of death." Antidepressants are generally effective in that most studies demonstrate at least a 50% decrease in symptoms for about 70% of the patients. In addition to antidepressants, specific structured psychotherapies have been shown to treat depression, especially in less severe, non-psychotic patients. "Sadly, too often these treatments are not used when they are needed, or are given at a dose or for a duration that is ineffective," they added.

Mental illness contributes a substantial burden of disease worldwide, and globally about 450 million people suffer from mental disorders, reported S. Marshall Williams, Ph.D., et al., in

---

1 Insel, Thomas R., M.D., and Charney, Dennis S., M.D., "Research on Major Depression: Strategies and Priorities," JAMA 289(23): 3167-3168, 2003.

the Journal of the American Medical Association (JAMA). For example, depression has emerged as a risk factor for such chronic illnesses as high blood pressure, diabetes, and cardiovascular disease.[1]

One fourth of the world's population will develop a mental or
behavioral disorder at some time during their lives. In fact, mental disorders account for about 25% of disability in the United
States, Canada, and Western Europe, and they are a leading cause
of premature death. In the U.S., about 22% of the adult population has one or more diagnosable mental disorders in a given year.
"The estimated lifetime prevalence for mental disorders among the
U.S. adult population are about 29% for anxiety disorders; 25%
for impulse-control disorders; 21% for mood disorders: 15% for
substance-abuse disorders; and 46% for any of 3 diseases," the researchers added. "However, mental illness costs the U.S. an estimated $150 billion, excluding the cost of research."

Every year, over 17 million Americans experience the pain of
clinical depression, according to the Complete Guide to Pain Relief. Women with depression are said to outnumber men 2 to 1.
That is, some type of depression affects 20% of women, 10% of men,
along with 5% of adolescents during their lifetime. And, according
to the World Health Organization, the percentages can be tabulated worldwide.[2]

"The causes of depression are unknown, but researchers are convinced that there is a genetic component, since it tends to run in
families," the article in JAMA added. "One type, seasonal affective
disorder (SAD), occurs during the winter months, when there are
fewer daylight hours. Patients with this type of depression tend to
live in northern areas and invariably develop it annually."

DEPRESSION IN THE ELDERLY

Depression in the elderly is often underdiagnosed and undertreated, and too often caregivers, family members, and the person
who is suffering assume that the illness is an inevitable part of the
aging process. According to Miriam Cohen, PhD, "The unwitting
acceptance by society of depression as 'natural' to aging closes the
door to effective intervention, especially since it may prevent the
older person who is suffering from seeking help. Failure to realize
that the older person's despair is an illness deprives that person of

---

1 Williams, S. Marshall, Ph.D., et al. "The Role of Public Health in Mental Health Problems,"
   JAMA 294(18): 2293, 2005.
2 Kalyn, Wayne, editorial director. The Complete Guide to Pain Relief. Pleasantville, NY: The
   Reader's Digest Association, Inc., 2000, pp. 355-356.

not only insight into his or her condition, but, more importantly, relief from it."[1]

Since the 1950s, antidepressant drugs have constituted the major method of treating depression. Compliance with the medication regimen is essential, and several different types of antidepressants are thought to be equally effective. However, the drugs have different side effects, which are more or less acceptable to different people, depending on their medical problems as well as their personal coping capacities, Cohen adds. "Physicians have had the most experience with tricyclic antidepressants — tricyclic refers to the drugs' chemical structure." Nortriptyline (Pamelor), desipramine (Norpramin), amitriptyline (Elavil), and imipramine (Tofranil) are examples.

Elderly patients are especially sensitive to the side effects of antidepressants, which may produce confusion or delirium if drug doses are too high. Many drugs in addition to antidepressants have anticholinergic effects, and, since elderly people often take more than 1 drug, care must be taken that the anticholinergic effects of multiple drugs do not result in a confusional state, says Cohen. (Anticholinergic refers to the opposing or blocking the physiological action of acetylcholine, a neurotransmitter.) In an overdose, tricyclic antidepressants are potentially lethal. The most common manifestations of an overdose are a rapid heartbeat and low blood pressure. Life-threatening cardiac arrhythmias can also occur. "Other antidepressants that have been available for several decades are the monoamine oxidase (MAO) inhibitors," she notes. "These include isocarioazid (Marplan), phenelzine (Nardil), and tranylcypromine (Parnate)." These antidepressants halt the action of the brain enzyme monoamine oxidase, and they may be effective in those who have not responded to other medications, or those who have atypical depression symptoms.

MAO inhibitors are not prescribed as frequently as the other medications, because severe hypertensive and hypotensive crises can occur if foods containing tyramine — some cheeses, aged or fermented foods, fava beans, chicken livers, wines, and some alcoholic beverages — are not carefully avoided, Cohen says.

The newest classes of antidepressants are referred to as the selective serotonin reuptake inhibitors, so called because of their hypothesized mechanism of action — inhibiting activity of the neurotransmitter serotonin. Drugs in this group include sertraline

---

1 Cohen, Miriam, Ph.D. "Special Report: Mind, Mood, and Medication in Later Life,"' Medical and Health Annual. Chicago, IL: Encyclopaedia Britannica, Inc., 1994, pp. 229ff.

(Zoloft), fluoxetine (Prozac), and paroxetine (Paxil). The side effects include nausea, diarrhea, agitation, and sexual dysfunction. Other antidepressants that cannot be grouped into a single class include trazodone (Desyrel), bupropion (Wellbutrin), amoxapine (Asendin), and Maprotiline (Ludiomil).

"It is now recognized that a significant decline in cognitive function is not an inevitable part of aging, but rather it is the result of disease," Cohen says. "Forgetfulness is the first symptom of Alzheimer's disease."

SOME SIGNS OF DEPRESSION

Depression takes many forms. To cite further from S. Marshall Williams, Ph.D., writing in JAMA,[1] the most common type symptoms of the most common type of clinical depression include:

- A persistently depressed mood.
- Diminished interest in or enjoyment of pleasurable activities, such as sex.
- Significant changes in weight.
- Insomnia or excessive sleeping.
- Hyperactivity or lethargy.
- Fatigue almost daily.
- Feelings of worthlessness or inappropriate guilt.
- Inability to concentrate or make decisions.
- Recurrent thoughts about suicide or death.

"Sadness is part of everyday life and should not be confused with clinical depression," he said. "As defined by the American Psychiatric Association, it occurs when 5 or more of the symptoms just listed affect someone most of the time for about 2 weeks."

On occasion, depression develops without any obvious precipitating factors, or it can appear to a response to an environmental problem, such as the loss of a job or loved one. Another factor in depression is a hormonal condition, such as thyroid disease. "The most reliable indicators of major depression are lethargy, changes in sleep patterns and appetite, feelings of helplessness, low self-esteem, and a profound inability to make decisions," the publication reported.

Manic depression, or bipolar disorder, is characterized by alternating periods of depression and euphoria. This can be initiated by a serious psychological breakdown.

---

1 Williams, S. Marshall, Ph.D., et al. "The Role of Public Health in Mental Health Problems," JAMA 294(18): 2293, 2005.

Symptoms of Major Depression

Having at least 5 of these symptoms nearly every day for at least 2 weeks:

- Feeling sad and empty.
- Decreased interest or pleasure in activities.
- Appetite change with weight loss or weight gain.
- Decreased or increased sleeping.
- Fatigue or loss of energy.
- Feeling worthless or guilty.
- Being either agitated or slowed down.
- Difficulty thinking or concentrating.
- Recurrent thoughts of death or suicide.

There are various types of depression, including the following:

- Bipolar disorder (manic-depressive disorder), which involves episodes of major depression and episodes of abnormally elevated mood called mania (severe) or hypomania (less severe).
- Dysthymia, which are mild depression symptoms lasting for at least 2 years.
- Postpartum depression, which is mother's depression following the birth of her baby.
- Seasonal affective disorder, which is major depression occurring regularly in seasons with low sunlight.

Treatments for depression include:

- Medications. Several types of antidepressant medications can be effective, but they must be taken for several weeks before they begin to work.
- Psychotherapy. A number of "talking therapies" have proven to be effective. They involve evaluating and changing the thoughts, attitudes, and relationship problems associated with depression.
- Bright light. Daily exposure to bright light can be helpful for seasonal depression.
- Electroconvulsive therapy. These treatments involve the passage of electric current through the brain while the patient is under anesthesia. The treatments are usually given 3 times a week for several weeks.

An analysis reported in Archives of General Psychiatry found that a nationally representative U.S. sample suggests that overeating and oversleeping can be used to identify an atypical depression subgroup that is distinct from other depressed patients in terms of demographics, psychiatric comorbidities and abuse history.[1]

When compared with nonatypical depression, atypical depression was associated with a greater percentage of women and an earlier age of onset. The atypical patients also reported higher rates of most depressive symptoms, suicidal thoughts and attempts, psychiatric comorbidity — panic attacks, social phobias, and drug dependence — disability and restricted activity days, use of some health-care services, paternal depression, and childhood neglect and sexual abuse.

Transmission to menopause has long been considered a period of increased risk of depressive symptoms, according to a research team in Archives of General Psychiatry. However, it has not been determined whether this period is one of increased risk for major depressive disorder, especially for women who have not had previous bouts with depression.[2] Physical symptoms associated with the menopausal transition and mood changes seen during this period may affect many women as they age, and it may be a significant burden of illness, the researchers added.

Traditionally thought of as an episodic, remitting illness, major depression disorder often has a chronic course, with protracted episodes of incomplete remission episodes, according to Martin B. Keller, M.D., of Brown University in Providence, Rhode Island, and colleagues at other facilities.[3] At any given time, an estimated 3% of the U.S. population suffers from chronic depression, and chronic forms of the disorder are associated with more marked impairments in psychosocial function and work performance, increased health care utilization, and more frequent suicide attempts and hospitalizations, than acute depression. "Because they frequently begin early in life, and are often lifelong, chronic forms of depression account for an inordinate proportion of the enormous burden of illness associated with depression." In their study, they randomly assigned 681 adults with a chronic nonpsychiatric major depressive disorder to 12 weeks of outpatient treatment with nefazodone (Serzone) with a maximal dose of 600 mg/day, the cognitive be-

---

1 Matza, Louis S., et al. "Depression with Atypical Features in the National Comorbidity Survey: Classification, Description, and Consequences," Archives of General Psychiatry 60: 817-826, 2003.

2 Cohen, L. S., et al. "Risk for New Onset of Depression During the Menopausal Transition: The Harvard Study of Moods and Cycles," Archives of General Psychiatry 63: 385-390, 2006.

3 Keller, Martin B., M.D., et al. "A Comparison of Nefazodone, The Cognitive Behavioral-Analysis System of Psychotherapy, and Their Combination for the Treatment of Chronic Depression," The New England Journal of Medicine 342: 1462-1470, 2000.

havioral analysis system of psychotherapy (16 to 20 sessions) or both.

At the beginning of the study, all patients had scores of at least 20 on the 24-item Hamilton Rating Scale for Depression, which indicated clinically significant depression. "Remission was defined as a score of 8 or less at weeks 10 and 12," the research team added. "For patients who did not have remission, a satisfactory response was defined as a reduction in the score by at least 50% from the beginning of the study and a score of 15 or less."

While the rates of withdrawal were similar in the 3 groups, adverse events in the drug group were consistent with the known side effects of the drug, that is, headache, somnolence, dry mouth, nausea, and dizziness. "We found that the combination of pharmacotherapy (nefazodone) and the cognitive behavioral analysis system of psychotherapy was significantly more efficacious than either treatment alone for outpatients with chronic forms of depression." The rates of response to either treatment alone were similar to the rates reported in previous trials of antidepressants for the treatment of chronic forms of depression in outpatients, indicating that at least one form of psychotherapy is effective in treating these patients. However, nefazodone produced effects more rapidly than did the psychotherapy.

A report by the Agency for Healthcare Research and Quality shows that almost one fourth of about 32 million stays in 2004 in U.S. community hospitals for adult patients involved such mental health disorders as depression, bipolar disorder, schizophrenia, or substance abuse-related disorders, according to Tracy Hampton, Ph.D., in the Journal of the American Medical Association.[1]

About 1.9 million of the stays were for those who were hospitalized mostly because of a mental health or substance abuse problem. In the other 5.7 million stays, patients were admitted for another condition but were also diagnosed as having a mental health or substance abuse disorder. Medicare covered almost half of the stays, Medicaid paid for 18%, and about 8% were not insured, Hampton said.

The biological mechanisms by which depression and type 2 diabetes are associated remain unclear, however, a study by Sherita Hill Golden, M.D., of Johns Hopkins University in Baltimore, Maryland, and colleagues at other facilities, contributes to a grow-

---

1 Hampton, Tracy, Ph.D. "Mental Health of Inpatients," JAMA 297(20): 2188, 2007.

ing body of literature that indicates a bidirectional association between the 2 serious long-term diseases.[1]

This connection was partially explained by lifestyle factors, impaired fasting glucose levels, and untreated type 2 diabetes. Treated type 2 diabetics showed a positive association with depressed symptoms.

"Future studies should determine whether interventions aimed at modifying behavioral factors associated with depression will complement current type 2 diabetes prevention strategies," the researchers continued. "However, these findings suggest that clinicians should be aware of increased risk of elevated depressive symptoms in those with treated type 2 diabetes, and consider routine screening for depressive symptoms among these patients."

It would be appealing to attempt to categorize depression in terms of monoamine-depletion forms that are perhaps related to genes coding for enzymes involved in neurotransmission and cortisol-related forms that are characterized by a more long-term course, hippocampal atrophy, and a history of psychosocial stress, according to R. H. Belmaker, M.D., and Galila Agam, Ph.D., of the Ben Gurion University in the Negev in Beersheba, Israel.[2] However, they continue, the clinical data do not fall into such neat categories, since monoamine-based antidepressants are most effective in those with severe depression when cortisol levels remain high after the administration of dexamethasone, a respiratory corticosteroid to treat inflammation and other conditions.

"Major depressive disorder is likely to have a number of causes," the researchers added. "Middle-aged and elderly patients with depression may have a disorder related to cardiovascular disease and originating from endothelial dysfunction. In patients with an anxious and depressive personality, depression may be due to genetically determined personality factors or adverse childhood experiences."

They added that avoidance of premature closure on any one scientific theory of the mechanism of depression will best serve the search for new, more effective treatments. It is possible that the pathogenesis of acute depression is different from that of recurrent or chronic depression, which is characterized by long-term declines in function and cognition. "Mood can be elevated by stimulants, by brain stimulating, or by ketamine, an anesthetic that af-

---

1 Golden, Sherita Hill, M.D., et al. "Examining a Bidirectional Association Between Depressive Symptoms and Diabetes," JAMA 299(23): 2751-2759, 2008.
2 Belmaker, R. H., M.D., and Agam, Galila, Ph.D. "Major Depressive Disorder," New England Journal of Medicine 358: 55-68, 2008.

fects mood, etc., or by depressed by monoamine depletion in recovered patients, for short periods, but longer-term improvement may require reduction of the abnormal glucocorticoid function induced by stress or increases in brain neurotrophic factors," the researchers added.

DEPRESSION AND THE HEART

Depression is present in 1 of 5 outpatients with coronary heart disease, and in 1 of 3 outpatients with congestive heart failure, and yet the majority of cases are not recognized or appropriately treated, according to Mary A. Whooley, M.D., of the Veterans Medical Center and University of California, San Francisco Medical Center in California.[1] "While it is not known whether treating depression improves cardiovascular outcome, antidepressant treatment with selective serotonin reuptake inhibitors (SSRIs) is generally safe, alleviating depression and improving quality of life," Whooley said.

Depression has been associated with the development of congestive heart failure (CHF) and with adverse outcomes in patients with CHF, Whooley continued. In a study examining incidence of CHF among 4,500 patients who were enrolled in the Systolic Hypertension in the Elderly Program, the cumulative evidence of CHF in the depressed patients was 16%, whereas the incidence was only 7% in the nondepressed group.

Cardiac rehabilitation has several important components, including training patients to exercise, to eat healthy foods, to adhere to preventive medications, and to reduce psychological stress. Cardiac rehabilitation is known to improve cardiovascular outcomes, and its psychological components may be partly responsible for these benefits, Whooley continued. She went on to say that, given its potential benefits for smoking cessation, bupropion is an excellent first choice for cardiac patients who smoke. However, it can slightly increase blood pressure.

An increased prevalence of low bone mineral density (BMD) has been observed in patients with major depressive disorders (MDD), especially among women, according to Archives of Internal Medicine.[2]

The researchers recruited participants in their study from July 1, 2001 to February 29, 2003, which measured baseline BMD in 89

1 Whooley, Mary A., M.D. "Depression and Cardiovascular Disease: Healing the Broken-Hearted," JAMA 295(24): 2874-2881, 2006.

2 Eskandari, F., et al. "Low Bone Mass in Premenopausal Women with Depression," Archives of Internal Medicine 167(21): 2329-2336, 2007.

premenopausal women with MDD, and 44 healthy controls. The prevalence of low BMD was greater for those with MDD when compared to controls at the neck of the femur, total hip, and tended to be greater at the lumbar spine.

It has been found that 10% of mentally ill elderly have major depression, reported Linda Ganzini, M.D., and colleagues, at the Portland Veterans Affairs Medical Center in Oregon.[1] The research team added that 43 classes of medications have been implicated in drug-induced depression, including reserpine, beta-blockers, levodopa, corticosteroids, and antipsychotics.

There appears to be no evidence that age is an independent risk factor for drug-induced depression. Actually, drug-induced depression can be misdiagnosed in the elderly, since they have frequent occurrences of other mental problems. Regular inquiries into the symptoms of mood disorders in geriatric patients should be made, as well as to how drugs may affect their development.

SOME TRIGGERS AND TREATMENTS FOR DEPRESSION

Medications: Certain anti-inflammatory, analgesic, antimicrobial, cardiovascular, and central nervous system medications, and hormones can trigger depression.[2]

Magnet therapy: In evaluating 12 patients with depression, it was found that when they were given magnet therapy for 2 weeks, their depression improved satisfactorily, more than when they were given a placebo treatment for a separate 2-week period, according to the American Journal of Psychiatry.[3] The magnet therapy involved application of magnets to the same area of the head daily over 10 days during a 2-week trial. The research team sent an electrical pulse through the magnet during a 2-second interval to activate the electromagnetic field. The magnet therapy reduced depression scores by an average of 5 points, the researchers said. Those who were given a placebo had their scores worsened by 3 points.

The rapid generation and then abolition of the magnetic field causes nerve cells to depolarize in the cortex, which may be linked

---

1 Ganzini, Linda, M.D., et al. "Drug-Induced Depression in the Aged: What Can Be Done?" *Drags and Aging* 3(2): 147-158, 1993.

2 Reynolds, Charles F., III, M.D. "Recognition and Differentiation of Elderly Depression in the Clinical Setting," *Geriatrics* 50: S6-S15, 1995.

3 La Voie, Angela. "Magnets May Help Battle Depression," *American Journal of Psychiatry* 154: 1752-1756, 1997.

to circuits to deeper structures that may cause a change in brain activity that helps to improve mood, the researchers added.

Cholesterol: In evaluating 29,133 men, ranging in age from 50 to 69, and followed for 5 to 8 years, low blood levels of total cholesterol were associated with low mood and subsequent heightened risk of hospital treatment due to major depressive symptoms, and of death and suicide, according to the British Journal of Psychiatry.[1]

Dental fillings: In a study reported in the Journal of Orthomolecular Medicine, 11 manic depressive patients had their amalgams fillings removed, while 9 controls with amalgams were told they were being given a sealant. Of the 87 scales on the Minnesota Multiphasic Personality Inventory-2, the amalgam removal group improved significantly more in 47 of them.[2]

The researchers found that depression and hypomania scores improved significantly as did anxiety, anger, schizophrenia, paranoia, and many other conditions. Scores on the Million Clinical Multiaxial Inventory II improved more significantly in the scales of avoidance, dependence, and antisocial and borderline behavior, when compared to the sealant/placebo group.

The Clinical Personality Pattern category and the severe Personality Pathology category also revealed significantly more improvement in the amalgam removal group.

In addition, the amalgam removal group reported a 42% decrease in the number of somatic health problems after amalgam removal, compared to an 8% increase in somatic symptoms in the placebo/sealant patients, the researchers added.

Psychotherapy: In an article in Archives of General Psychiatry, a research team reported that patients showed significant improvements in depression and a positive effect following 16 weeks of telephone-administered treatments.[3] This study confirms that several studies have shown that telephone administered cognitive-behavior therapy (T-CBT) is superior to forms of no treatment controls. Telephone psychotherapy was conducted in the pa-

---

1   Partonen, T., M.D., et al. "Association of Low Blood Serum Total Cholesterol with Major Depression and Suicide," British Journal of Psychiatry 175: 259-262, 1999.

2   Siblerud, Robert L., MS, et al. "Psychometric Evidence That Dental Amalgam Mercury May Be An Etiological Factor in Manic Depression," Journal of Orthomolecular Medicine 13(1): 31-41, 1998.

3   Mohr, D.C., et al. "Telephone-Administered Psychotherapy for Depression," Archives of General Psychiatry 62: 1007-1014, 2005.

tients' homes. Treatment gains were maintained during 12 months of follow-up.

WHAT TO DO ABOUT DEPRESSION: VITAMINS AND DIETARY
SUPPLEMENTS

Vitamin B6

Mental symptoms have been known for many years to be a distinct feature of celiac disease in patients of all ages, according to Claes Hallert of Linkoping University in Sweden. Vitamin B6 is generally malabsorbed by celiac disease patients, and the vitamin was given at 80 mg/day to 12 celiac patients for 6 months.[1] After retesting by the Minnesota Multiphasic Personality Inventory (MMPI) questionnaire, a substantial improvement was shown in the MMPI group. Such an improvement has not been observed in celiac disease patients on a gluten-free diet alone, Hallert said.

A depressed mood in celiac patients may be, in part, nutritional in origin, and responsive to vitamin B6 therapy, since the vitamin is important in the conversion of 5-hydroxytryptophan, through decarboxylation, to serotonin. Vitamin B6 is also important in the conversion of L-dopa to dopamine, which is subsequently converted to noradrenaline, Hallert added.

As reported in the Scandinavian Journal of Gastroenterology, 12 patients — 8 men and 4 women — ranging in age up to 63 years — with celiac disease, were contrasted with surgical patients who acted as controls.[2]

Following 1 year after gluten withdrawal, the celiac patients showed depressive symptoms, in spite of evidence of no changes in depressive symptoms. When retested 3 years later, after being given 80 mg/day of vitamin B6 orally, there was a drop in the "depression score" from 70 to 56, which became normalized like other pretreatment abnormalities in the Minnesota Multiphasic Personality Inventory.

The researchers added that their study suggests that there is a causal relationship between celiac disease and depressive symptoms, which were normalized with vitamin B6 therapy.

---

1   Hallert Claes. "Depression In Coeliac Disease," Epilepsy and Other Neurological Diseases in Coeliac Disease," 28: 211-217, 1997.

2   Hallert Claes, et al. "Reversal of Psychopathology in Adult Coeliac Disease with the Aid of Pyridoxine (Vitamin B6)," Scandinavian Journal of Gastroenterology 18: 299-304, 1983.

Vitamin B12

In an article in the American Journal of Psychiatry, a research team found a significant vitamin B12 deficiency in 14.9% of the 478 nondepressed patients; 17% of 100 mainly depressed patients; and 27% of severely depressed subject.[1]

It was reported that those with a vitamin B12 deficiency were 2.05 times as likely to be severely depressed as those who did not have a deficiency of the vitamin.

Researchers reported in the Quarterly Journal of Medicine that cases of psychiatric disorders that are due to a B12 deficiency, have been undiagnosed through medical, neurological, and psychiatric units before being referred to a physician, sometimes years later, who have frank pernicious anemia.[2]

A vitamin B12 deficiency may occur in the absence of subacute combined degeneration of the spinal cord or any abnormality of the peripheral blood and marrow. In psychiatry, general medicine, and neurology, it is important to note that a normal peripheral blood and marrow biopsy does not exclude a vitamin B12 deficiency, the researchers said.

Folic Acid

A research team evaluated 26 men and 69 women, ranging in age up to 73, who were suffering from major depressive disorders, or the relationship between blood levels of folic acid and depressive symptoms, compared with 34 men and 26 women who were normal controls.[3]

It was reported that there were significantly lower blood and red blood cell folate concentrations in those with major depressive disorders, than in the normal controls.

Lower blood levels of the B vitamin were associated with more severe depression, the researchers added. There was no association between serum and red blood cell folate considerations and endogenticity of depression or the presence of weight loss.

The researchers added that those with lower plasma folic acid levels had significantly higher self-related morbidity than those

1 Penninx, B. W., et al. "Vitamin B12 Deficiency and Depression in Physically Disabled Older Women: Epidemiologic Evidence from the Women's Health and Aging Study," American Journal of Psychiatry 157(5): 715-721, May 2000.

2 Strachan, R. W., et al. "Psychiatric Syndromes Due to Avitaminosis B12 with Normal Blood and Marrow," Quarterly Journal of Medicine 34(135): 307-313, 1965.

3 Abou-Saleh, M.T., et al. "Serum and Red Blood Cell Folate in Depression," Acta Psychiatrica Scandinavica 80: 78-82, 1989.

with higher concentrations. They also had less favorable response to antidepressant therapy than those with higher levels.

In addition, both plasma and red blood cell folate concentrations were significantly lower in drug-free, acutely ill depressive subjects than in the controls.

Don't Forget Vitamin D

A vitamin D deficiency is now considered a worldwide pandemic.

In a study of 1,282 community residents, 65 to 95, in the Netherlands,[1] it was found that levels of vitamin D — 25(OH)D — in the blood were 14% lower in 169 patients with mild depression, and 14% lower in 26 patients with major depressive disorder, compared to 1,087 controls, levels of parathyroid hormone (PTH) were 5 and 33% higher, respectively.

The results reveal an association of depression status and severity with decreased blood, levels of vitamin D and increased serum PTH levels in older people. Produced by the parathyroid glands, PTH helps to control the level of calcium in the blood. Even small variations can impair muscle and nerve function.

DHEA

As reported in Biological Psychiatry, 3 men and 3 women, ranging in age from 51 to 72, with documented depression, were given 30 to 90 mg/day of oral dehydroepiandrosterone (DHEA) for 4 weeks. The doses above 30 mg/day were divided into 2 or 3 doses.[2]

The researchers reported that depression ratings and memory performance were significantly improved in the volunteers. In fact, one patient, who received the therapy for 6 months, her depression ratings improved 48 to 72%, and her semantic memory preference improved 63%.

Unfortunately, after treatment was halted, the measurement parameters returned to the levels at the beginning of the study. The researchers confirmed that depression ratings and memory performance were directly related to increases in blood levels of DHEA, DHEA sulfate, and to an increase in their ratios with plasma cortisol levels.

---

1 Hoogendijk, W. J. G., et al. "Depression Is Associated with Decreased 25-Hydroxyvitamin D and Increased Parathyroid Hormone Levels in Older Adults," Archives of General Psychiatry 65(5): 508-512, 2008.
2 Wolkowitz, O. M., et al. "Dehydroepiandrostsrone (DHEA) Treatment of Depression," Biological Psychiatry 41: 311-318, 1997.

Cortisol/hydrocortisone is a steroid hormone secreted by the adrenal glands, which secrete epinephrine and norepinephrine. In a study described in the American Journal of Psychiatry, 22 patients with major depression, who were either medication-free or on stabilized antidepressant regimens, were given 90 mg/day of DHEA or a placebo for 6 weeks in a double-blind trial.[1] The DHEA therapy was associated with a significantly greater reduction in Hamilton Depression Scale ratings than was placebo, according to Owen M. Wolkowitz, M.D., and colleagues. Five of the 11 patients treated with DHEA, compared with none of the 11 given a placebo, showed a 50% decrease or greater in depressive symptoms. The volunteers were instructed to take 30 mg/day of DHEA for the first 2 weeks, then 30 mg twice daily for 2 weeks, then 30 mg 3 times a day for the final 2 weeks.

Carnitine

At Catholic University of The Sacred Heart in Rome, Italy, a research team evaluated 24 geriatric patients who were hospitalized with depressive syndrome.[2] In the study, reported in Drugs, Experimental and Clinical Research, the researchers gave half of the patients acetyl-L-carnitine for 1 month and a placebo thereafter. The remainder were given a placebo, followed by acetyl-L-carnitine afterward.

The researchers reported that the carnitine therapy was highly effective and significantly effective, since depressive tendencies were significantly modified in most treatment groups. However, general somatic symptoms, anxiety, asthenia (loss of strength), and sleep disturbances were not affected.

The research team added that their research confirms that L-carnitine was especially effective in those showing more serious clinical symptoms. No side effects were recorded.

Researchers at Servizio Psichiatrico in Torino, Italy, evaluated the antidepressant activity of acetyl-L-carnitine versus a placebo in 28 depressed patients. They reported that there was a significantly higher clinical biological efficacy for the carnitine therapy when compared with placebo.[3]

1 Wolkowitz, O. M., M.D., et al. "Double-Blind Treatment of Major Depression with Dehydroepiandrosterone," American Journal of Psychiatry 156(4): 646-649, April 1999.
2 Tempesta, E., et al. "L-Acetylcarnitine in depressed Elderly Subjects: A Cross-Over Study Versus Placebo," Drugs, Experimental and Clinical Research 13(7): 417-423, 1987.
3 Gecele, Michela, et al. "Acetyl-L-Carnitine in Aged Subjects with Major Depression: Clinical Efficacy and Effects on the Circadian Rhythm of Cortisol," Dementia 2: 333-337, 1991.

Omega-3 Fatty Acids

A research team at the University of Sheffield in the United Kingdom compared 10 depressed patients with 14 healthy, matched controls. It was found that there was a significant reduction in red blood cell count, and membrane omega-3 fatty acids in the depressed patients, which was not due to caloric intake.[1] However, the severity of depression correlated negatively with red blood count levels and with dietary intake of omega-3 fatty acids (fish oils, etc).

Docosahexaenoic acid (DHA) emerged as a significant predictor of depression in multiple regression analysis across the whole study population, the researchers reported in Journal of Affective Disorders.

The research team added that, in depressed patients, where the diet was low in omega-3 fatty acids, the red blood count membrane composition of omega-3 fatty acids was also reduced. This was not found in the controls.

An imbalance in the ratio of omega-3 and omega-6 fatty acids (vegetable oils) may contribute to depressive symptoms, according to Nutrition Reviews, Dieting has also been associated with alterations in mood, the researchers added.[2]

In addition, heightened depressive symptoms have been associated with low blood levels of cholesterol. They added that serotonin and its precursor, trypthophan, are very important in the neurobiology of depression.

Food restriction may contribute to inadequate consumption of omega-3 fatty acids, and a study involving healthy women found that both low dietary intake of long-chain omega-3 fatty acids and higher levels of body dissatisfaction together were significantly associated with severe depression.

The research team went on to say that extremely low-fat diets, which are prescribed for lowering cholesterol and/or disease prevention effects, tend to replace saturated fats with omega-6 polyunsaturated fatty acids, which increase the omega-6/omega-3 fatty acid ratio in the diet. This may potentiate a relative deficiency in omega-3 fatty acids, and the balance between the fatty acids may modulate the metabolism of biogenic amines.

1   Edwards, Rhian, et al. "Omega-3 Polyunsaturated Fatty Acid Levels in the Diet and in Red Blood Cell Membranes of Depressed Patients," Journal of Affective Disorders 48: 149-155, 1998.

2   Bruinsma, K. A., et al. "Dieting, Essential Fatty Acid Intake, and Depression," Nutrition Reviews 53(4): 98-108, April 2000.

SAM-e

In evaluating 48 patients with major depression, a research team at Ospedale Crist Re in Rome, Italy, each was given 4 weeks of treatment with S-adenosyl-L-methionine (SAM-e). The medication was given intravenously and intramuscularly at 400 mg/day, while outpatients received 800 mg/day orally.[1] Evaluations were documented using the Beck's Depression Inventory by comparing scores at the beginning of the study and on day 28 of the therapy. The researchers reported in Current Therapeutic Research that SAM-e is effective and relatively safe in depressed patients who have associated internal illnesses. It is said to have antidepressant activities by its interaction with monoamines through a common metabolic pathway which involves methylation reactions.

In 80 depressed postmenopausal women, 45 to 59 years of age, they were involved with a 30-day, double-blind trial using 1,600 mg/day of SAM-e or a placebo.[2] The researchers reported a significantly greater improvement in depressive scores in the group treated with SAM-e vs placebo from day 10 of the study. Side effects were minimal.

Writing in the Journal of Neurology, Neurosurgery and Psychiatry, researchers evaluated 30 depressed patients in a double-blind study of intravenous SAM-e at 200 mg/day or intravenous placebo daily for 14 days. Four patients with Alzheimer's dementia were given oral SAM-e at 1,200 mg daily as 400 mg 3 times daily.[3] The researchers found that SAM-e, either orally or intravenously, was associated with increases in cerebrospinal fluid (CSF), indicating that the substance crosses the blood-brain barrier.

These data provide a rational basis for the antidepressant effects of SAM-e, the researchers said. CSF-SAM was low in a group of patients with Alzheimer's dementia, which suggests a possible disturbance of methylation in Alzheimer's patients. Methylation is the addition of methyl groups in biochemistry.

SAM-e is the major methyl donor in important methylation reactions in the brain, according to a research team in Lancet. The methylation process in the nervous system may have an important influence on mood and some affective disorders.[4]

1 Criconia, Anna Marie, et al. "Results of S-adenosyl-L-methionine in Patients with Major Depression and Internal Illness," Current Therapeutic Research 55(6): 666-674, June 1994.

2 Salmaggi, R., et al. "Double-Blind, Placebo-Controlled Study of S-Adenosyl-L-Methionine in Depressed Postmenopausal Women," Psychother. Psychosom. 59: 34-40, 1993.

3 Bottiglei, T., et al. "Cerebrospinal Fluid S-Adenosylmethionine in Depression and Dementia: Effects of Treatment with Parenteral and Oral S-Adenosylmethionine," Journal of Neurology, Neurosurgery and Psychiatry 53: 1096-1098, 1990.

4 Reynolds, E. H., et al. "Methylation and Mood," Lancet July 28, 1984, pp. 196-198.

The antidepressive actions of SAM-e and the neuropsychiatric symptoms that are evidenced with a severe folic acid deficiency suggest that methylation is an important process in affective disorders. A deficiency of the B vitamins is also common in dementia.

The research team added that folic acid and SAM-e may be of benefit in certain types of depressive syndromes. For example, SAM-e, methionine, the amino acid, and folic acid may be involved in the reticular activating and limbic systems, which affect mood and related functions, such as drive and arousal. This might explain why methionine loading may activate these systems, resulting in the deteriorating sometimes noted in schizophrenia.

As reported in Current Therapeutic Research, Italian researchers evaluated 40 alcoholic patients with major depression, who received 200 mg/day of SAM-e intravenously, and 400 mg twice daily orally.[1]

It was found that significant improvement was seen in most psychometric testing, beginning on day 14 and continuing through the end of the study.

Standard antidepressant therapy is often unsuccessful in treating depression in these chronic alcoholic patients, but SAM-e was well tolerated and was also effective, the researchers added.

St. John's Wort

In evaluating 3,250 patients with depression from 663 private practitioners — 76% women, ranging in age from 20 to 90 — who participated in a 4-week trial of a St. John's wort extract at 300 mg 3 times daily. The results showed in about 30% of the patients a normalizing or improvement in their depressive condition.[2] Some 49% of the patients were mildly depressed, 46% intermediately depressed, and 5% severely depressed.

Side effects were reported in 2.4% of the patients, and 1.5% discontinued the study. Side effects included gastrointestinal irritation, allergic reactions — which is common with plant extracts in susceptible people — tiredness, and restlessness.

As reported in Patient Care, 2 to 4 g/day of St. John's wort may be a benefit in anxiety, depressive moods, skin inflammation, blood

1   Agricola, R., et al. "S-Adenosyl-L-Methionine in the Treatment of Major Depression Complicating Chronic Alcoholism," Current Therapeutic Research 55(1): 83-91, January 1994.

2   Woelk, H., et al. "Benefits and Risks of the Hypericum Extract LI-160: Drug Monitoring Study with 3,250 Patients," Journal of Geriatrics, Psychiatry and Neurology 7(Suppl. 1): S34-S38, 1994.

injuries, wounds, and burns. It has been shown to be a mild antidepressant, sedative, and anxiolytic, (it relieves anxiety).[1]

Fatty oil-preparations may have benefit as typical anti-inflammatory agents. The tannin content of the herb can lead to digestive complaints, and may cause problems when ingested in large amounts, the researchers added.

As reported in Phytomedicine, a research team from the University of Exeter in the United Kingdom evaluated 14 studies using St. John's wort for depression in relation to placebo, and 4 studies against standard medication. The results showed that Hypericum perforatum (St. John's wort) is superior to placebo in alleviating the symptoms of depression using the quantified Hamilton Scale.[2] The researchers added that the herb is equally as effective as a standard medication and there are few side effects. It is safe and effective for symptomatic treatment of various forms of depression, they continued.

In an article in the British Medical Journal, Klaus Linde and colleagues at Ludwig-Maximillian-Universitat in Munich, Germany, reported on a meta-analysis (a compilation of studies) of 23 randomized trials involving 1,737 patients, who had mild to moderately severe depression. Fifteen of the studies were placebo-controlled, and 8 compared Hypericum (the active ingredient) with another drug treatment.[3]

The research team reported that the herb's extracts were significantly superior to placebo and similarly effective as standard antidepressants. Two volunteers dropped out of the study because of side effects from the herb, and 7 who were on standard antidepressants.

As we know, some patients are allergic to plant extracts, and 19.8% of the patients in this study noted side effects, compared with 52.8% who were given standard antidepressants.

The researchers concluded that the extracts of hypericum are more effective than placebo for the treatment of mild to moderately severe depressive disorders.

The daily dose of hypericum and the dose of total extracts varied between 0.4 and 2.7 mg and 300 and 1,000 mg, respectively.

1 Benjamin, S. D. "St. John's Wort and Depression," Patient Care, August 15, 1999, p. 33.

2 Ernst, E., et al, "St. John's Wort, An Antidepressant: A Systematic, Criteria-Based Review," Phytomedicine 2(1): 67-71, 1995.

3 Linde, Klaus, et al. "St. John's Wort for Depression — an Overview and Meta-Analysis of Randomized Clinical Trials," British Medical Journal 313: 253-258, 1996.

Lithium

As reported in Psychosomatics, a 72-year-old man was treated with antidepressant medications, which brought a good clinical response. Three weeks following treatment, he developed hepatitis and all therapy was stopped. His depressive symptoms returned within 4 weeks.[1]

After several weeks, he was placed on lithium carbonate at 300 mg 3 times daily, and 10 days later he showed improvement. He continued to improve, and the dosage was reduced to 300 mg/day.

Within 6 days of the lower dosage, the depressive symptoms increased substantially. The lithium dosage was increased to 900 mg/day, and the patient responded.

On June 22, 1973, the gifted theatrical producer and director Josh Logan appeared on the "Today" show on television to recount his lifelong battle with Manic-Depressive Syndrome. This condition involves a period of elation in which the patient is talking wildly, working feverishly, doing all kinds of crazy things in a loud, uncontrolled spirit of gaiety, followed by a period of depression so severe that suicide is contemplated.[2]

He told on the program how Ronald R. Fieve, M.D., a psychiatrist, had prescribed lithium, and his depression was gone, along with the wild swings from elation to depression.

During World War II in the United States, lithium was used as a salt substitute, therefore, a physician prescribing lithium needs to take this into consideration, since many people need to curb their salt intake.

Ginkgo Biloba

According to an article in the Journal of Orthomolecular Medicine, a patient who had had symptoms of unipolar depression for over 30 years, was given 135 mg of Ginkgo biloba extract. The dosage was 33 mg in the morning, and 17 mg thereafter every 2 hours. At night the patient was given 2 valerian tablets, with each tablet containing 110 mg of 5.5:1 valerian root extract and 30 mg of 3:1 hops extract. The patient also took small amounts of zinc and vitamin B6.[3]

1 Lieberman, J. A., et al. "Acute Antidepressant Effect of Lithium in Unipolar Depression," Psychosomatics 25(12): 932-933, 1984.

2 Adams, Ruth, and Murray, Frank. Minerals: Kill or Cure? New York: Larchmont Books, 1974, p. 185.

3 Seaiey, R., B.Sc. "Surviving Unipolar Depression — The effectiveness of Ginkgo Biloba," The Journal of Orthomolecular Medicine 11(3): 168-172, 1996.

Following 10 months of therapy, the patient felt remarkably better. The researcher suggested that the Ginkgo biloba extract may work by inhibition of biogenic amines, helping to maintain brain neurotransmitters, inhibition of enzyme activities, inhibition of COMT and MAO, which lead to increased concentrations of catecholamines, enhanced release of catecholamines and other neurotransmitters and activities of N-methyl D-aspartate (NIMDA)-type glutamate receptors.

Phosphatidylserine (PS)

Ten elderly women, ranging in age from 70 to 81, who had been depressed between 6 months and 12 years, were given a 150-day course of placebo at 3 capsules/day, followed by phosphatidylserine at 300 mg/day for 45 days, in which two 100 mg capsules were taken at 8 a.m. and 1 at noon.[1] Before and after the placebo course, and at the end of the PS therapy, patients were given the 17-item Hamilton Rating Score for Depression. As reported in Acta Psychiatrica Scandinavia, the PS therapy resulted in a consistent improvement in depressive symptoms, memory, and behavior. The depressive symptoms did not change after the placebo trial, but were significantly reduced after the PS therapy, the researchers said.

Thyroxine

At the Klinikum Benjamin Franklin in Berlin, Germany, researchers evaluated 17 severely ill, therapy-resistant euthyroid (normally functioning thyroid gland) patients with major depression, who had been depressed for a mean of 11.5 months, in spite of treatment with antidepressants.[2] The patients were studied for the effect of thyroxine (an active iodine compound) added to their antidepressant medication, at a dose that was increased to a mean of 482 mcg/day. The Hamilton Rating Scale for Depression declined from 26.6 prior to the addition of T4 (thyroxine) to 11.6 at the end of 8 weeks of therapy. The researchers reported that 8 patients fulfilled the criteria for full remission within 8 weeks, and 2 others fully remitted within 12 weeks. Seven patients did not remit or become less severe.

Of the 10 remitting patients maintained on high-dose T4, and followed for a mean of 27.2 months, 7 of the 10 patients had an

1 Maggioni, M., et al. "Effects of Phosphatidylserine Therapy in Geriatric Patients with Depressive Disorders," Acta Psychiatrica Scandinavica 81: 265-270, 1990.

2 Bauer, Michael, M.D., Ph.D. "Treatment of Refractory Depression with High-Dose Thyroxine," Neuropsychopharmacology 18(6): 444-455, 1998.

excellent outcome, and 2 had milder and shorter episodes during T4 augmentation treatment, while 1 failed to benefit from the T4 treatments during the follow-up period. There were minimal side effects, the researchers reported.

FIGHTING DEPRESSION WITH LIGHT THERAPY

Light therapy is both a very old and a very new treatment for depression, according to Raymond Lam, M.D., and colleagues at the University of British Columbia in Canada. In the second century A.D., the physician Aretaeus recommended that "Lethargies are to be laid in the light, and exposed to the rays of the sun."[1]

The modern use of light as a treatment for depression arose in the early 1980s from the investigations of circadian rhythm disturbances in seasonal and non-seasonal mood disorders, Lam added.

While most studies have used treatments of at least 2 hours of daily exposure to 2,500 lux light, more recent studies have shown that 10,000 lux-light boxes require only 30 minutes of daily exposure to produce similar response rates, and this treatment is used widely in clinical practice.

The optimal timing of light therapy during the day continues to be somewhat controversial, Lam said. Response to light therapy usually occurs within 1 week of treatment, and almost certainly after 2 weeks. The therapy is normally not used in spring and summer. However, some patients with seasonal affective disorder (SAD) experience mood slumps during a period of dark, rainy weather and resume light therapy.

Side effects of light therapy are mild, but they may include insomnia, headache, eye strain, visual blurring, agitation, and nausea.

The current protocol of 10,000 lux light for 30 minutes a day shows response rates in SAD of 60 to 80%. The protocol for the diagnosis of SAD includes a trial of light therapy of 10,000 lux for 30 minutes daily for 7 to 14 days. If there is a full response, then continue until spring and summer, Lam added.

If there is partial response, increase to 60 minutes of daily exposure over 7 to 14 days. If there is still no response, continue switching to evening light exposure for 7 to 14 days. If there is partial response, the practitioner may add medications, Lam continued.

At University Hospital in Vancouver, Canada, Raymond W. Lam, M.D., just mentioned, evaluated 54 depressed, drug-free out-

---

1 Lam, Raymond W., M.D., et al. "Light Therapy for Depressive Disorders: Indications and Efficacy," Mood Disorders, Systematic Medication Management 25: 215-234, 1997.

patients with seasonal affective disorder, who were given 2 weeks of 2,500 lux cool-white fluorescent light exposure from 6 to 8 a.m.[1]

This light therapy significantly reduced depression scores. The specific symptoms of hypersomnia and hyperphagia are predictors of a positive response to morning bright light therapy and seasonal affective disorder, he said. In hypersomnia, sleep periods are very long. Hyperphagia is over-eating.

In 96 depressed patients with SAD, they were randomly assigned to 1 of 3 treatments for 4 weeks of light therapy, reported Archives of General Psychiatry. Each treatment was 1.5 hours/day, which included morning light (start time at 6 a.m.), evening light (start time about 9 p.m.), or a morning placebo (start time about 6 a.m.).[2]

The bright light was about 6,000 lux and was produced by light boxes, while the placebos were sham negative-ion generators. After 3 weeks of treatment, the morning light produced more of a complete or almost complete remission than did the placebo.

While bright light therapy had an antidepressant effect beyond the placebo effect, it took about 3 weeks for a significant effect to occur. However, bright light produced more full remissions than did placebo, the researchers said.

As reported in Acta Psychiatrica Scandinavica, 61 patients with winter depression, whose ages ranged up to 70, were studied using lightbox treatment. Eighty percent of the participants were women.[3]

The patients were randomly assigned to either lightbox treatment with 1,500-2,500 lux of white light for 2 hours in the morning for 6 days on an out-patient basis, or dawn stimulation treatment at home with 60 to 90 minutes of light augmentation time to 100-300 lux for 2 weeks.

Results showed a 40% improvement in the dawn stimulation group, and a 57.4% improvement in the lightbox group. The majority of volunteers in both groups maintained their improvement during the 9-week follow-up period, the researchers said.

A lux is a unit of light or illumination and is also called candle-meter or meter-candle light. This corresponds to a luminous flux of 1 lumen per square meter of surface.

1 Lam, Raymond W., M.D. "Morning Light Therapy for Winter Depression: Predictors of Response," Acta Psychiatrica Scandinavica 89: 97-101, 1994.

2 Eastman, C. I., et al. "Bright Light Treatment of Winter Depression: A Placebo-Controlled Trial," Archives of General Psychiatry 55: 883-889, 1998.

3 Lingjaerde, O., et al. "Dawn Stimulation vs. Lightbox Treatment in Winter Depression: A Comparative Study," Acta Psychiatrica Scandinavica 98: 73-80, 1998.

EXERCISE AND DEPRESSION

In an article in Archives of Internal Medicine, 156 men and women with major depressive disorder, who were over 50 years of age, were randomly assigned to either an aerobic exercise program, the antidepressant sertraline hydrochloride zoloft or a combination of exercise and, the medication. After 16 weeks, the groups did not differ substantially on various depression assessment tests.[1]

However, those receiving combination therapy exhibited less severe depressive symptoms initially, and showed a more rapid response than those with initially more severe depressive symptoms.

An exercise training program may be considered an alternative to antidepressants for the treatment of depression in older patients, reported James A. Blumenthal, Ph.D.

While antidepressants have a more rapid initial therapeutic response, after 16 weeks of treatment, exercise was as effective in reducing depression, Blumenthal added.

The exercise program consisted of 3 supervised exercise sessions weekly for 16 weeks, where volunteers trained at 70 to 85% of their heart rate reserve. Each aerobic session began with a 10-minute warm-up exercise period, followed by 30 minutes of continuous walking or jogging at an intensity that would maintain heart rate within the assigned training range. The exercise session was followed by a 5-minute cool-down session.

Although Blumenthal did not mention it, the Alexander Technique is an excellent way to warm up, in that movements are so slight you can hardly see them. It is counterproductive to jerk your muscles around like piano wire, as so many exercisers do.

Exercise is a form of meditation, which allows for a quiet time and working out aggression, according to Bryan Stamford, Ph.D., of Minneapolis, Minnesota. It can increase alertness and creativity, release energy, enhance sleep, and it may cause positive changes in brain chemicals, he reported in The Physician and Sports Medicine.[2]

In evaluating 43 male and female volunteers — ranging in age up to 60 years of age — they were assigned to a training group, which for 9 weeks underwent a program of systemic aerobic exercises consisting of 1 hour of training with an instructor 3 times a

---

1   Blumenthal, James A., Ph.D. "Effects of Exercise Training on Older Patients with Major Depression," Archives of Internal Medicine 159: 2349-2356, 1999.
2   Stamford, Bryan, Ph.D. "The Role of Exercise in Fighting Depression," The Physician and Sports Medicine 23(12): 79-80, December 1995.

week at 50 to 70% of their maximum aerobic capacity, or to an occupational therapy control group.[1]

The researchers reported that there was a significant reduction in depression scores, and an increase in maximum oxygen uptake in the aerobic exercising group. This suggests that moderate exercise with an increase in maximum oxygen uptake of 15 to 30% was enough to obtain an antidepressive effect.

Every country can and should begin now to improve its efforts to treat those with mental illness, reported Gro Harlem Brundtland, M.D., director general of the World Health Organisation.[2]

In fact, a WHO survey found that 40% of the 185 countries surveyed have no national health policy; 30% have no programs to improve mental health conditions; and 25% have no specific mental health legislation. And over 37% of the countries have no community care facilities. Brundtland continued, "The global toll of mental illness and neurological disorders is staggering. Neuropsychiatric disorders account for 31% of the disability in the world. For example, 450 million people have a mental or neurological disorder. Of these, 121 million have depression, and 50 million have epilepsy. Every year, 1 million people commit suicide, and 10 million to 20 million attempt suicide."

A great deal of the suffering is unnecessary, she said. For instance, 60% of those with major depression can fully recover if treated. But, in industrialized and developing countries, less than 25% of those affected receive treatment, for reasons that include stigma, discrimination, scarce resources, lack of skills in primary health care, and deficient public health policies. "Solutions based on scientific evidence are available and affordable," she added. "Through recent advances in neuroscience, neuroimaging, genetics, and behavioral sciences, we know more about brain functioning and behavior than ever before, and breakthroughs in therapy and medication have occurred.

Electroconvulsive therapy (ECT) was developed based on the observation of patients with depression who had epileptic-like seizures, reported Treating Mental Disorders.[3]

Following a physical exam, the patient undergoes 6 to 12 treatments, during which time sleep is induced with a medication, as

1 Martinsen, E. W., et al. "Effects of Aerobic Exercise on Depressions: A Controlled Study," British Medical Journal, July 13, 1985, p. 291.
2 Brundtland, Gro Harlem, M.D. "Mental Health: New Understanding, New Hope," JAMA 286(19): 2391, 2001.
3 Nathan, Peter E., et al. Treating Mental Disorders. New York: Oxford University Press, 1999, pp. 108-109.

well as to relax the muscles. The electric stimulus is then delivered through electrodes attached to the head. The procedure usually takes about 15 minutes.

"The use of ECT is effective but primarily in the treatment of depression that is thought to be the result of physiological causes, such as an imbalance in brain chemistry," the publication said. ECT is recommended after patients have not responded to, or can't tolerate the side effects of antidepressants, and after these patients haven't improved with other therapies.

Writing in the Journal of the American Medical Association, M. Fink and M. A. Taylor[1] reported that the effect of ECT on memory is "circumscribed and mostly transient," and that there is only a "modest cognitive advantage of high-dose unilateral ECT." Responding to the article, Anne B. Donahue, JD, of Vermont State House in Montpelier, said that some forms of ECT are associated with an increased risk of persistent long-term effects on cognitive performance in community settings.[2] "In a cohort study, bilateral ECT was associated with broader and more severe short-term and long-term cognitive effects than right unilateral ECT, and that adverse cognitive effects could persist for an extended period, and only receipt of bilateral treatment distinguished the group with marked and persistent retrograde amnesia."

In addition, she continued, a small study found that during the interictal (the period between convulsions) stage of bilateral ECT, enhanced left frontotemporal theta activity was correlated with retrograde amnesia, suggesting that left medial temporal lobe structures are involved in the pathophysiology of ECT-induced memory effects. (Named for the eighth letter of the Greek alphabet, theta rhythm is a rather high amplitude brain wave pattern.)

VITAMIN D TO THE RESCUE

In a study at the Intermountain Medical Center in Murray, Utah, which involved 7,358 patients, 50 years of age or older, they were diagnosed with coronary artery disease, myocardial infarction, congestive heart failure, cerebrovascular accident, transient ischemic accident, arterial fibrillation or peripheral vascular disease, but with no history of depression.

The results indicated an inverse association between vitamin D level and the risk of depression.

1 Fink, M., and Taylor, M. A. "Electroconvulsive Therapy Evidence and Challenges," JAMA 298(3): 330-332, 2007.

2 Donahue, Anne B, JD. "Electroconvulsive Therapy and Memory Loss," JAMA 298(16): 1862, 2007.

After adjusting for potential cofounders, the researchers said that very low, low, and normal vitamin D levels were significantly associated with an increased risk of depression, compared to those getting optimum levels of the vitamin.

The study strengthens the hypothesis of an association between vitamin D intake and depression, the researchers added.[1]

B Vitamins May Ease Depression

At the University of Western Australia in Perth, a research team conducted a double-blind study involving 273 stroke survivors.[2] They reported that long-term supplementation with B vitamins may be associated with a reduced risk of major depression in stroke survivors.

The patients were randomized to be given vitamin B supplements or a placebo. The protocol consisted of 2 mg/day of folic acid; 2.5 mg/day of vitamin B6; and 0.5 mg/day of vitamin B12 for one to 10.5 years.

The researchers reported that those in the treatment group showed a 52% reduced risk of major depression, compared to those given the look-alike pill. "If these findings can be validated externally, B-vitamin supplementation offers hope as an effective, safe, and affordable intervention to reduce the burden of post-stroke depression," the researchers said.

Omega-3 Fatty Acids Ease Depressive Symptoms

Researchers at the University of Pavia in Italy conducted a double-blind study involving 46 women, ranging in age from 66 to 95 years, who had been diagnosed with depression. They concluded that supplementation with long-chain omega-3 polyunsaturated fatty acids may improve depressive symptoms and the quality of life.[3]

The women were randomized to one of two groups for the 8-week study. The treatment group received 2.5 g/day of omega-3 fatty acids with 1.67 g of eicosapentaenoic acid (EPA) and 0.83 g of docosahexaenoic acid (DHA), while the controls were given a

---

1 Muhlestein, J. R., et al. "Association of Vitamin D Levels with Incident Depression Among a General Cardiovascular Population," American Heart Journal 159(6): 1037-1043, 2010.

2 Almeida, O. P., et al. "B-Vitamins Reduce the Long-Term Risk of Depression After Stroke. The LITATOPS-DEP Trial," Annals of Neurology 68(4): 503-510, 2010.

3 Rondanelli, M., et al. "Effect of Omega-3 Fatty Acids Supplementation on Depressive Symptoms and On Health-Related Quality of Life in the Treatment of Elderly Women and Depression: A Double-Blind, Placebo-Controlled, Randomized Trial," Journal of the American College of Nutrition 29(1): 55-64, 2010.

placebo. At the end of the study, depressive symptoms — evaluated by the Geriatric Depression Scale — and quality of life — evaluated using the Short-Form 36-Item Health Survey — significantly improved in the treatment group, when compared to those given a placebo.

4. Understanding the Human Brain

Although modern medicine has an enormous array of measuring instruments, computers, and laser technology, and it has made fascinating strides toward eliminating many of the maladies that affect the human body, it has discovered nothing to match the overwhelming complexity of the human brain and nervous system, explained the Columbia University College of Physicians and Surgeons Complete Home Medical Guide.[1]

This intimidating mass of gray matter, white matter, and electrical impulses, combined with the sprawl of the peripheral nerves interacting with the muscular system, creates an awe-inspiring synthesis of thought, emotion, and action with no apparent limits. "Research has not unraveled all of the brain's complexities," the publication continued, "but attempts to fathom the depths of such a complex structure have given rise to a wealth of understanding."

The brain is part of the central nervous system, which also includes the spinal cord, both of which are encased in bone for protection. The brain is confined within the skull, while the spinal cord is held within a canal that is surrounded by the vertebrae of the spine. The peripheral nervous system comprises the nerve roots, as well as the nerves that supply the muscles and various organ systems.

"The spinal cord is connected to the brain by the brainstem, which consists of the medulla, the pons, and the midbrain, all of

---

1   Tapley, Donald F., M.D., et al., medical editors. The Columbia University College of
    Physicians and Surgeons Complete Home Medical Guide. New York: Crown Publishers,
    Inc., 1985, pp. 588ff.

which maintains such vital bodily functions as breathing and circulation," the publication said. "Paired cranial nerves exit from the brainstem to control eye movements, muscles, and sensation of the face, taste, swallowing, and tongue movements."

Situated above the brainstem are the largest components of the brain, the cerebrum and the cerebellum. The cerebrum is segregated into left and right hemispheres, which, in turn, are divided into lobes.

"The cerebral hemispheres control such functions as speech, memory, and intelligence," the publication continued. "Some of these functions, such as speech, are controlled by specific areas, and others, such as memory, are apparently controlled by the cerebral hemispheres. Under the cerebral hemispheres is the cerebellum, which controls subconscious activities, such as coordinating movements and maintaining balance."

Inside the brain, at the top of the brainstem, are other necessary structures, such as the hypothalamus, which is a major endocrine regulatory center that influences sleep, appetite, and sexual desire, and the thalamus, which is a critical relay station that links the cerebral hemispheres to the other parts of the nervous system.

The publication went on to report that, feeding the brain and its various components with oxygen and nutrients are 2 main sets of blood vessels, the paired carotid and vertebral arteries. These structures subdivide into smaller blood vessels which supply different parts of the brain. When the blood supply is interrupted, or when a blood vessel hemorrhages, a stroke will develop.

"The brain and spinal cord are covered with 3 layers of membranes called meninges, and they float in a cerebrospinal fluid, which is a waterlike bath that cushions the soft brain structures from injury against the encasing bones," the publication said.

Disorders of the brain and spinal cord are treated by neurologists, neurosurgeons, physicians, and those with specialized, advanced training. These maladies range from the simple to the complex.

One of the complications that specialists have to treat is dementia, a term used to describe a progressive and usually irreversible loss in intellectual function that eventually impairs a person's ability to work and socialize. Some of the functions that are affected are memory, learning, ability, judgment, rational thought, personality, and the capacity for abstract thought.

"The most common cause of dementia is Alzheimer's disease, which is responsible for 20% of those confined to nursing homes and other chronic care facilities," the publication added. "Alzheimer's disease is caused by an unexplained degeneration of nerve cells. Research has linked this degeneration to a disturbance in nerve cell networks that utilize the neurotransmitter acetylcholine."[1]

Alzheimer's begins insidiously with mild forgetfulness and mood changes, often depression. Mental abilities continue to deteriorate so that the patient is unable to work, loses their way in familiar surroundings, and they often repeat conversations endlessly. Apathy alternates with irrational behavior, but the patient cannot be reasoned with.

"Eventually," the publication said, "the victim becomes completely incapacitated, unable to be left alone, and speech fails so that even the most basic needs cannot be communicated."

Another typical cause of dementia is cerebrovascular disease, and those who have suffered multiple strokes affecting large parts of both cerebral hemispheres become demented in a condition known as multi-infarct dementia. Brain tumors, severe or multiple head injuries (such as those caused by sports), and several uncommon infectious diseases of the brain that are less frequent causes of dementia.

Emerging evidence suggests that proteins associated with the immune system may play additional roles in normal brain development and in the healthy adult brain, according to Bridget M. Kuehn in the February 13, 2008 issue of the Journal of the American Medical Association. Studies also suggest that perturbations of these roles may underlie some neurological diseases.[2]

"Contrary to dogma that the blood-brain barrier protects the brain from the immune system by acting as a barricade to its components, scientists have found that certain key immune system proteins are, in fact, expressed and active in healthy brains, Kuehn said.

Ben A. Barres, M.D., Ph.D., of the Stanford University School of Medicine in Palo Alto, California, said that scientists have known for many years that proteins involved in the classic complement cascade, a key component of the innate immune system, were present in the brain, and these proteins may play a role in the brain's response to injury.

Scientists have reported that the protein that initiates the cascade — the Clq protein — was not expressed in healthy adult brains. "When Barres and his colleagues conducted a gene chip ex-

---

1   ibid, pp 592-593.
2   Kuehn, Bridget M. "Scientists Probe Immune System's Role in Brain Function and Neurological Disease," JAMA 299(6): 619-620, 2008.

periment designed to determine which neuronal genes were regulated by astrocytes (star-shaped cells of brain and spinal cord), they were surprised to find that only the gene encoding the Clq protein was strongly controlled by these glial cells," Kuehn added. "They realised the neurons they were studying were from developing brains, and further studies revealed that Clq is expressed at synapses throughout the developing brain." (A synapse is the point where a nervous impulse passes from one neuron to another).

The fact that Clq was found at the synapses (junctures) only during the period of development, when selective synapse pruning is shaping the structure of the brain, coupled with Clq's known immune system role in tagging items for elimination, led the researchers to the hypothesis that Clq helps tag weak or inappropriate synapses for elimination during normal development, Kuehn added.

Barres said that evidence also points to a role of Clq in neurodegenerative diseases. The protein is elevated in many such diseases. As an example, expression of Clq is upregulated 70-fold in Alzheimer's disease.

It has been hypothesized from an evolutionary standpoint that a nutritionally-rich diet is necessary for the maintenance of the metabolically active brain, according to Perspectives in Biology and Medicine. However, the brain is metabolically expensive, since it requires 20% of the total resting oxygen consumption in the body.[1]

Meat may be important in the diet because it is a source of essential fatty acids, and, in ample supply, essential as well as other unsaturated fatty acids in meat may have provided a survival advantage, with a 3-fold increase in the size of the human brain within 3 million years of evolution, reported Frank D. Mann of Scottsdale, Arizona.

He went on to say that a diet rich in animal fat would have increased the intake and hepatic liver synthesis of cholesterol, which may have been important in the development of a large brain.

Cholesterol is an important constituent of cell membranes and it is necessary for the formation of nerve fibers and the repair of the brain. Cholesterol is needed for brain repair, and hemorrhagic stroke may be caused, in part, by a low-fat diet, Mann said.

The body requires 2,000 mg/day of cholesterol to survive. If this amount is not obtained from the diet, the body simply manufac-

---

1 Mann, Frank B. "Animal Fat and Cholesterol May Have Helped Primitive Man Evolve a Large Brain," Perspectives in Biology and Medicine 41(3): 417-425, Spring 1998.

tures the rest. Cholesterol is necessary for the functioning of sex hormones, for the conversion of vitamin D from the sun, and other uses.

The brain contains the highest level of vitamin C in the body, and active uptake mechanisms in the choroid plexus and cell membrane maintain intracellular levels at 16 to 25 times higher than blood levels of the vitamin, reported the Institute of Neurology in London, England.[1]

Extracellular brain levels of the vitamin are lowest during sleep, and highest with prolonged activity and stress. The transfer of proteins that take up glutamate, an amino acid, do so in exchange for vitamin C. That is, the uptake of glutamate results in the release of the vitamin.

It is not surprising that brain levels of vitamin C are highest during prolonged stress. All animals, birds, reptiles — except man, guinea pigs, some apes, and a fruit-eating bat in India — manufacture their own vitamin C as needed, and, when stressed, pump out loads of the vitamin. If the egg had vitamin C, it would be the world's perfect food. It does not contain vitamin C because the hen makes her own.

Vitamin C is a competitive antagonist at dopamine receptors, and it antagonizes the effect of amphetamines and enhances the effects of the antipsychotic drug haloperiodol Haldol, explained John H. Smythies.

Ascorbate (vitamin C) therapy in early Parkinson's disease delays the need to give L-Dopa by 2 years, Smythies continued. And there is a clear case for the use of vitamin C in schizophrenia, autism, and Parkinson's disease.

Ethanol (alcohol) results in oxidative stress in the brain and raises the level of dopamine metabolites and lowers vitamin C in the brain.

Smythies added that stroke, hypoxia, ischemia, or seizure activity and trauma all lead to a massive release of glutamate in the brain, resulting in a 6- to 8-fold increase in extracellular brain vitamin C, which may be a defense mechanism against reperfusion. A number of vitamins and minerals reduce vulnerability to oxygen-derived free radicals, reperfusion injury, and so forth. Glutamate is an ester of glutamic acid, an amino acid or form of protein. Hypoxia is redued oxygen supply.

---

1 Smythies, John R, "The Role of Ascorbate in Brain Therapeutic Implications," Journal of the Royal Society of Medicine 89(5): 241, May 1996.

In the brain, on a dry weight basis, white matter and myelin comprise 50 to 70% lipids/fats, and gray matter — mostly neuronal cells — is about 40% fats, according to Harold W. Cook, Ph.D., of Dalhouse University in Halifax, Nova Scotia, Canada.[1]

The lipid content of the brain is definitely greater than most other body organs, including the liver, kidney, and heart, which is less than 25%, he said.

The total phospholipids of the brain have a ratio of omega-3 to omega-6 fatty acids of about 1:1, compared to 1:4 in the liver, heart, and kidney. The brain is much less acceptable than the liver to dietary fluctuations, he said. Omega-3 fatty acids are derived from fish oils, while omega-6s come from vegetable sources.

People who have experienced a major depression in the previous 10 years in late middle age are twice as likely as those who haven't to develop problems with concentration, memory, or problem-solving ability after the age of 65, according to Shirley S. Wang in the July 3, 2007 issue of the Wall Street Journal.[2]

Depression is also associated with shrinkage of the part of the brain related to memory, and studies show that a significant number of older people will not recover their mental sharpness even if their mood recovers, she continued.

"Not everyone who gets depressed ends up with dementia," Wang added. "And in some patients, depression may be a consequence of rather than a cause of conditions such as Alzheimer's disease. However, many doctors suggest this link with cognitive impairment provides yet another reason to seek treatment for depression."

Some scientists believe that depression weakens the brain by bathing it in damaging chemicals called glucocorticoids, which are produced during periods of stress, Wang said. These chemicals, such as Cortisol, may erode pathways between neurons — nerve cells that transmit messages — and, if this erosion occurs along with a pre-existing brain abnormality, it may accelerate cognitive problems.

"The pre-existing signs of Alzheimer's disease that researchers focus on are 'amyloid plaques' and 'neurofibrillary tangles,' which are brain deposits that signal apoptosis or cell death," Wang continued. "In 2 separate reports published in the past year, researchers injected glucocorticoids into mice that had predispositions to

1 Cook, Harold W., Ph.D. "Brain Metabolism and Alpha-Linolenic Acid During Development," Nutrition 7(6): 440-442, November/December 1991.

2 Wang, Shirley S. "How Depression Weakens the Brain," The Wall Street Journal, July 3, 2007, pp. D1, D6.

Alzheimer's, and the Alzheimer's-related indicators increased in these animals, compared with mice that were not injected."

A research team at the Alzheimer's Disease Center at Rush University Medical Center in Chicago, Illinois, have found clues to a link between depression and disease. In their study tracking the mental health of almost 900 elderly people, the researchers autopsied the brains of over 200 patients who had died by 2006. They found signs of Alzheimer's in 98% of the brains, but fewer than half of the people had shown any evidence of dementia while they were living.

It was those who had experienced more distress in the years before their deaths, including depressive symptoms, who had shown more cognitive impairment, Wang said. It has been found that those with low levels of distress are better able to tolerate age-related changes in the brain, commented Robert S. Wilson, M.D., who is with the Rush Alzheimer's group.

In some people, Wang said, vascular medical conditions associated with inflammation of the blood vessels, such as hardening of the arteries, could generate both dementia and depression. And mood changes may simply be the first noticeable sign of Alzheimer's disease or other dementia.

There is some evidence that treating depression, either with medication or certain types of psychotherapy, not only benefits a patient's psychological well being, but also reduces the frequency or severity of future depression, and apparently it spares the brain from injury from the load of chronic stress, Wang said.

Silicon is important in the forming or maintaining healthy brains, bones, and blood vessels, and it may play a role in aging and diseases that affect the brain, according to a research team at the USDA Agricultural Research Center in Grand Forks, North Dakota.[1]

The substance may play an important role in the brain under stress conditions of low dietary calcium and high dietary aluminum, the researchers said. A deficiency may also play a role in the development of ischemic heart disease and high blood pressure.

The average daily intake of silicon ranges from 20 to 50 mcg/day, and the recommended daily intake is probably between 5 and 10 mcg/day.

The intake of silicon effects macromolecules, such as glycosaminoglycan, which is part of a protein-polysaccharide complex, col-

---

1 Seaborn, Carol D., Ph.D., and Nielsen, Forrest H., Ph.D. "Silicon A Nutritional Beneficence for Bones, Brains, and Blood Vessels," Nutrition Today, July/August 1993, pp. 13-18.

lagen, and elastin, which is required for healthy bones, brains, and blood vessels. It should probably be considered a nutrient of concern in human health because it can be enhanced by stressors such as low dietary calcium, high dietary aluminum, and low estrogen status, the researchers said.

Silicon is one of the most abundant elements on earth, and it is found in large amounts in soils and plants, according to Foods & Nutrition Encyclopedia. Although the early chemists considered silica an elementary substance, Antoine Lavoisier suspected, in 1787, that it was an oxide of an undiscovered element.[1]

In 1823, Jons J. Berzelius, the Swedish chemist, discovered the element, and the name silicon is derived from the Latin silex or silicis, meaning flint or hard.

The main sources of silicon in the diet are the fibrous parts of whole grains, liver, lungs, kidneys, and brains of animals. However, much of the silicon in whole grains is lost during processing.

A person dies when the brain function ceases, the heart stops beating, and breathing and blood circulation cease, reported Janet M. Torpy, M.D., in the May 14, 2008 issue of the Journal of the American Medical Association. Because life-support techniques have become so advanced, it is possible that even in the face of fatal injury or unrecoverable illness, the heart can be kept beating with medication and respiration (breathing) can be artificially performed with a ventilator.[2]

"Brain death, as understood in U.S. law and medical practice, occurs when there is no function of the entire brain," Torpy added. "The brainstem is the area of the brain that controls breathing and circulation, and, therefore, controls essential life function."

When the brain, including the brainstem, has ceased to function, the individual is truly dead by medical and legal standards. Clinical criteria for determining brain death include:

No response to any stimulus — no movement, withdrawal grimace, or blinking.

No breathing efforts when taken off the ventilator (the apnea test).

Pupils dilated and not responsive to light.

No gag reflex, no corneal reflex (blinking when the surface of the eye is touched), and absence of other specific reflexes.

These tests are used:

---

1   Ensminger, A., et al. Foods and Nutrition Encyclopedia. Clovis, CA: Pegus Press, 1983, pp. 1993-1994.
2   Torpy, Janet M., M.D. "Brain Death," JAMA 299(18): 2232, 2008.

Computed tomography (CT) scans of the brain may reveal abnormalities, such as bleeding (hemorrhage), massive stroke, brain injury, or severe brain swelling (edema).

Electroencephalography (EEG) records electrical brain activity. No EEG activity suggests the brain is dead.

Cerebral radionucide injection shows no uptake of the radioactive material in the brain when a person is brain dead.

When Ariel Sharon, then Israel's prime minister, was taken to a hospital on December 18, 2005, he was susceptible to blood clots that could be swept from the heart to his brain, resulting in a major stroke.[1] While anticlotting drugs might have protected him, brain scans showed microbleeds, which are pinpoint drops of blood that leaked from blood vessels in the brain. Doctors feared that an anticlotting drug might turn a new microbleed into a life-threatening hemorrhaic stroke.

"Until recently, microbleeds were all but unknown," reporter Gina Kolata said. "Now, with improved scans, they are turning up consistently. In fact, one recent study found them in the brains of 1 out of 5 people 60 and older. Questions now arise. Just because something turns up on an M.R.I. scan, is it significant? If it may or may not be significant, what to do about it?"

When the microbleeds are on the outer surface of the brain, they often seem associated with a condition in which blood vessels are damaged by the protein amyloid, Kolata continued. This is the same protein that piles up in the brains of patients with Alzheimer's disease. And the microbleeds from amyloid can be associated with dementia.

For over a decade, Monique M. B. Breteler, M.D., a neuroepidemiologist at Erasmus University in Rotterdam, and her colleagues, have been following a group of Rotterdam residents 45 and older. They found in evaluating almost 4,000 volunteers that over 20% have evidence of microbleeds. The older the person, the more likely of microbleeds. For example, this condition was found in 18% of 60-year-olds, and almost 40% in those over 80.

Steven M. Greenberg, M.D., of Massachusetts General Hospital in Boston, discussed a 74-year-old patient, who experienced an episode in which part of his face went numb, then his hand, and then the numbness faded and he felt fine. The patient had an abnormal heart rhythm, which meant that anticlotting drugs might help him avoid a stroke caused by blood clots in the heart. But an

---

1 Kolata, Gina. "A Quandary on Blood Drops in the Brain," The New York Times, July 1, 2008, pp. F1, F4.

95

M.R.I. found microbleeds on the surface of the brain, meaning they were probably associated with amyloid. This meant that anticlotting drugs like warfarin could be dangerous.

Dr. Greenberg decided to forego warfarin, and instead suggested that the patient use baby aspirin, with its mild anticlotting properties. So far the patient has done well, Kolata reported.

The cerebral cortex, the outer layer of the brain involved with reasoning, planning, and self-awareness, has a central clearinghouse of activity below the crown of the head that is widely connected to more specialized regions in a large network similar to a subway map, reported Benedict Carey in the July 1, 2008 Issue of the New York Times.[1]

The report, published in PLoS Biology, an online journal, provides the most complete rough draft of the cortex's electrical architecture, the cluster of interconnecting nodes and hubs that help guide thinking and behavior, Carey added.

The study also provides an illuminating demonstration of how new imaging techniques focused on the brain's white matter — the connections between cells instead on the neurons themselves — are filling in a dimension of human brain function that has been somewhat obscure.

"This is about the coolest paper I have seen in a long time, and forward-looking in terms of where the science is going," said Marcus E. Raichle, M.D., of Washington University in St. Louis, Missouri. "They've found in the brain what looks like a hub map of the airline system for the United States."

In the study, a research team from the University of Lausanne in Switzerland, Harvard University and Indiana University in the United States, evaluated the brains of 5 healthy male volunteers. The protocol used a new technique — diffusion spectrum imaging — which allows scientists to estimate the density and orientation of the connections running through specific brain locations.

"Using a computer analysis of the results, the researchers ranked the busiest spots on the cortex in order, by the number of connections they had," Carey continued. "Finally, they plotted those spots back onto the brain maps of the 5 volunteers."

The research team reported that the hubs clustered in each man's brain, in a region about the size of a palm, were centered atop the cortex like a small skullcap.

Added Olaf Sporns, M.D., of Indiana University in Indianapolis, "we haven't had a comprehensive map of the brain showing what is

---

1 Carey, Benedict. "Scientists Identify the Brain's Activity Hub," ibid, p. F6.

connected to what, and you really need the whole thing before you can ask certain questions, like what happens if activity is clogged up at one of the hubs? How does that affect functioning?"

Top 10 Brain Nutrients

Although acetyl-L-carnitine is Robert Crayhon's favorite brain booster, he has 9 other candidates:[1]

Acetyl-L-carnitine is most important for maintaining optimal brain health. Recommendation: 250 to 1,000 mg/day.

Phosphatidylserine (PS): A crucial partner with carnitine for optimal brain health. Recommendation: 100 to 300 mg/day.

EPA and DHA. DHA is probably the most important to get. Recommendation: 500 to 1,000 mg/day of the two fatty acids combined.

Magnesium: Crucial for the health of the brain. Recommendation: 400 mg/day.

Folic acid and vitamin B12: The two B vitamins work together and resolve many cases of depression and dementia. Recommendation: 400 to 2,000 mcg/day of each.

Zinc: Brain requires sufficient amounts of this mineral. Recommendation: 25 mg/day with 2 mg/day of copper sebacate.

Vitamin E: It helps to slow the progression of Alzheimer's disease and Parkinson's disease. Recommendation: 400 IU/day.

Vitamin B6: Needed for nerve-cell communication. Recommendation: 50 mg/day.

CoQ10: It keeps nerve cells energized and protected. Recommendation: 50 to 100 mg/day.

Phosphatidylcholine (PC): It helps overall nerve-cell function. Recommendation: 500 to 1,000 mg/day.

---

1 Crayhon, Robert, M.S. The Carnitine Miracle. New York: M. Evans and Co., Inc. 1998, pp. 159-160.

5. Your Brain: Use It or Lose It

Researchers are optimistic about the potential of the aging brain, since evidence has challenged long-held beliefs by demonstrating that the brain can grow new nerve cells, according to Roni Caryn Rabin.[1]

"For a long time, we assumed that we're born with all the nerve cells that we are ever going to have, and that the brain is not capable of generating new ones because, once these cells die, we cannot replace them," said Molly V. Wagster of the Neuropsychology of Aging branch of the National Institutes of Health in Washington, D.C. "However, those assumptions have been challenged and put by the wayside."

Wagster added that new nerve cells have occurred in older rats, monkeys, and humans. Most of the areas that show neurogenesis and have been investigated so far are important for learning and memory, especially in the hippocampus.

"Scientists do not yet have all of the answers, but studies of older people who have maintained their mental acuity provide some clues," Rabin reported. "They tend to be socially connected, with strong ties to relatives, friends, and community. They are often both physically healthy and physically active, and they tend to be engaged in stimulating or intellectually challenging activities."

A number of interventional studies have introduced older adults to exercise regimens and have reported remarkable results, Rabin added.

---

1 Rabin, Roni Caryn. "For a Sharp Brain, Stimulation." The New York Times, May 13, 2008, p. H4.

For example, a research team at the University of Illinois at Urbana-Champaign recruited a group of sedentary adults, ranging in age from 60 to 75, and assigned them to an aerobic exercise program. The participants met 3 times a week to walk, while a control group did anaerobic stretching and toning.

The researchers measured the group's cognitive function before and after the 6-month program, and they reported improvements among those who had done the walking.

"Six months of exercise will buy you a 15 to 20% improvement in memory, decision making ability, and attention," said Arthur F. Kramer, a professor of psychology at the Illinois school. "It will also buy you increases in the volume of various brain regions in the prefrontal and temporal cortex, as well as more efficient neuronetworks that supply the kind of cognition we examined."

Seeking stimulation through interesting work, volunteer opportunities, or continuing education is beneficial, Rabin continued. Travel, read, take up a new language or learn to play a musical instrument. Staying socially connected is also associated with brain health, as is managing stress effectively.

She quoted Bruce E. McEwen, who heads the neuroendocrinology lab at Rockefeller University in New York, as saying that chronic stress can lead to the rewiring of areas of the brain that are involved in emotion, memory, and decision-making. The brain becomes more biased toward more anxiety, more depression, less flexibility in terms of decision making, and it becomes less able to store information.

The brain, like other parts of the body, changes with age, and those changes can impede clear thinking and memory, reported Jane E. Brody in the December 11, 2007 issue of the New York Times. But many older people seem to remain sharp as a tack well into their 80s and beyond. While their pace nay have slowed, they continue to work, travel, attend plays and concerts, play cards and board games, study foreign languages, design buildings, work with computers, write books, do puzzles, knit or perform other mentally challenging tasks that can befuddle younger people.[1]

However, when these mentally alert people die, autopsies often reveal extensive brain abnormalities like those in patients with Alzheimer's disease, Brody added.

This prompted Nikolaos Scarmeas, M.D., and Yaskov Stern of Columbia Presbyterian Medical Center in New York to recall that,

---

1 Brody, Jane E. "Mental Reserves Keep Brains Agile," The New York Times, December 11, 2007, p. F7.

in 1988, a study of cognitively normal elderly women, showed that they had advanced Alzheimer's disease pathology in their brains. Other studies indicated that up to two-thirds of people with autopsy findings of AD were cognitively intact when they died.

Something must account for the disjunction between the degree of brain damage and its outcome, the New York researchers wondered. They suggest that it is "cognitive reserve."

"Cognitive reserve, in this theory, refers to the brain's ability to develop and maintain extra neurons and connections between them via axons and dendrites," Brody continued. "Later in life, these connections may help compensate for the rise in dementia-related brain pathology that accompanies normal aging." (Dendrites are two types of branching processes of nerve cells.)

Ongoing studies suggest that there are several ways to improve the brain's viability, although it is best to start early to build up cognitive reserves, and that this account can be replenished even later in life, Brody continued. For example, cognitive reserve is greater in these who complete higher levels of education.

"The more intellectual challenges to the brain early in life, the more neurons and connections the brain is likely to develop and perhaps maintain into later years," she said. "Several studies of normal aging have found that higher levels of educational attainment were associated with slower cognitive and functional decline."

However, brain stimulation does not have to stop with a diploma, experts say. Better-educated people may go on to choose more intellectually demanding occupations and pursue brain-stimulating hobbies, resulting in a form of lifelong learning.

Cathryn Jakobson Ramin wrote that, if you are doing the same thing over and over, without introducing new mental challenges, it won't be beneficial. In a word, "use it or lose it." The brain requires continued stresses to maintain or enhance its strength.[1]

Brody added that Scarmeas published a lengthy study in 2001 of cognitively healthy elderly New Yorkers, and, on average, those who pursued the most leisure activities of an intellectual or social nature, had a 38% lower risk of developing dementia. The more activities, the lower the risk.

A research team at the University of Kentucky in Lexington, headed by David A. Snowdon, Ph.D., evaluated 93 nuns who were born before 1917, for their relationship between linguistic ability in

---

1 Ramin, Cathryn Jakobson. Carved in Sand: When Attention Fails and Memory Fades in Midlife, Harper; 1 edition (April 3, 2007).

early life to cognitive function and Alzheimer's disease in later life, reported the Journal of the American Medical Association.[1]

Low idea density early in life had a stronger and more consistent association with poor cognitive function than did lower grammatical complexity, Snowdon said.

In evaluating neuropathology in 14 sisters who had died, Alzheimer's disease was found in all those with low idea density in early life, and in none of the nuns with high idea density. The low linguistic ability early in life was a strong predictor of poor cognitive function in Alzheimer's disease later in life, he added.

When older people can no longer remember names at a cocktail party, they may think their brainpower is waning, but a number of studies suggest that this assumption may be wrong," said Sara Reistad-Long in the New York Times.[2] Instead, she said, the aging brain is simply taking in more data and trying to sift through a clutter of information, often to its long-term benefit. "Some brains do deteriorate with age, such as Alzheimer's disease, but, for most of aging adults, the researchers say that much of what occurs is a gradually widening focus of attention that makes it more difficult to latch onto just one fact, like a name or a telephone number."

Shelley H. Carson, M.D., of Harvard University in Boston, Massachusetts, said that distractibility may not in itself be a bad thing. It just may increase the amount of information available to the conscious mind. In studies where volunteers were asked to read passages that are interrupted with unexpected words or phrases, those 60 and older work more slowly than college students. While college students plow through the text regardless of what the out-of-place words mean, older people tend to slow down when the words are related to the topic. This suggests that they are not just stumbling over the extra information, but are taking it in and processing it.

When both groups were later asked questions for which the out-of-place words might be answers, the older people tended to respond much better than the students, Reistad-Long continued.

She quoted Jacqui Smith, M.D., of the University of Michigan at Ann Arbor, as saying that, "these findings are consistent with the context we are building for what wisdom is. If older people are taking in more information from a situation, and they are able

---

1 Snowdon, David A., Ph.D. "Linguistic Ability in Early Life and Cognitive Function and Alzheimer's Disease in Later Life," JAMA 275(7): 528-532, 1996.

2 Reistad-Long, Sara. "Older Brain Really May Be a Wiser Brain," The New York Times, May 20, 2008, p. F5.

to combine it with their comparatively greater store of general knowledge, they are going to have a nice advantage."

According to a research team at the University of Michigan at Ann Arbor, the elderly are not growing older but are growing sharper. They concluded that researchers have found that older Americans were less likely to experience memory loss and other cognitive problems than they were a decade before, according to Eric Nagourney in the New York Times.[1]

The study, originally published in Alzheimer's and Dementia, found that when the thinking skills of 7,000 people were tested in 2003 and compared with those in a similar group in 1993, there was a significant improvement. Only 8.7% of the newer group had problems with memory or performing mental calculations, compared with 12.2% in the earlier group.

The improvement suggests that the combined impact of recent trends in medical, lifestyle, demographic, and social factors, have been positive for the cognitive health of older Americans, Nagourney reported.

Another reason for the decline, said Kenneth M. Langa, M.D., is that people in 2003 had more schooling and were more likely to participate in intellectually stimulating activities in later life.

"Research has shown that people who are better educated may develop more of what is known as cognitive reserve, giving them more of a cushion when illness and age take their toll," Nagourney said.

High amounts of leisure time have been associated with a reduced risk of Alzheimer's disease, according to Archives of Neurology. In fact, greater participation in prediagnosis leisure activities, especially intellectual pursuits, was associated with faster cognitive decline, supporting the hypothesis that the disease course in AD may vary as a function of cognitive reserve.[2]

The study involved 283 patients with incident Alzheimer's disease, with a mean age of 79 years. The study included Hispanics (56.2%) and African-Americans (31.1%).

In another article in Archives of Neurology, mild cognitive impairment in 577 individuals was associated with race (African-Americans), low educational level, low Modified Mini-Mental State Examination, and Digit Symbol Test Scores, cortical atrophy,

---

1 Nagourney, Eric. "Dementia Percentages Decline in Elderly," The New York Times, February 26, 2008, p. F8.
2 Heizner, E. P., et al. "Leisure Activity and Cognitive Decline in Incident Alzheimer Disease," Archives of Neurology 63(12): 1749-1754, 2007.

magnetic resonance imaging (MRI) identified infarcts, and measurements of depression.[1]

Apathy in Alzheimer's disease is associated with a reduced metabolic activity in the bilateral anterior cingulate gyrus (a bundle of fibers in white matter) and medial orbitofrontal cortex (in the center), and it may be associated with reduced activity in the medial thalamus (a large oval mass of gray matter), according to Archives of Neurology. Apathy is best described as indifference or absence of interest in the environment. It is often the initial sign of cerebral disease.[2]

The study reinforces the confluence of evidence from other investigational studies in implicating medial frontal dysfunction and related neuronal circuits in the neurobiology of apathy in Alzheimer's disease and other neuropsychiatry diseases. Neurons are the functional units of the nervous system, which is composed of the entire nerve apparatus, brain, and spinal cord.

A study at the University of Washington in Seattle evaluated dementia and Alzheimer's disease in a group of 2,356 volunteers. The study began in 1994, and follow-up interviews by phone were conducted every 2 years, reported Archives of Neurology.[3]

The research team evaluated 215 cases of dementia, and 151 cases of Alzheimer's disease. They determined that AD rates rise from 2.8 per 1,000 person-years (those 65 to 69 years old), to 56.1 per 1,000 person-years in the older than 90-year group.

While sex was not a factor, the researchers determined that educational level (over 15 years versus less than 12 years) was associated with a decreased risk of Alzheimer's disease.

The research team also concluded that their dementia and Alzheimer's disease incidence rates are consistent with recent U.S. and European studies, thus providing clinicians and researchers with new information concerning the reproductibility of incidence estimates. An increased risk was associated with age, the apolipoprotein E (ApoE) genotype, and low baseline cognitive screening test scores.

"Educational level was inversely associated with the risk of dementia, and it was positively associated with the baseline (beginning of the study) cognitive test score," the researchers added.

1 Lopez, Oscar L., M.D., et al. "Risk Factors for Mild Cognitive Impairment in the Cardiovascular Health Study Cognition: Part 2," Archives of Neurology 60: 1394-1399, 2003.

2 Marshall, G. A., et al. "Positron Emission Tomography Metabolic Correlates of Apathy in Alzheimer Disease," Archives of Neurology 611: 1015-1020, 2007.

3 Kukull, Walter A., M.D., et al. "Dementia and Alzheimer's Disease Incidence: A Prospective Cohort Study," Archives of Neurology 59: 1737-1746, 2002.

"Thus, detection of AD by the screening test could also be influenced by educational level."

Several large community-based studies have examined the factors that predict which people are likely to maintain a good memory, language skills, and overall cognitive function as they age, according to Marilyn Albert, Ph.D., of the Johns Hopkins University School of Medicine in Baltimore, Maryland. She was interviewed by Bridget M. Kuehn in the February 1, 2006 issue of the Journal of the American Medical Association.[1]

In spite of geographic and cultural differences of the populations studied, they have all reached similar conclusions about the lifestyle factors that seem to contribute to maintaining healthy cognitive functioning into advanced age.

The various community studies have identified a relatively small set of factors that appear to predict who will function well over time, Albert said. Those include physical activity, mental activity, social engagement, and good vascular health.

Albert went on to say that rodents have been put into running wheels and compared with animals who were more sedentary. It is rather clear that the exercised animals have better memory. They also have changes in the levels of various chemicals that are involved with maintenance and repair in the brain.

"The chemical that has repeatedly been found to be increased following exercise is called brain-derived neurotrophic factor (BDNF)," Albert continued. "Also, some studies have indicated that there is increased neurogenesis as a result of physical activity."

Albert went on to say that we need to pay attention to controlling vascular risks, and we now know that increased blood pressure, diabetes, high cholesterol, smoking, and increased weight are bad for the vessels of the heart, and they are also bad for the vessels in the brain.

"The other findings suggest that physical and mental activities might be directly beneficial for the brain, and that people ought to consider changing their lifestyle to be sure to incorporate them, if they haven't already," Albert said.

High levels of high-density lipoprotein cholesterol (HDL) — the so-called good cholesterol — may help to prevent a decline in memory, reported Eric Nagourney.[2] A research team headed by Archana Singh-Manoux, M.D., said that people with high levels of HDL did better on memory tests than those with lower levels.

---

1   Kuehn, Bridget M. "Studies Explore Strategies for Staying Sharp," JAMA 295(5): 287, 2006.
2   Nagourney, Eric. "Good Cholesterol, Good Memory," The New York Times, July 1, 2008, p. F6.

While it was not addressed in this article, dietary fish and ome-ga-3 fatty acids are some of the natural ways to increase HDL-cholesterol."The researchers checked the cholesterol levels of more than 3,000 British civil servants and gave them memory tests at an average age of 55, and retested them again when they were 61," Na-gourney said. "For the tests, volunteers were read a list of 20 words and then asked to write down as many as they could remember within 2 minutes." Not only did volunteers with higher HDL do better than the others tested, those whose HDL levels declined be-tween tests also saw a decline in their performance.

The original study appeared in an issue of Arteriosclerosis, Thrombosis, and Vascular Biology, a publication of the American Heart Association.

Even frail adults living at home who participate in a moderate activity program can experience distinct benefits in their physical and mental functioning capacities, according to Christine K. Cas-sel, M.D., of the Oregon Health Sciences University School of Med-icine in Portland.[1] Working to understand healthy brain functions has overlapped with understanding diseases of the brain, which together could lead to major new approaches to prevent, amelio-rate, or successfully reverse memory loss associated with healthy aging, and with pathological progressive neurological decline. "Cognitive and emotional function is vital to independence, pro-ductivity, and quality of life, and the debilitation associated with Alzheimer disease is among the most feared of aging-related condi-tions." The brain is arguably the major organ of interest as people age, and the report by Ball, et al.[2] demonstrates the effectiveness of simple cognitive exercises to improve memory. The implication of this finding for healthy aging is enormous.

Having a mentally challenging occupation and higher levels of education appears to buffer the effects of brain changes and dam-age caused by Alzheimer's disease, according to Joan Stephenson, Ph.D.[3]

Italian scientists[4] tested memory and cognitive skills of 242 people with Alzheimer's disease, 72 with mild cognitive impair-ment, and 144 controls. In addition, they used brain imaging to measure participants' brain glucose metabolism to determine the

---

1 Cassel, Christine K., M.D. "Use It or Lose It: Activity May Be the Best Treatment for Aging," JAMA 288(18): 2333-2335, 2002.
2 Ball, K., et al. "Effects of Cognitive Training Intervention with Older Adults: A Randomised Controlled Trial," JAMA 288(18): 2271-2281, 2002.
3 Stephenson, Joan, Ph.D. "Alzheimer Disease Protection," JAMA 300(19): 2239, 2008.
4 Garibotto, V., et al., Neurology 71(17): 1342-1349, 2008.

extent of Alzheimer's disease pathological changes. "Among those with AD or mild cognitive impairment that progressed to AD during the study, those who had more education and mentally taxing jobs had significantly more changes and damage in the brain for a given level of memory impairment," Stephenson said. "In other words, AD-related tissue damage might impair memory more quickly in those with less intellectual stimulation."

The scientists found no association among healthy controls, or those with mild cognitive impairment who did not develop AD during the study. Added the researchers, "This study suggests that education and occupation may be proxies for brain function reserve, reducing the severity and delaying the clinical expression of AD pathology."

It is not surprising that mentally stimulating activities in old age appear to compress the cognitive morbidity associated with Alzheimer's disease by slowing cognitive decline before dementia sets in, thus hastening its development thereafter, according to a research team at the Rush Alzheimer's Disease Center, Rush University Medical Center in Chicago, Illinois.[1]

Time magazine discussed a 15-year, ongoing study that David Snowdon, Ph.S., has undertaken,[2] as he peers into the minds, memories, and — when they die — the brains of the School Sisters of Notre Dame at the convent on Good Counsel Hill in Minnesota. Snowdon, who is with the University of Kentucky at Lexington, is trying to understand why some of the nuns get Alzheimer's disease and some do not. The study investigates nutrition, lifestyle habits, exercise, etc., to track how the brain deteriorates with age.

"To ensure that the sisters' generous gift to science will continue to educate others, Snowdon is attempting to have the brain bank and archive records permanently endowed," reported Michael D. Lemonick and Alice Park. "That way, future generations will continue to benefit from lessons that women like Sisters Ada, Roselle, and Nicolette are teaching all of us about how to age with grace and good health."

When the article was written, here is the status of the participants:

Nuns, ages 75 to 102, who volunteered to join the Nun Study in 1986: 675.

Nuns who have died: 334.

1 Wilson, R. S., et al. "Cognitive Activity and the Cognitive Morbidity of Alzheimer's Disease," Neurology 75(11): 990-996, 2010.

2 Lemonick, Michael D., and Park, Alice. "How One Scientist and 678 Sisters Are Helping Unlock the Secrets of Alzheimer's," Time, May 14, 2001, pp. 54-64.

Brain autopsies that have been performed: More than 300.
Nuns, ages 84 to 106, who have survived: 344.
Nuns who are symptom free: About 100

NINE WAYS TO AVOID MENTAL DECLINE

Here are 9 ways to preserve mental functioning, and keep your brain at its optimal functioning level, even as you age:[1]

Be selective with your attention. Focus your attention on things you want to learn, and remember to learn and remember and minimize distractions. (Jean Martin, Ph.D., of Mount Sinai School of Medicine in New York)

Stimulate your brain. Read, go to museums, or play a musical instrument. Do word puzzles, play chess, card and board games. (Margaret Sewell, Ph.D., of Mount Sinai)

Recognize and treat depression. This has a toxic effect on attention. Depression masks its effects as sadness, changes in sleep patterns or appetite, irritability, or lack of interest in activities you used to enjoy. (Dr. Martin)

Stay physically active. Exercise has a direct benefit on improving performance on cognitive tests, as well as managing other risk factors. Whether you walk, bike, swim, go to the gym, do yard or house-work, it all contributes to a healthier brain.

Follow a healthful diet. Avoid packaged foods like cookies' and crackers. Select healthful fats that benefit your brain, such as olive and canola oils, and fatty fish like salmon and mackerel.

Interact with others. Don't become socially isolated. Volunteer at the library, join a church group, or babysit your grandchildren.

Get adequate nutrition. Malnutrition and vitamin deficiencies can lead to cognitive impairment. Make sure you do not have a vitamin B12 deficiency, which can be easily rectified. (Dr. Sewell)

Use tools that compensate for decline. Develop skills that aid memory, such as writing things down and making lists. As an example, take paper and pen to doctor's appointments, and ask the doctor to repeat information that you don't understand. (Dr. Martin)

Get enough sleep. Your brain needs adequate rest to function well. If you have problems sleeping, ask your doctor on how to improve your sleep habits.

---

1   "9 Ways to Keep Mental Decline at Bay," Focus on Healthy Aging, Mount Sinai School of Medicine, Volume 9G, undated.

6. Importance of Sleep

It is an old wives' tale that, as we grow older, less sleep is required. Research shows that older people who sleep 8 hours or more have fewer complaints. It may be more difficult for older people to get the necessary sleep, and those who do not sleep well suffer from tension and nervous exhaustion. In fact, some of the problems of the aged may simply be due to a lack of sleep, according to The Book of Health.[1]

Since the amount of sleep required varies with each individual, no arbitrary number of hours of sleep can be set. The prime requisite is that one should sleep enough to awaken rested and refreshed.

"In some people, sleeplessness may cause frustration, irritation, and nervousness," the publication added. "Often a glass of wine or warm milk help to induce sleep. Chronic constipation may be a factor in insomnia, and changes in eating habits and fluid intake may be necessary."

Electroencephalogram (EEG) recordings of the electrical impulses produced by the brain during sleep show that there are 2 distinct types of sleep, that is, REM (rapid eye movement), and NREM (nonrapid eye movement) sleep, reported the American Medical Association Home Medical Encyclopedia. They alternate in cycles lasting roughly 90 minutes throughout the night.[2]

---

1 Clark, Randolph Lee, M.D., and Cumley, Russell W., Ph.D., editors. The Book of Health. New York: Van Nostrand Reinhold Co., 1974, pp. 635ff.

2 Clayman, Charles B., M.D., medical editor. The American Medical Association Home Medical Encyclopedia. New York: Random House, 1989, pp. 914ff.

NREM sleep, which accounts for the major part of sleep, starts with drowsiness, brain waves become increasingly deeper and slower until brain activity and metabolism fall to their lowest level. Dreams are infrequent.

"In REM sleep," the publication added, "the brain suddenly becomes more electrically active — with a wave pattern resembling that of an awake person — and its temperature and blood flow increase. The eyes move rapidly, and dreaming, often with elaborate story lines, occurs. REM sleep, also called paradoxical sleep, periodically interrupts NREM sleep."

The initial REM period usually takes place 90 to 100 minutes after the onset of sleep, and it lasts about 5 to 10 minutes. REM sleep periods grow progressively longer as sleep continues, and the last of the night's 4 to 5 REM sleep periods may last about an hour, the publication said.

Sleep disturbances cause human misery and ill health at any age, but among the elderly these disturbances are commonplace, according to Miriam Cohen, Ph.D. The quality and quantity of sleep, the maintenance and depth of sleep, and the ability to sleep is a consolidated fashion all diminish with age.[1]

"The age-related changes in sleep in many cases are independent of any medical or psychiatric disorders," Cohen said. "In addition, sleep disorders in the elderly may be caused by transient illnesses, poor sleep habits, pain, chronic illness, dementia, affective disorders or milder mood disturbances, breathing problems during sleep (apnea, snoring, etc.), prescribed and over-the-counter drugs — including appetite suppressants, antihistamines-corticosteroids, cardiovascular drugs, hormones, etc. — and periodic leg jerks (nocturnal myoclonus)."

Benzodiazepines are the most widely prescribed group of sedative-hypnotic drugs for sleep disorders, she added. These include flurazepam (Dalmane), temazepam (Restoril), triazolam (Halcion), and lorazepam (Ativan). Their rapid sedative action — meaning the patient falls asleep sooner — and rapid elimination from the body — the patient does not suffer a "hangover" or prolonged sedation, are the reasons for the popularity of these drugs.

While the benzodiazepines are generally safe, they can cause sensory-motor impairments, Cohen continued. Excessive doses decrease energy, clear thinking, libido and sexual performance. If

---

1 Cohen, Miriam, Ph.D. "Special Report: Mind, Mood, and Medication in Later Life," *Medical and Health Annual*. Chicago, IL: Encyclopaedia Britannica, Inc., 1994, pp. 229ff.

the drugs are taken for an extended period, dependence can occur, and the potential for abuse develops.

"Dependence manifests itself most acutely when the elderly person stops taking the drug, and he/she develops withdrawal symptoms," Cohen said. "These include anxiety, agitation, and the desire to relieve these symptoms by resuming the drugs. If the physician gradually reduces the dose over a period of several weeks, withdrawal symptoms are minimized."

When faced with a distraught older patient who is unable to sleep, the physician is tempted to prescribe a drug, but most geriatric specialists agree that the use of sedative-hypnotic agents for chronic sleep disturbances should be postponed until other measures have been tried, Cohen said.

These include increasing daytime activities; regularizing and curtailing the number of hours spent in bed; assuming that the environment for sleep is optimal in terms of noise, light, temperature, and bedding; using the bedroom exclusively for sleeping — not for watching TV, working, etc. — avoiding coffee, tea, nicotine, alcohol, and certain OTC medications that contain stimulating substances; and determining whether diet and prescription medications for other conditions are contributing to the sleep problems.

"Since biblical times," Cohen continued, "warm milk, which contains the amino acid L-tryptophan, has been recognized as a natural sedative. Alcohol is frequently used by elderly people to facilitate sleep, and some doctors recommend a glass of wine or shot of brandy before bedtime. In general, however, it tends to deepen sleep for the first few hours, but then disrupts it later in the night."

Over-the-counter sleeping aids are generally not a good choice for older people. The active agent in most of these medications — Sominex, Nytol, Compoz — is an antihistamine, and antihistamines may put the older patient at risk for delirium. In addition, sleeping aids generally do not include special usage and design instructions for the elderly, Cohen said.

Obstructive sleep apnea (OSA) imposes considerable risks of developing cardiovascular disease abnormalities because of the repetitive cycles of snoring, airway collapse, and awakening, according to Tracy Hampton, Ph.D., in the June 25, 2008 issue of the Journal of the American Medical Association.[1]

One reason for this increased risk is that low blood oxygen levels during these cycles induces harmful responses, such as high

---

1 Hampton, Tracy, Ph.D. "Sleep Apnea Linked to Cardiovascular Risk," JAMA 299(24): 2841, 2008.

blood pressure in the vasculature (the blood vessel network of an organ).

OSA is frequently underdiagnosed but recognizing the condition is important because it has been linked to increased blood pressure and risk of stroke, said Mary Morrell, Ph.D., of the Royal Brompton Hospital in London, England, speaking at the American Thoracic Society's 2008 International Conference in Toronto, Canada.

"This sleep disorder may pose a special danger for those who have already experienced a stroke, according to an analysis of 132 Swedish patients who were followed for 10 years after having had a stroke," Hampton added. "The study showed that OSA increased patients' risk of dying by up to 76%, an elevated risk that was independent of smoking, body mass index, high blood pressure, diabetes, atrial fibrillation (rapid heartbeat)."

A recent study headed by Ferran Barbe, M.D., of the Biomedical Research Institute in Lleida, Spain, found that treatment with continuous positive airway pressure (CPAP) may also lower blood pressure among those with OSA and high blood pressure, Hampton reported. CPAP is said to be the most effective treatment for OSA when such conservative measures as getting sufficient sleep, abstaining from alcohol and sedative use, and losing weight are not effective.

The Spanish study involved 394 patients with hypertension and non-sleepy OSA (a mild form that does not affect daytime alertness), who were randomized to receive CPAP or no treatment. It was reported that, on average, patients who used a CPAP machine experienced a 2 mmHg drop in both systolic (beating) and diastolic (resting) blood pressure after 1 year when compared with the controls.

"Our study suggests that CPAP can be used not only to treat the symptoms of sleep apnea, but also to reduce cardiovascular risk in those with apneic or breathing problems," Barbe said.

Sleep apnea is a complication of obesity that in many cases is not recognized, but may be life-threatening, according to Richard L. Atkinson, M.D. With increasing overweight an individual finds it more and more difficult to breathe, especially while sleeping, and some obese people have periods during sleep when they stop breathing.[1]

---

1   Atkinson, Richard L., M.D. "Obesity," *Medical and Health Annual.* Chicago, IL: Encyclopaedia Britannica, Inc., 1995, p. 339.

"When this happens, the oxygen level in the blood drops, and the carbon dioxide level rises," Atkinson said. "This alerts the brain and the person must wake up to start breathing again. Some people may wake up as many as 600 times in a night."

Without a good night's sleep, sleep apnea sufferers become confused and sleepy during the day, have severe nightmares, and even develop hallucinations. The excess carbon dioxide buildup is thought to lead to high blood pressure, and eventually some of these people develop congestive heart failure. If the cardiac condition is left untreated, the mortality rate is about 70% in 5 years.

"Fortunately, weight loss improves or even cures most of these conditions," Atkinson added. "Some studies show that even modest weight loss may produce dramatic improvements in risk factors associated with obesity."

The prevalence of sleep-related breathing disorder (SRBD) and insomnia symptoms increases considerably with advancing age, reported a research team in the Archives of Internal Medicine. Having both insomnia symptoms and SRBD was associated with significantly lower daytime functioning, and longer psychomotor reaction times compared with those who had neither condition.[1]

Because insomnia and comorbid with SRBD is associated with the greatest functional impairment, and SRBD is commonly found in the elderly population, health care providers should also consider SRBD in elderly patients with insomnia symptoms, the researchers added.

A body mass index of 30 or higher, neck circumference greater than 15.5 inches, and a history of loud snoring or stop-breathing episodes, chokes or struggles with breath, were independently predictive of SRBD in those with insomnia symptoms.

At the Yale University School of Medicine in New Haven, Connecticut, 175 people, 70 years of age or older, were admitted to a general medical unit for observation, reported the Journal of the American Geriatric Society.[2] A nonpharmacologic sleep protocol consisted of a back rub, a warm (non-alcoholic) drink, and relaxation tapes were administered by nursing personnel to patients who had complained about having trouble going to sleep, or who requested a sedative-hypnotic drug. A cohort of 111 patients received the drug-free sleep protocol, and 74% complied with the

1 Gooneratne, N. S., et al. "Consequences of Comorbid Insomnia Symptoms and Sleep-Related Breathing Disorder in Elderly Subjects," Archives of Internal Medicine 166: 1732-1738, 2006.
2 McDowell, Jane M., M.S.N., R.N., et al. "A Nonpharmacologic Sleep Protocol for Hospitalized Older Patients," Journal of the American Geriatric Society 46(6): 700-705, 1998.

therapy. (Chronic sedative hypnotic users were more likely to refuse this protocol than nonusers.)

The quality of sleep correlated strongly with the number of parts of the protocol received, which suggested a dose-response relationship with the highest correlation for those who received 2 to 3 parts of the therapy, reported Sharon K. Inoyue, M.D., the lead researcher.

Part 1 of the protocol consisted of 5 minutes of slow-stroke back massage, consisting of slow rhythmic stroking on both sides of the spinous processes, from the crown of the head to the sacral area, with the patients in a side-lying position. Part 2 consisted of a warm drink of either milk or herbal tea. Part 3 consisted of listening to relaxation tapes of classical music or nature sounds played on either a head-set or a bedside cassette tape player.

If the protocol was ineffective after 1 hour, the nurse could continue with the usual care. The sleep protocol reduced sedative hypnotic drug use from 54 to 31%, and the sleep protocol had a stronger association with the quality of sleep.

Sleep physicians are extremely reluctant to prescribe sedatives for insomnia, except in the event of an obvious trauma, such as the death of a spouse, and even then only for a very temporary period, according to Suzan Jaffe, Ph.D., of the Sleep Program at Hollywood Medical Center in Florida. Improper withdrawal from sleeping pills can cause the insomnia the prescriptions were designed to treat.[1] She advises only occasional use of over-the-counter sleeping pills, since we don't know the long-term effects of them. They are certainly not benign, and certain ingredients that can cause addiction.

Melatonin

At the Sleep Laboratory at the Bruce Rapport Faculty of Medicine in Haifa, Israel, researchers evaluated 4 groups of elderly patients.[2]

The first group was 80 independently living patients with insomnia, mean age of 73.

The second was 15 patients with insomnia, mean age of 82, who had lived a minimum of 6 months in a nursing home.

Twenty-five patients without sleeping disorders, a mean age of 71.4 years, who were living independently in the community.

---

1 Feinstein, Alice, editor. Symptoms: Their Causes and Cures. Emmaus, PA: Rodale Press, Inc., 1994, p. 276.

2 Haimov, I., et al. "Sleep Disorders and Melatonin Rhythms in Elderly People," Bairish Medical Journal 309: 167, 1994.

Twelve young men, mean age of 20, without sleep disorders.

The research team found a correlation between disturbances of rhythm of 6-sulphatoxymelatonin excretion and poor sleep quality in elderly patients. All patients correlation between disturbances of 6-sulphatoxymelatonin with insomnia had significantly lower sleep efficiency and a higher activity level during sleep.

The peak excretion of 6-sulphatoxymelatonin in the elderly patients was 49% lower than in the younger volunteers, even though the peak in the elderly subjects without sleep disorders did not differ significantly from those in younger participants.

This data suggests a relationship between deficiency of melatonin or disruption of its rhythms and an increased prevalence of sleep disorders with advancing age.

The authors suggest that a lack of exposure to bright light in institutions may lead to a reduction of 6-sulphatoxymelatonin excretion in old age. Melatonin deficiency seems to be a key component in the incidence of sleep disorders in elderly people, and melatonin replacement therapy may be of benefit. The pineal gland, a small cone-shaped structure in the brain, secretes melatonin after the sun goes down, and the secretion reaches a peak around midnight, then wanes through the remainder of the night. It is also available as a supplement. Scientists also refer to it as N-acetyl-5-methoxytryptamine.

In a 3-week Israeli study, 9 volunteers — 68 to 80 years of age, who were otherwise healthy but suffering from insomnia — were given 2 mg of melatonin. The amount of time it took to fall asleep was cut from 40 to 15 minutes.[1] The patients slept longer without waking up, and reported a more refreshing sleep. The research study was successfully duplicated in 30 additional patients.

An evaluation of 8 women and 6 men, with an average age of 61, who were hospitalized in an intensive care unit (ICU) for more than 4 days, showed that lack of sleep was a severe problem in these patients, who were evaluated by actigraphy.[2] The researchers reported that the nocturnal peak melatonin secretion was not present, therefore, melatonin supplements may improve sleep in ICU patients.

---

1 Shaffer, Marjorie. "Melatonin Could Help Elderly Sleep Better," Medical Tribune, July 22, 1993, p. 15.

2 Shilo, L., et al. "Patients in the Intensive Care Unit Suffer from Severe Lack of Sleep Associated with Loss of Normal Melatonin Secretion Pattern," American Journal of Medical Science 317(5): 278-281, 1999.

As reported in The Lancet, researchers in another study gave 0.3 mg of melatonin to 9 elderly insomniacs, ranging in age from 51 to 78 years of age for 3 consecutive days or a placebo.[1]

It was found that melatonin greatly reduced the number of movements per night, latency of sleep onset, awakenings per night, and improved subjective sleep quality without increased morning sleepiness. The dose did not affect core body temperature. Physiologic oral doses of melatonin can promote and sustain sleep in elderly insomniacs, reported Richard J. Wurtman, Ph.D., and Irina Zhdanova of the Massachusetts Institute of Technology in Cambridge.

Patients may become dependent on benzodiazepine therapy for insomnia; however, melatonin therapy for discontinuation showed benefit as an adjunct in the weaning process and sleep-maintenance alternative to benzodiazepine therapy, reported Harold J. Bursztajn, M.D.[2] For clinicians who treat patients with benzodiazepine-dependent problems, and who suffer from insomnia, melatonin therapy as an alternative to benzodiazepine dependence may be of benefit.

Compared with placebo, oral doses of 0.3 mg or 1.0 mg of melatonin decreased sleep onset latency and latency to Stage 2 sleep, and it did not suppress rapid eye movement (REM) sleep or delay its onset, according to Clinical Pharmacology and Therapy.[3]

At Tel-Aviv University in Israel, researchers evaluated 12 elderly insomniacs, and it was found that 6-sulphatoxymelatonin measured during the night was lower than normal and/or delayed compared with elderly noninsomniacs.[4] They were given 2 mg/night of controlled-release melatonin with placebo for 3 weeks in a double-blind trial, which showed that sleep efficiency was significantly greater after melatonin therapy than after placebo.

5-HTP

A relatively new supplement, 5-hydroxytryptophan (5-HTP), is said to be a natural alternative to Prozac, according to Earl Mindell, R.Ph., Ph.D. Like Prozac and other drugs known as selective

---

1   Wurtman, Richard J., Ph.D., and Zhdanova, Irina. "Improvement of Sleep Quality by Melatonin," The Lancet 346: 1491, December 2, 1995.

2   Bursztajn, Harold J., M.D. "Melatonin Therapy: From Benzodiazepine-Dependent Insomnia in Authenticity and Autonomy," Archives of Internal Medicine 159: 2393-2395, November 8, 1999.

3   Zhdanova, I. V., et al. "Sleep-Inducing Effects of Low Doses of Melatonin Ingested in the Evening," Clinical Pharmacology and Therapy 57(5): 552-558, 1995.

4   Garfinkel, D., et al. "Improvement of Sleep Quality in Elderly People by Controlled-Release Melatonin," Lancet 346: 541-544, August 26, 1995.

serotonin reuptake inhibitors, 5-HTP enhances the activity of se-rotonin, the hormone produced by the brain that is involved in mood, sleep, and appetite.[1] "Low levels of serotonin are associat-ed with depression, anxiety, and sleep disorders," Mindell added. "Drugs such as Prozac prevent the brain cells from using up sero-tinin too quickly, thereby causing a deficiency. However, 5-HTP works somewhat differently in that it increases the cell's produc-tion of serotonin, which boosts serotonin levels. 5-HTP is some-what similar to tryptophan supplements, which were popular in the 1980s as a sleep aid. They were recalled by the Food and Drug Administration in 1988 after a tainted batch from a Japanese man-ufacturer caused serious side effects, including several deaths."

There is no indication that 5-HTP is dangerous. In one Swiss study, depressed patients were given either 100 mg of 5-HTP 3 times daily or 150 mg of fluvoxamine maleate, an SSRI (Selective Serotonin Reuptake Inhibitor) antidepressant. "Starting at week 2 and continuing through week 6, both groups reported significant improvement on standard depression rating scales, however, those taking 5-HTP seemed to have made more progress than those tak-ing the prescription drug," Mindell continued.

Other studies have shown that 5-HTP not only is an effective antidepressant, but also it can help to suppress appetite, a boon for those who need to lose weight. An Italian study reported that patients taking the supplement reduced their carbohydrate in-take and they felt satisfied sooner than did a group taking a place-bo, Mindell said. "When you boost your level of serotonin, you are also increasing your level of melatonin, which can result in a better night's sleep," Mindell added. "If 5-HTP is similar to an SSRI, why not take the SSRI? For one thing, prescription antidepressants are more expensive, and they often cause some unpleasant side effects, such as dry mouth, anxiety, and loss of libido. These side effects are not felt with 5-HTP."

Mindell recommends up to 2 50 mg capsules daily on an emp-ty stomach.

Magnesium

Researchers have suggested that a low magnesium level can lead to shallow sleep and more nighttime awakenings. According to James G. Penland, Ph.D., of the USDA/Grand Forks Human Nu-trition Center in North Dakota, "Low magnesium status means

---

1 Mindell, Earl, R.Ph., Ph.D. Earl Mindell's Supplement Bible. New York: Simon & Schuster, 1998, pp. 71-72.

that your magnesium intake is very low on a daily basis, probably less than 200 mg/day."[1] "This deficiency isn't uncommon, especially among people with reduced caloric intakes, such as the elderly and those on weight-loss diets." Even if magnesium levels are normal, certain medications can keep your body from absorbing the mineral efficiently, he reported. The most common offenders are probably diuretics (water pills) that are prescribed for high blood pressure. Penland said that 400 mg/day of the mineral should be sufficient to prevent sleep problems. However, if you have heart or kidney problems, consult your doctor before taking magnesium supplements.

Valerian

In a double-blind trial, eight mild insomniac patients were given either 450 mg or 900 mg of an aqueous extract of valerian root (Valeriana officianalis), or a placebo.[2] Results showed a significant decrease in sleep latency (dormancy) with 450 mg of the extract when compared with the placebo. However, the larger dosage did not produce any further benefit in sleep latency.

In 10 patients, 450 and 900 mg of an aqueous valerian extract, when given daily, reduced perceived sleep latency and wake time after sleep onset, according to Psychopharmacology.[3]

Valerian, when given at dosages ranging from 500 mg to 12 g prior to bedtime, or sometimes in divided doses 3 times daily, is used as a sedative and hypnotic, according to Eric Heiligenstein, M.D., a Madison, Wisconsin physician.[4]

A research team in Switzerland gave 200 mg of an aqueous solution of valerian twice daily, compared with a placebo and a proprietary OTC preparation of the herb, to 128 volunteers with sleep problems.[5] The herbal preparation produced a significant decrease in subjectively evaluated sleep latency scores, and a significant improvement in sleep quality. With the OTC proprietary valerian solution, patients felt more sleepy than normal the next morning. However, the aqueous extract improved sleep quality of poor or ir-

1   Feinstein, Alice, editor. Prevention's Healing with Vitamins. Emmaus, PA: Rodale Press, Inc., 1996, pp. 339-340.

2   Leatherwood, P. D., M.D., and Chauffard, F. "Aqueous Extract of Valerian Reduces Latency to Fall Asleep in Men," Planta Medica, 1995, pp. 144-148.

3   Baiderer, G., and Borbely, A. A. "Effect of Valerian on Human Sleep," Psychopharmacology 87: 406-409, 1985.

4   Heiligenstein, Eric, M.D., et al. "Over-the-Counter Psychotropics: A Review of Melatonin, St. John's Wort, Valerian, and Kava-Kava," Journal of the American College of Health 46: 271-276, 1998.

5   Leatherwood, P. D., M.D., et al. "Aqueous Extract of Valerian Root (Valeriana Officinalis L.) Improves Sleep Quality in Men," Pharmac. Biochem. Behavior. 17(1): 65-71, 1982.

regular sleepers without causing a hangover the next morning, the researchers added.

Exercise

In a 10-week randomized trial of 32 volunteers, ranging in age from 60 to 84, who began a supervised weight training program 3 times weekly, compared to an attention-control group, this brought a significant improvement in all subjective sleep-quality and depression measures, according to a research team at the Human Nutrition Research Center on Aging in Boston, Massachusetts.[1]

Depression measures were reduced by almost 2-fold when compared with the control group. Also, the quality of life subscale significantly improved with exercise. Weight lifting was effective in improving subjective sleep quality, depression, strength, and quality of life, according to Maria A. Fiatarone, M.D., the lead researcher.

There are conflicting data on the effect of acute and chronic exercise on sleep, according to Karia A. Kubitz, M.D., of Kansas State University in Manhattan. Acute and chronic exercise can increase slow wave sleep and total sleep time, but it may also decrease sleep onset latency and REM sleep, she added.[2]

Morning exercise is not likely to compromise sleep regardless of its intensity and duration, and mild to moderate exercise late in the afternoon may actually improve sleep, reported Helen S. Driver, M.D., and Sheila R. Taylor of the University of Witwatersrand in South Africa.[3] They added that high intensity, long duration exercise close to bedtime or exercise which is different to the patient may disturb or disrupt sleep patterns.

Caffeine

At the Center for Devices and Radiological Health in Rockville, Maryland, a research team evaluated the impact of caffeine and medications containing the drug on sleep complaints in a community population of people 67 years of age or older. The prevalence of caffeinated medications use by the patients was 5.4%.[4]

---

1 Singh, Nalin A., et al. "Sleep, Sleep Deprivation, and Daytime Activities: A Randomized Controlled Trial of the Effect of Exercise on Sleep," Sleep 20(2): 95-101, 1997.

2 Kubitz, Karla J., M.D., et al. "The Effects of Acute and Chronic Exercise on Sleep: A Meta-Analytic Review," Sports Medicine 21(4): 277-291, 1996.

3 Driver, Helen S., M.D., and Taylor, Sheila R. "Sleep Disturbances and Exercise," Sports Medicine 21(1): 1-6, 1996.

4 Brown, S. Lori, Ph.D., et al. "Occult Caffeine As a Source of Sleep Problems in an Older Population," Journal of the American Geriatric Society 43: 860-864, 1995.

Those reporting the use of any caffeine-containing medications were at an increased risk of having trouble falling asleep with an odds ratio of 1.79. However, there was no significant risk of other reported nighttime or daytime sleep problems associated with the use of caffeine-containing drugs. After adjusting for variables, the patients using caffeine-containing medications still showed a significantly increased risk of having trouble falling asleep.

The authors concluded that the use of caffeine-containing medications is associated with sleep disorders, and they urged health-care providers to be aware of the situation. Older patients should be encouraged to read labels on medications and select drugs that are caffeine free when possible.

7. A Prudent Diet Is Important

The number of older people is growing rapidly worldwide, with over 580 million people older than 60, and the number is expected to grow to 1,000 million by 2020, according to Kim T. B. Knoops, M.Sc. and colleagues. With the increase in life expectancy, the leading causes of death have shifted dramatically from infectious diseases to noncommunicable illnesses, and from younger to older individuals.[1] In industrialized countries, about 75% of the deaths in those older than 65 are now due to cardiovascular diseases and cancer. "Regardless of predisposing factors, diet and lifestyle influence morbidity and mortality during the course of life.... Because of a cumulative effect of adverse factors throughout life, it is especially important for older people to adopt diet and lifestyle practices that minimize their risk of death from morbidity, and maximize their prospects for healthful aging."

Their study analyzed the association of individual and combined dietary patterns and lifestyle factors (alcohol and smoking use, physical activity, etc.) in elderly men and women from 11 European countries in the Healthy Aging: A Longitudinal Study in Europe (HALE) population. The study supports the hypothesis that participants who follow a Mediterranean-type diet and maintain a healthful lifestyle are less likely to die from all-cause and cause-specific mortality, even at ages 70 to 90. They concluded that "a Mediterranean diet, rich in plant foods in combination with non-smoking, moderate alcohol consumption, and at least 30 minutes

---

1 Knoops, Kim T. B., M.Sc, et al. "Mediterranean Diet, Lifestyle Factors, and 10-Year Mortality in Elderly European Men and Women: The HALE Project," JAMA. 292(12): 1433-1439, 2004.

of physical exercise per day, is associated with a significantly lower mortality, even in old age."

Some studies have revealed that cognitive deterioration in the elderly is associated with deficiencies of micronutrients and macronutrients. Some vascular risk factors and cardiovascular diseases have been implicated in vascular dementia and Alzheimer's disease.[1] The inverse association between cognitive decline and the ratio of omega-3 and omega-6 fatty acids in erythrocyte membranes dovetails with results obtained in some studies that assessed fatty acid intake in the participants. Omega-3s are found in fish oils, while omega-6s are in vegetable oils.

In 1995, erythrocyte (red blood cell) membrane fatty acid composition was measured in 246 men and women, ranging in age from 63 to 74 (in the Etude du Vieillissement Arterial (EVA) cohort (group). During a 4-year follow-up, cognitive abilities were assessed with the Mini-Mental State Examination.

It was found that both stearic acid (saturated) and total omega-6 polyunsaturated fatty acids were associated with a greater risk of cognitive decline. Conversely, a higher proportion of total omega-3 fatty acids was associated with a lower risk of cognitive decline.

The inverse association between cognitive decline and the ratio of omega-3 fatty acids to omega-6 fatty acids in red blood cell membranes agrees with results obtained in some studies that assessed fatty acid intake in the volunteers.

Note that Americans tend to consume more omega-6s than they do omega-3s. "While we need both fatty acids, we need to keep a balance between them. Too many omega-6s and not enough omega-3s can result in the body's eicosanoids getting out of balance... Fatty acids strongly influence membrane fluidity," the researchers continued. The central nervous system (brain and spinal cord) has the second highest concentration of fats after adipose tissue, and these brain lipids contain high amounts of long-chain polyunsaturated fatty acids (PUFAs), especially arachidonic acid and docosahexaenoic acid (DHA).

These 2 PUFAs, which are the main constituents of neural cell membrane phospholipids, belong to the omega-6 and omega-3 PUFA families, and they can only be obtained from the diet.

"Intakes of linoleic acid and alpha-linolenic acid, both of which are especially important during periods of brain growth and devel-

---

1 Heude, Barbara, et al. "Cognitive Decline and Fatty Acid Composition of Erythrocyte Membranes — the EVA Study," *American Journal of Clinical Nutrition* 77: 803-808, 2003.

opment, have received considerable attention," the research team continued. "Lack of sufficient quantities of these fatty acids is a limiting factor in brain development."

They went on to add that one cross-sectional study reported data on fatty acid analysis of blood plasma in patients with Alzheimer's disease, other types of dementia, and cognitive impairment compared with controls. Low concentrations of omega-3 fatty acids appear to be risk factors for cognitive impairment and dementia.

The study provides new epidemiological arguments for the potential influence of PUFA intake on cognitive deterioration, and possibly on the early development of Alzheimer's disease.

Although data is lacking on aged animals, supplementation with long-chain omega-3 PUFAs was shown to improve environmental adaptation ability in young mice.

Metabolism of arachidonic acid, the most abundant omega-6 PUFA in red blood cells, gives rise to inflammatory mediators, whereas omega-3 PUFAs, found in fish, act as arachidonic acid antagonists, the researchers said. Thus, omega-3 PUFAs have anti-inflammatory properties and may decrease the production of pro-inflammatory cytokines in humans. Cytokines are hormone-like proteins which regulate immune responses, and are involved in cell-to-cell communication.

"In fact," they continued, "neuroinflammation seems to be a central feature of Alzheimer's disease and many compounds, such as various cytokines and prostaglandins, have been identified in brain tissue from AD patients. These compounds are known to promote and sustain inflammatory responses. Some epidemiologic studies have suggested that nonsteroidal anti-inflammatory drugs (NSAIDs) might reduce the risk of AD."

At the National Institute of Public Health and Environment in Bilthoven, The Netherlands, a research team evaluated 939 men, ranging in age from 69 to 89, who participated in the Zutphen Elderly Study.[1] The men were evaluated for cognitive impairment and cognitive decline for 3 years, and a high linoleic acid intake was associated with cognitive impairment after adjusting for variables. However, high intake of omega-3 fatty acids was not associated with cognitive impairment, Linoleic acid is available in safflower oil, soybean oil, sunflower oil, corn oil, and margarine.

---

1 Kalmijn, S., et al. "Polyunsaturated Fatty Acids, Antioxidants, and Cognitive Function in Very Old Men," American Journal of Epidemiology 145(1): 33-41, 1997.

On the other hand, high fish consumption tended to be inversely associated with cognitive impairment and cognitive decline, the researchers added.

Essential fatty acids are important in membrane fluidity, membrane-associated activities, functional proteins, and in the production of signaling molecules from oxygenated linoleic and alpha-linolenic acid derivatives, according to an article in Lipids.[1]

Changes in dietary polyunsaturated fatty acid intake can influence neuronal membranes and neurotransmission. There may be a link between Alzheimer's disease and an essential fatty acid deficiency, as well as an aluminum build-up, and one researcher has described how this may be prevented by dietary manipulation.[2] Senile plaques and associated neurofibrillary tangles are probably the cause of AD, and the principal component of senile plaques is the beta-amyloid of protein. In Alzheimer's disease, there is significant modification in the essential fatty acid composition, and there appears to be a reduction in essential fatty acids, along with a corresponding increase in saturated fatty acids (meat, milk, eggs, butter, etc.) This results in increased permeability of cellular membranes and a reduction in membrane fluidity. Consequently, the cellular membranes of Alzheimer's diseased brains might be penetrated by the enzyme that could cut the beta-amyloid precursor protein (beta-APP). This could release a large fragment of this protein into the extracellular space with the beta-amyloid section intact.

The same researcher says that essential fatty acid deficiency also reduces prostaglandins, and they may be involved in the pathogenesis of AD. Essential fatty acids, such as linoleic acid, cannot be made by the body and must be supplied by the diet.

The Western diet contains large amounts of saturated fatty acids, plus partially hydrogenated vegetable oils containing trans-fats. Some experts suggest that the relative essential fatty acid deficiency in the Western diet is the cause of many common Western diseases. The deficiency of essential fatty acids is derived from the relationship between essential fatty acids in the diet, and certain non-essential fatty acids. An example are long-chain saturated fatty acids and trans isomers of fatty acids.

Aside from the relative deficiency of essential fatty acids in the Western diet, the consumption of aluminum may be another contributing factor in AD. Aluminum has been found in the neurons,

---

1 Fernstrom, J. D. "Effects of Dietary Polyunsaturated Fatty Acids on Neuronal Function," Lipids 34: 161-169, February 1999.
2 Newman, P. E. "Could Diet Be One of the Causal Factors of Alzheimer's Disease?" Medical Hypothesis 39: 123-126, 1992.

glial cells, dense cores of senile plaques, diffuse plaques, and neu-rofibrillary tangles of AD brains.

Another study of AD patients compared 7 patients admitted to hospital with Alzheimer's disease, to 6 functionally ill non-AD controls. There was a greater concentration of the metal in the blood and serum of the AD group that was showing up 3 weeks after admission. Desferrioxamine has been prescribed to AD patients showing a 3-fold increase in the urine and aluminum excretion, as well as slowing of the deterioration in general function when compared to controls.

There are probably other causes of Alzheimer's disease, such as viruses, neurotoxic metals, trace elements, neurotoxins of biological origin, immune deficiency, illness, and the natural aging process. But, while these conditions are beyond an individual's control, the researcher underscores the fact that prevention of fatty acid deficiency and the accumulation of aluminum, can be modified through dietary intakes. He recommends that these modifications should begin as early in life as possible, and that the individual maintain a healthy ratio of essential fatty acids to trans-fatty acids.

Homocysteine is a usually benign amino acid that is normally processed by the body, but it can build up to toxic levels in the bloodstream and cause serious health problems. Over 20 case-control and cross-sectional studies which involved over 15,000 patients, support the role of elevated homocysteine levels in vascular disease, according to Archives of Neurology.[1] The publication said that one meta-analysis estimated that 10% of the risk of coronary artery disease in the general population is due to elevated homocysteine.

In another study, elevated blood levels of the substance were associated with Alzheimer's disease. It was found that the upper third of the serum homocysteine distribution had at least a 2-fold increased risk of developing Alzheimer's. There was also an inverse relationship between blood levels of folic acid, the B vitamin, and vitamin B12 and the risk of AD.

High levels of homocysteine may be a second biochemical factor, the other being ApoE-4 levels, which increases the risk of both vascular disease and Alzheimer's. However, the authors of that study did not find an association between AD and the C677-T mutation in methylenterahydrofolate reductase, which is a com-

---

1   Diaz-Arrestia, Ramon, M.D., Ph.D. "Homocysteinemia: A New Risk Factor for Alzheimer Disease?" Archives of Neurology 55: 1407-1408, 1998.

mon mutation that is known to result in elevations of homocysteine and produce hardening of the arteries, especially in those with marginal folic acid intake.

Homocysteine has attracted attention because it is a potentially easily reversible risk factor, according to Ramon Diaz-Arrastia, M.D., Ph.D., of the University of Texas-Southwestern Medical Center in Dallas. He says that polyvitamin therapy with folic acid, vitamin B6, and vitamin B12 is effective in lowering homocysteine levels in most people. Therefore, neurologists may want to add measurements of homocysteine levels to their battery of tests that are routinely done in usually futile searches for reversible factors that predispose to dementia.

Docosahexaenoic acid (DHA) is the major fatty acid of neurological and retinal membranes, and it makes up over 30% of the structural lipid/fat of the neuron, and it is especially concentrated in synaptosomal membranes. Neurons are functional units of the nervous system, consisting of nerve cells and other structures. Symptoms are membrane-bound sacs that break away when brain tissue is homogenized (blended) under controlled conditions.[1]

Elevating circulating levels of DHA through dietary intervention has resulted in improvement in a variety of conditions, including dyslexia, Alzheimer's disease, and adrenoleukodystrophy (ALD), which is a neurological disturbance, often affecting young men, due to myelin degeneration in the white matter of the brain.

In evaluating 1,188 elderly volunteers — with a mean age of 75 — a 2-fold higher frequency of Alzheimer's disease was found in those from the lower half of the DHA distribution. Those with at least one ApoE-4 gene had a 4-fold greater risk of Alzheimer's disease and, in women, a 4-fold greater risk of low scores on the Mini-Mental State Exam in the subsequent 10 years if they were also in the lower half of the DHA distribution.

Docosahexaenoic acid, which belongs to the omega-3 family of fatty acids, is a large polyunsaturated fatty acid that is concentrated in cold-water ocean fish and their oils. Together with eicosapentaenoic acid (EPA), DHA is said to reduce blood fats associated with cholesterol and blood clot formation.

Low levels of circulating phosphatidylcholine-DHA may be a significant risk factor for low scores on the Mini-Mental State Exam, and in the development of Alzheimer's disease in the elderly, reported D. J. Kyle and colleagues.

---

1 Kyle, B. J., et al. "Low Serum Docosahexaenoic Acid Is a Significant Risk Factor for Alzheimer's Dementia," Lipids 34: S245, 1999.

Phosphatidylcholine (PC) or lecithin is one of the most popular dietary supplements that is said to enhance memory, protect against heart disease, increase energy levels, and other uses. However, lecithin sold over-the-counter is not pure PC but a mixture of phospholipids, Lecithin is available in red meat, eggs, liver, soybeans, peanut butter, apples and other foods, and it is sold over-the-counter as lecithin granules. Two tablespoons of granule lecithin daily supplies 1,725 to 3,450 mg of phosphatidylcholine and 250 to 500 mg of choline, a vitamin B cousin.

The richest sources of DHA are salmon, mackerel, and herring. Cod and flounder have lesser amounts.

Poor nutrition and stunted growth during childhood may increase the risk of Alzheimer's disease and other cognitive impairments, according to tests conducted on 3,733 elderly Japanese-Americans.[1]

As reported in Pediatrics, the study group involved Japanese-American men who had emigrated to Hawaii as adults, after experiencing malnutrition during childhood in Japan. Researchers reported that decreasing height was linked to an increase in poor mental performance.

In addition, Alzheimer's was more prevalent in the shortest group of men, 4.7% of whom had the disease, compared to an Alzheimer's affliction rate of 2.9% in the tallest group of men. A deficit in height due to childhood malnutrition may indicate deficits in brain development, the authors reported.

When a dietitian at a Toledo, Ohio nursing home noticed that the Alzheimer's patients were losing an unhealthy amount of weight, she reduced the number of foods in their diets that required the use of utensils — meats that needed cutting — and added things like meatloaf sandwiches, which were easy to handle, reported Prevention's Healing with Vitamins.[2]

When a food and nutrition professor at Bowling Green State University in Ohio reviewed the patients' records, it was found that the dietary changes helped the patients to maintain their weight. The new foods also decreased frustration, increased morale, and, as a result, increased consumption of food, one of the best sources of important vitamins and minerals.

Diet contributes to the development of Alzheimer's disease through modulation of oxidative stress and inflammation. Inflam-

---

1 "Alzheimer's Disease and Poor Nutrition," Pediatrics 28(36): 7, September 18, 1998.
2 Feinstein, Alice, editor. Prevention's Healing with Vitamins. Emmaus, PA: Rodale Press, Inc., 1996, p. 85.

mation can originate from oxidative stress as well as from the se-
ries 2 prostaglandins.[1]

Total dietary fat is a high risk factor for AD, while high monounsaturated fatty acids found in the Mediterranean diet have been
shown to reduce cognitive decline. Fish reduces the risk of developing Alzheimer's disease, and linolenic acid, an omega-3 fatty acid also found in nuts, seeds (flaxseed) have been inversely related to AD.

Concerning Alzheimer's, the diet later in life appears to be more
important than a diet earlier in life. For example, the diet 4 years
prior to the onset of AD showed the best results. Also, a diet rich in
cereals and grains is strongly inversely related to AD. Further, the
genetic predisposition to AD through apoprotein E (ApoE) and
diet are both important in the etiology of the disease.

Vitamin E supplements have been shown to reduce the risk of
Alzheimer's, since it protects lipids/fats against nitric oxide-initi-
ated peroxidative damage. An excess of nitric oxide, which is a free
radical, is toxic to brain cells. A colorless, free-radical gas, NO is
thought to affect immune reactions and memory.

Lipid peroxides are fats and cholesterol that are susceptible to
free-radical damage, and when damaged they form toxic derivatives called lipid peroxides. Antioxidants can block the formation
of these toxic compounds. Lipid peroxidation is an interaction between fats and oxygen, which can lead to the destruction of cells.

As mentioned earlier, elevated levels of homocysteine — which
can be inactivated with B6, B12, and folic acid — have been associated with Alzheimer's disease, and high levels of LDL-cholesterol
(the bad kind) have been found in the blood of AD patients, Grant
said.

In 278 nondemented elderly people, 65 to 84 years of age, an
inverse relationship was found between monounsaturated fatty
acid energy intake and cognitive decline.[2] The research team found
a significant inverse association between monounsaturated fatty
acid intake, and Digit Cancellation Test scores.

In an elderly population in Southern Italy, with a typical Mediterranean diet and a high intake of monounsaturated fatty acids, this appeared to protect against age-related cognitive decline.
The Mediterranean diet consists chiefly of fresh fruits, vegetables,
grains, and olive oil.

---

1   Grant, W. B. "Dietary Links to Alzheimer's Disease," Journal of Alzheimer's Disease 1: 197-
    201, 1999.
2   Soifrizzi, V., et al. "High Monounsaturated Fatty Acid Intake Protects Against Age-Related
    Cognitive Decline," Neurology 52(1): 1563-1569, May 1999.

DHA, one of the fatty acids in fish, is an important structural component of gray matter in brain cells, explained Ken Babal, C.N., in Seafood Sense. Consequently, the more fish you eat, the more DHA ends up in your brain.[1] "Autopsies of patients with advanced Alzheimer's disease have shown that their brains had about 30% less DHA in various areas, compared with the brains of those of the same age without the disease." Babal discussed a study which analyzed the fish-eating patterns of over 800 men and women, ranging in age from 54 to 94, living in nursing homes, then checked for the occurrence of Alzheimer's disease 4 years later. While 131 patients had developed Alzheimer's, the frequent fish-eaters — those who ate at least 1 fish meal weekly — had a 60% lower risk rate than those who never — or hardly ever — ate fish. The study's authors reported that, among the omega-3 fatty acids in fish, DHA was the strongest protector against Alzheimer's disease, while EPA seemingly had no influence, and alpha-linolenic acid only served those of a specific genotype.

Fish consumption has been shown to reduce the risk of developing Alzheimer's disease by possibly reducing the inflammation to the cerebrovascular system, according to W. B. Grant. Also, frequent consumption of nonsteroidal anti-inflammatory drugs (NSAIDs) can reduce the risk of AD.[2]

However, it is noted that fish can bioaccumulate toxins, which include heavy metals and pesticides. Since world fish stocks are being rapidly depleted, it is important to know the sources of your fish, and possibly finding other sources of omega-3 fatty acids.

A research team in Paris, France, examined 2 types of weight loss that is seen in Alzheimer's disease. The first is a severe weight loss that is correlated with a reduction in daily caloric intake and with an increased difficulty in performing the activities of daily living.[3] The second type of weight loss, which is slow and progressive, although clinically significant, is not associated with either a decrease in caloric intake or an inflammatory condition. The researchers added that vitamin deficiencies in Alzheimer's including vitamin B6, vitamin B12, and folic acid; elevated homocysteine levels; antioxidant deficiencies — especially vitamin E — along with

---

1 Babal, Ken, C. N. Seafood Sense. Laguna Beach, CA: Basic Health Publications, Inc., 2005, p. 47.

2 Grant, W. B. "Fish Consumption, Cancer, and Alzheimer's Disease," American Journal of Clinical Nutrition 71: 599-603, 2000.

3 Gayonnet, S., et al. "Alzheimer's Disease and Nutrition. Review of Neurology (Paris) 155(5): 343-349, 1999.

iron and zinc; may influence memory capacity and have an effect on cognitive impairment.

Top Antioxidants in Foods

Eating plenty of spinach and blueberries, produce that is high in "ORAC," may help to slow the processes associated with aging in both body and brain. ORAC is an antioxidant assay (oxygen radical absorbance capacity). Two human studies reported that eating high-ORAC fruits and vegetables or simply doubling intake of fruits and vegetables naturally high in antioxidants, raise the antioxidant power of the blood between 13 and 25%.

Foods High in ORAC[1]	ORAC Units per 100 Grams or 1 Serving
Fruits	
Prunes	5,770
Raisins	2,830
Blueberries	2,400
Blackberries	2,036
Strawberries	1,540
Raspberries	1,220
Plums	949
Oranges	750
Red grapes	739
Cherries	670
Vegetables	
Kale	1,770
Spinach	1,260
Brussels sprouts	980
Alfalfa sprouts	930
Broccoli florets	880
Beets	840
Red bell peppers	710
Onions	450
Corn	400
Eggplant	390

Nutritionists continually urge us to eat more salmon, since it is a rich source of omega-3 fatty acid. However, unless you live in Washington, Oregon, Canada, and other pristine locations where wild salmon is plentiful, you are probably being short-changed with the ubiquitous farm-raised salmon. Salmon is also rich in vitamin D, which is deficient in many diets around the world.

Michael F. Holick, M.D., and Tai C. Chen, of the Boston University Medical Center in Massachusetts, reported that their new study revealed that wild-caught salmon had on average 500 to

1,000 IU of vitamin D in 100 grams or a typical serving of 3.5 ounces.[1] By contrast, farmed salmon contained around 100 to 250 IU of vitamin D per serving. "The most likely reason is that vitamin D is plentiful in the food chain, but is not plentiful in the pelleted diet fed to farm-raised salmon," they added. Dr. Holick and his associate added that a vitamin D deficiency is now a worldwide pandemic, which is impacting on people's health. "The major cause of a vitamin D deficiency is the lack of appreciation that sun exposure in moderation is a major source of vitamin D for most humans. However, very few foods naturally contain vitamin D, and foods that are fortified with vitamin D are often inadequate to satisfy either a child's or an adult's vitamin D requirement."

In the absence of adequate sun exposure, at least 800 to 1,000 IU/day of vitamin D3 may be necessary to achieve this in children and adults, they continued. To compound the problem, farmed salmon have significantly higher concentrations of environmental contaminants, such as polychlorinated biphenyls (PCBs) than their wild counterparts, Tracy Hampton, Ph.D, reported in the Journal of the American Medical Association. These data were derived from samples of 700 salmon from around the world.[2] She quoted Terry Troxell, Ph.D., of the FDA's Center for Food Safety and Applied Nutrition as saying that "over 90% of farmed salmon consumed in the United States comes from North and South America, so these fish have maybe 20 parts per billion (ppb) of PCBs, and that's before the skin is removed, which contains a lot of fat, where the contaminants are." Troxell added that scientists analyzed raw, not cooked, fish, and that cooking would reduce the levels of PCBs by about 30%. The source of contamination is probably from the farmed salmon's diet of fish oils and fish meal, obtained primarily from small pelagic (ocean water) fish that can have high contaminant concentrations, Hampton added.

"We are not telling people to stop eating fish — even farmed salmon — but do not eat them so frequently," advised David Carpenter, M.D., of the University of Albany in Rochester, New York, one of the investigators. Carpenter and his colleagues also reported that European-raised salmon contain significantly higher concentrations of chemicals, such as PCBs, dioxins, dieldrin, and other organochlorine contaminants than farmed salmon from North and South America.

1   Holick, Michael F., M.D., and Chen, Tai C. "Vitamin D Deficiency: A Worldwide Problem with Health Consequences," American Journal of Clinical Nutrition 87: 1080S-1088S, 2008.
2   Hampton, Tracy, Ph.D. "Farmed, "Wild Salmon Pollutants Probed," JAMA 291(8): 929-930, 2004.

Levels of PCBs in fish sold in the U.S. have fallen significantly over the years, and most of the fish are not from areas reported in the investigation, which initially appeared in Science magazine in 2004. "Carpenter and his colleagues said that, although PCB contamination levels found in farmed and wild salmon do not exceed FDA guidelines, under EPA guidelines, no more than 1 or 2 meals per month of farmed salmon should be consumed," Hampton continued. "Even so, the EPA guidelines are based on the amount of PCBs thought to be able to cause only 1 additional cancer case in 100,000 people over a 70-year lifetime."

The fly in the gumbo is: How do you know where the salmon you are eating came from?

A vitamin D deficiency is common in older people, and it has a reported prevalence of 30 to 90%, depending on the definition used, according to Marjolein Visser and colleagues at Vrije University in Amsterdam, Netherlands. This frequency in older people is partly due to their lower sunlight exposure, and the reduced capacity of older skin to synthesize vitamin D3 under the influence of UV light.[1]

A poor nutritional intake also contributes to a lower vitamin D status in older people, the researchers added. Thus, the high prevalence of vitamin D deficiency in nursing home patients may be the consequence of their poor physical health and functioning.

"Low levels of vitamin D have been associated with osteoporosis, obesity, diabetes, and cardiovascular disease, and these associations offer an additional explanation for the associations between lower vitamin D concentrations and nursing home admissions, because these diseases increase the risk of functional limitations, disability, and cognitive impairment in old age," the researchers said.

The research team went on to say that it is known that vitamin D supplementation in older people increases 25(OH)D and 1,25-hydroxyvitamin D concentrations, and supplementation could be appropriate in settings of nutritional adequacy and frailty. However, spending more time outdoors will also improve vitamin D status. Regular outdoor walking[2] has already been shown to reduce the risk of mobility decline. In addition, beneficial effects of

---

1 Visser, Marjolein, et al. "Low Serum Concentrations of 25-Hydroxyvitamin D in Older Persons and the Risk of Nursing Home Admission," American Journal of Clinical Nutrition 84: 616-622, 2006.

2 Visser, Marjolein, et al. "Activity Type and Intensity and Risk of Morbidity Limitation: The Mediating Role of Muscle Parameters," Journal of the American Geriatrics Society 53: 762-770, 2005.

physical activity on cognitive functioning and chronic disease in older people have been reported.[1]

The Dutch researchers added that lower blood levels of 25(OH) D concentrations in older men and women are associated with a greater risk of future nursing home admissions, and may also be associated with a greater mortality risk. These results could indicate that lower vitamin D concentrations may specifically affect the level of independence in old age.

The proportion of North Americans with cognitive impairment is increasing as the population ages, therefore, it is important to understand environmental factors, such as nutrition, that may help to prevent or reduce such deficits.[2] Current evidence suggests that poor glucose regulation is associated with poor cognitive performance, and that the consumption of dietary carbohydrates can improve memory in certain situations. Unfortunately, research involving other macronutrients on cognitive function is lacking. "Compared with placebo, a 50-gram glucose drink improves memory-performance 15 to 20 minutes after it is drunk, most consistently in those who have relatively poor memories and glucose regulation," according to researchers.

Actually, blood glucose concentrations between 8 and 10 mmol/l may be optimal for improved memory, and the effects are most robust on tests of declarative memory (conscious recollections of facts and events), which is mediated by the medial temporal lobes and related structures. The researchers added that carbohydrate foods improved memory in the healthy elderly, although the effects were not related to changes in blood glucose.

They also found that barley, which only raised blood glucose to 6.7 mmol/l, improved memory similarly to glucose and potatoes, which raised blood glucose around 9.5 mmol/l. "These results suggest that the ingestion of energy, rather than changes in blood glucose concentration, may be involved in the mechanism mediating enhancements in cognitive performance after carbohydrate intake," they continued. In their glucose studies, however, few conclusions were apparent concerning the effects of protein and fat on cognition. But several studies showed that eating breakfast can improve cognitive performance, when compared to those who did not eat that meal.

---

1 Weuve, J., et al. "Physical Activity, Including Walking, and Cognitive Function in Older Women," JAMA 292: 454-461, 2004.
2 Kaplan, Randall J., M.D., et al. "Dietary Protein, Carbohydrate, and Fat Enhance Memory Performance in the Healthy Elderly," American Journal of Clinical Nutrition 74: 687-693, 2001.

Their study involved 11 men and 11 women ranging in age from 61 to 79, who, after fasting overnight, consumed either a 300 ml drink containing pure protein (whey), carbohydrate (glucose), or fat (safflower oil), or a nonenergy placebo on 4 consecutive mornings. Cognitive tests were then given 15 to 60 minutes after drinking the liquids. "The ingestion of pure protein, carbohydrate, and fat all improved memory performance 15 minutes after ingestion in healthy elderly people," the researchers said. "In contrast with the common hypothesis that blood glucose concentrations must be elevated for memory to be impaired, these data suggest that the ingestion of energy, in the absence of elevations in blood glucose, can improve memory. In addition, such macronutrients may potentially affect cognition by additional unique mechanisms."

While low-calorie sweeteners are a dietary staple for many people trying to maintain or lose weight, an emerging body of evidence shows that these substances offer little help to dieters, and they may even help promote weight gain, reported the Journal of the American Medical Association.[1] "A 2007 review found that laboratory, epidemiological, and clinical studies examining effects of low-calorie sweeteners presented an unclear picture of their usefulness." Some studies have suggested that low-calorie sweeteners may actually increase appetite for sweet foods, promote overeating, and lead to weight gain. Other studies demonstrate that artificial sweeteners blunt the body's energy expenditure mechanisms and activate taste pathways differently from sucrose/sugar. This may prompt dieters to rethink their weight-loss strategies.

The same article noted that another study revealed that sugar is more potent than low-calorie sweeteners in stimulating brain areas related to expectation and satisfaction, thereby turning off the desire for more sweetness. Other studies suggest that certain regions of the brain, such as the anterior insula, may be attractive targets for modulating food-reward sensations.

Excess body weight during midlife is associated with an increased risk of death, according to Kenneth F. Adams, Ph.D., and colleagues. They defined obesity as a body mass index (BMI) — the weight in kilograms divided by the square of the height of the individual in meters — of 30.0 or more. However, they admitted that the relation between overweight — a BMI of 25.0 and 29.9 — and the risk of death has been questioned.[2] The researchers exam-

---

1 Hampton, Tracy, Ph.D. "Sugar Substitutes Linked to Weight Gain," JAMA 299(18): 2137-2138, 2008.Z

2 Adams, Kenneth F., Ph.D., et al. "Overweight, Obesity, and Mortality in a Large Prospective Cohort of Persons 50 to 71 Years Old," New England Journal of Medicine 355: 763-768, 2006.

ined BMI in relation to the risk of death from any cause in 527,265 American men and women in the National Institutes of Health-AARP cohort, who were 50 to 71 years of age, who were enrolled in 1995–1996.

During the follow-up of 10 years through 2005, 61,317 participants (42,173 men and 19,144 women) had died. An initial analysis revealed an increased risk of death for the highest and lowest categories of BMI among both men and women, in all racial, ethnic, and age groups. In an analysis of BMI during middle age, among those who never smoked, the associations became stronger, with the risk of death increasing by 20 to 40% among overweight people, and by 2 to at least 3 times among obese people. The risk of death among underweight persons was attenuated.

"The biomedical foundation for an association between excess body fat and the risk of death is well established," the researchers said. "Medical complications of adiposity include high blood pressure, type 2 diabetes, cardiovascular disease, pulmonary disease, and cancer. Pathophysiologic processes that could plausibly mediate the connection between BMI and the risk of death include insulin resistance, lipid/fat abnormalities, hormonal alterations, and chronic inflammation. Within insulin resistance the body produces some insulin, but the body is unsure of how to respond to it. This is especially true of overweight people."

Regular consumption of tea, especially black or oolong tea, was associated with a lower risk of cognitive impairment and cognitive decline, reported Tze-Pin Ng, of the University of Singapore and colleagues at Alexandra Hospital.[1] The study involved community-dwelling Chinese over 55 years of age. The effects were most evident for black (fermented) and oolong (semi-fermented) teas, but no association was found between coffee intake and cognitive status.

Alzheimer's disease is so prevalent and so disastrous that definitive clinical trials to delay or prevent it must be carried out, reported William E. Connor and Sonja L. Connor of the Oregon Health and Science University in Portland.[2] In the meantime, because evidence exists that omega-3 fatty acids prevent episodes of sudden death, the American Heart Association has recommended that all

1 Ng, Tze-Pin, et al. "Tea Consumption and Cognitive Impairment and Decline in Cider Chinese Adults," American Journal of Clinical Nutrition 88: 224-231, 2008.

2 Connor, William E., and Connor, Sonja L. "The Importance of Fish and Docosahexaenoic Acid in Alzheimer Disease," American Journal of Clinical Nutrition 85: 929-930, 2007.

adults consume 2 fish meals each week.[1] "For people who are aller-gic to fish or who cannot obtain fish, we suggest the consumption of 1 fish-oil capsule (1,000 mg/day)." They added that the possibil-ity that the fatty acids DHA and EPA in fish and fish oil may delay the ravages of Alzheimer's disease is of great interest.

The Mediterranean Diet, supplemented with virgin olive oil or nuts, reduces the potency of cardiovascular risk factors and down-regulates cellular and humoral insufficiency pathways related to hardening of the arteries, according to Mari-Pau Mena of the Hos-pital Clinic in Barcelona, Spain, and colleagues at various facilities in that country.[2] "That these beneficial effects are observed in old-er people at high risk for cardiovascular disease suggests that it is never too late to change dietary habits to improve health status," the researchers said.

The Mediterranean Diet is characterized by an abundant in-take of vegetable products, a moderate consumption of fish and wine, and a low intake of meat, dairy, and industrial bakery prod-ucts. The cardioprotective effect of this diet has been attributed to its ability to improve conventional risk factors, such as adiposity, blood pressure, serum lipids, and insulin resistance, the research team added. Alternative mechanisms, such as an anti-inflamma-tory effect have also been postulated. A higher adherence to the Mediterranean diet is associated with a reduced risk of Alzheim-er's disease. However, this association does not seem to be medi-ated by vascular comorbidity.[3] The researchers said that this could be the result of either other histological mechanisms (oxidative or inflammatory) being implicated or measurement error of the vas-cular variables.

The study involved 194 patients with Alzheimer's disease, and 1,700 non-demented patients at a community-based cohort in New York City. The research team found that adherence to the Mediter-ranean Diet was associated with lower risk of Alzheimer's (odds ratio of 0.76). Compared with those in the lowest Mediterranean Diet tertile, those on the middle diet tertile had an odds ratio of 0.47, while those in the highest tertile had an odds ratio of 0.32.

1   Lichtenstein, A. H., et al. "American Heart Association Nutrition Committee. Diet and Lifestyle Recommendations Revision 2006: A Scientific Statement from the American Heart Association Nutrition Committee," 114: 82-96, 2006.

2   Mena, Mari-Pau, et al. "Inhibition of Circulating Immune Cell Activation: A Molecular Anti-inflammatory Effect of the Mediterranean Diet," American Journal of Clinical Nutrition 39: 248-256, 2009.

3   Scarmeas, N, et al. "Mediterranean Diet, Alzheimer's Disease, and Vascular Mediation," Archives of Neurology 63: 1709-1719, 2006.

And eating fewer calories may lead to better memory, reported Pam Belluck in the New York Times.[1] The study she cites seems to be the first to link calorie-restricted diets with improved memory in humans. Studies in animals have indicated memory improvement, but there is debate about the impact of calorie restriction on humans' cognitive function. The study involved 50 men and women, 50 to 72, who ranged from normal weight to overweight. Participants in one group ate food they normally ate, but were told to cut their calories by 30%, primarily by eating smaller portions. A second group of volunteers kept their calories the same, but were advised to increase the unsaturated (healthy) fat by 20%.

The participants were then tested by memorizing words. The calorie-restricted group averaged 20% improvement in memory performance. The other participants showed no significant change.

Memory improvement might be linked to a decrease in insulin and inflammation in the calorie-restricted participants, who lost 4 to 7 pounds.

Lower insulin levels might increase the sensitivity to receptors in the brain and improve insulin signaling, allowing memories to be maintained longer. Inflammation was thought to promote aggregation to toxic proteins and promote insulin resistance, so that decreased inflammation would help brain function.

In insulin resistance, many people with type 2 diabetes produce enough insulin, but their bodies do not respond to the action of insulin. This may happen if the person is overweight and has too many fat cells, which do not respond well to insulin. As people age, their body cells lose some of the ability to respond to insulin. Insulin resistance is linked to high blood pressure and high levels of fat in the blood. Insulin resistance may happen in those who take insulin injections. They may have to take high doses of insulin daily (200 units or more) to bring their blood sugar down to the normal range. This is also called insulin insensitivity.

The risk of developing Alzheimer's disease is 76% lower in those who drink the juice of pomegranate at least 3 times a week, compared to those who drink it less than once a week, probably because of the high levels of antioxidants called flavonoids in the juice. "These antioxidants neutralize free radicals, damaging molecules that attack cells and contribute to the formation of brain

---

1 Belluck, Pam. "Another Potential Benefit of Cutting Calories: Better Memory," New York Times, January 27, 2009. p. D3. Originally published in the Proceedings of the National Academy of Sciences in January 2009.

plaques...Pomegranate juice has already been shown to help prevent an Alzheimer's-like disease in mice."[1]

As reported in Archives of Neurology, 25(OH)D concentrations in a predominantly white Parkinson's disease cohort demonstrates a significantly higher prevalence of hypovitaminosis (vitamin insufficiency) in Parkinson's disease vs. both healthy controls and patients with Alzheimer's disease.[2] These data support a possible role of vitamin D insufficiency in Parkinson's disease. Additional studies are needed to determine the factors contributing to these differences and elucidate the potential role of vitamin D pathogenesis and clinical course of Parkinson's disease.

A higher adherence to the Mediterranean diet is associated with a trend for reduced risk of developing mild cognitive impairment, and with a reduced risk of this impairment conversion to AD.[3]

The study in a multiethnic community in New York involved 1,393 cognitively normal volunteers, 275 of whom developed mild cognitive impairment during a follow-up of 4.5 years.

Compared with those in the lowest Mediterranean diet adherence tertile, subjects in the middle tertile had 17% less risk of developing mild cognitive impairment, and those in the highest tertile had 28% less risk.

There were 482 people with mild cognitive impairment, of whom 106 developed Alzheimer's disease during follow-up. Compared with those with the lowest Mediterranean diet adherence tertile, those in the middle tertile had 45% less risk of developing AD, and those in the highest tertile had 48% less risk of developing AD.

The Mediterranean diet — high in vegetables, legumes, fruits, nuts, cereals, fish, olive oil and low in saturated fats — has been linked with a lower risk of Alzheimer's disease, reported James M. Ellison, M.D., of Harvard Medical School in Boston, Massachusetts.[4]

Daily administration of the omega-3 fatty acids docosahexaenoic acid and eicosapentaenoic acid (0.6 g.) for 6 months was associated with a significant decrease in expected decline of scores on the familiar Mini-Mental State Examination (MMSE) in a subgroup of people with very mild Alzheimer's disease. Their scores

---

1   Malt, Marianne, editor. Disease Free. Pleasantville, N. Y.: The Reader's Digest Association, Inc., 2009, p. 80.

2   Evatt, M. L., et al. "Prevalence of Vitamin D Insufficiency in Patients with Parkinson Disease and Alzheimer Disease," Archives of Neurology 65(10): 1348-1352, 2008.

3   Scarmeas, N., et al. "Mediterranean Diet and Mild Cognitive Impairment," Archives of Neurology 65(2): 216-225, 2009.

4   Ellison, James M., M.D. "A 60-Year-Old Woman with Mild Memory Impairment." JAMA 300(13): 1566-1574, 2008.

went down only 0.5 points compared with 2.6 point decline for placebo-treated people.

"Folic acid supplementation for 3 years conferred benefits in memory, processing speed, and sensorimotor speed in a Netherlands community cohort, but similar benefits were not found with a folate, B12, and B6 supplement given for 2 years in a cohort studied in the United States, where folate fortification of flour is mandatory," Ellison reported. He added that consistent physical exercise has been advocated for dementia risk reduction and shown to improve cognitive function in older people with subjective memory impairment or mild cognitive impairment.

It is currently difficult to generate predictive models that allow us to think about diet as a "treatment" in the modern sense of the word, explained Gordon W. Duff, M. D., et al., in the American Journal of Clinical Nutrition. Their observations were based on panel discussions at the Living Well to 100 Conference, which was held November 15-16, 2004, at Tufts University in Boston, Massachusetts.[1] There is no precision in dosing, and we possess surprisingly minimal knowledge of the effects of many specific nutrients on human biochemistry, or of potential interactions between bioactive nutrients. "In spite of this knowledge deficit," they added, "we have a model of prevention that enables us to find and treat an existing high risk patient, and also to identify the potentially high-risk patient and preserve health a priority. Such a model might incorporate multiple factors, including genetic make-up, nutrition, inflammation, and lifestyle behaviors. This concept embraces nutritional genomics. Nutrition, along with other behavior changes, and, when necessary, pharmacotherapy, may permit alterations in the health trajectory to foster healthy life." Understanding the roles of nutrition, genetics, and inflammation clearly requires interdisciplinary cooperation.

Developing partnerships among specialties should promote the goal of healthy living. "We need to come together as a science community and generate the evidence base to influence public policy and recommendations," they continued. "Although the challenges are real, we are approaching a time when we should seek to broaden our understanding of the potential value of nutrition and genetics in achieving healthy aging."

In a study at Columbia University Medical Center in New York, Nikolaos Scarmeas, M.D., and colleagues, reported that both a

---

1 Duff, Gordon W., et al. "The Future of Living Well to 100," American Journal of Clinical Nutrition 83(Supp.): 488S-490S, 2006.

higher Mediterranean-type diet and higher physical activity were independently associated with a reduced risk of Alzheimer's disease.[1] There was a gradual decrease of Alzheimer's disease risk with increasing physical activity and diet adherence, the researchers said. Compared with those with low physical activity plus low adherence to diet, high physical activity plus high diet adherence was associated with a 35 to 44% relative risk reduction in AD. "High physical activity in our cohort of 77-year-olds corresponded to about 1.3 hours of vigorous physical activity per week, 2.4 hours of moderate physical activity per week, or 4 hours of light physical activity per week, or a combination thereof," the researchers said. "Nevertheless, even this relatively small amount of physical activity was associated with a reduction in risk for developing AD."

In a study at Hanyang University in Seoul, Korea, the consumption of four to six servings of vegetables daily was found to be associated with a 32% reduced risk of stroke. For those who consumed over six servings daily had a 69% reduced risk of stroke, after adjusting for various potential cofactors.[2] The study involved 69 patients with first-event of stroke and 69 age, sex, and BMI-matched controls. "Our observational study suggests that the intake of fat and vegetables, rich sources of the vitamin B complex, calcium, and potassium may protect against stroke," the researchers said.

A research team at the University of Massachusetts at Lowell, in a study involving 21 institutionalized patients with moderate to severe Alzheimer's disease, found that the daily consumption of apple juice may improve behavioral symptoms.[3] The patients were given two 4-oz glasses of apple juice daily for one month. Caregivers reported an improvement in behavioral and psychotic symptoms associated with dementia, especially anxiety, agitation, and delusion. "This pilot study suggests that apple juice may be a useful supplement to augment pharmacological approaches for attenuating the decline in mood that accompanies progression of Alzheimer's, which may also reduce the caregiver burden," the researchers added.

At the National University of Singapore, researchers did a study involving 716 Chinese adults, 55 years of age and older, and

---

1 Scarmeas, Nikolaos, M.D., et al. "Physical Activity, Diet, and Risk of Alzheimer Disease," JAMA 302(6): 627-637, 2009.

2 Park, Y. "Intakes of Vegetables and Related Nutrients Such as Vitamin B Complex, Potassium, and Calcium, Are Correlated with Risk of Stroke in Korea," Nutrition Research and Practice 4(4): 303-310, August 2010.

3 Remington, R., et al. "Apple Juice Improved Behavioral But Not Cognitive Symptoms in Moderate-to-Late Stage Alzheimer's Disease in An Open-Label Pilot Study," American Journal of Alzheimer's Disease and Other Dementias 25(4): 367-371, 2010.

found an inverse relationship between tea consumption and cognitive performance.[1] After adjusting for potential cofounders, total consumption of tea was independently associated with better performance on global cognition, memory, information progressing speed, and other parameters. "We found a protective effect of tea consumption on cognitive function in community-living older Chinese adults," the researchers said. "However, the protective effect of tea consumption on cognitive function was not limited to any kind of tea."

A study at Tufts University, Boston, Massachusetts, which involved 2,834 Framingham Heart Study volunteers, consisted of 49% women between the ages of 32 and 83.[2] The intake of whole grains was found to be inversely associated with both subcutaneous adipose tissue and visceral adipose tissue. The intake of refined grains was positively related to the two just-named conditions.

In a study involving 39,765 men and 157,463 women, who were enrolled in the Professionals Follow-Up Study and the Nurses' Health Study I and II, a research team from the Harvard School of Public Health in Boston reported that substituting brown rice for white rice may reduce the risk of type 2 diabetes.[3] Five or more servings of white rice per week was associated with a 17% increased risk of type 2 diabetes, when compared with less than 1 serving per month. Most of the carbohydrate intake should come from whole grains rather than refined grains to prevent diabetes.

A higher intake of calcium from dairy products, and increased blood levels of vitamin D, are related to greater diet-induced weight loss, according to a research team from Ben-Gurion University of the Negev in Israel.[4] The 2-year study involved 322 volunteers with a mean age of 52 years. The calcium intake resulted in over 4.5 kilograms of weight loss in the preceding 6 months, and a similar reading was reported in the vitamin D takers at 6 months as well.

---

1 M Feng, L., et al. "Cognitive Function and Tea Consumption in Community Dwelling Older Chinese in Singapore," Journal of Nutritional Health and. Aging 14(6): 433-438, 2010.
2 McKeown, N. M., et al. "Whole and Refined-Grain Intakes Are Differently Associated with Abdominal Visceral and Subcutaneous Adiposity in Healthy Adults: The Framingham Heart Study," American Journal of Clinical Nutrition 92(5): 1165-1167, 2010.
3 Sun, Q., et al. "White Rice, Brown Rice, and Risk of Type 2 Diabetes in U.S. Men and Women," Archives of Internal Medicine 170(11): 961-969, 2010.
4 Shahar, D. R., et al. "Dairy Calcium Intake, Serum Vitamin D, and Successful Weight Loss," American Journal of Clinical Nutrition 92(5): 1017-1022, 2010.

8. Don't Forget to Exercise

Regular exercise during midlife may reduce the risk of developing Alzheimer's disease or other dementias later in life, according to a research team in Sweden and Finland.[1] The research involved 2,000 volunteers — ranging in age from 65 to 79 — who had previously been surveyed (at a mean age of 50.6 years) about their leisure-time activity. The original survey was to ascertain cardiovascular risk factors. In all, 1,449 agreed to be studied again (mean age of 71.6 years).

Those who exercised at least twice a week for 20 to 30 minutes during midlife were at least 50% less likely to develop Alzheimer's disease or other dementia when compared with those who were more sedentary, even after adjustments for vascular disorders, smoking, ApoE genotype, and other factors. The association was even stronger among those who had the ApoE gene variant. Those who inherit at least one copy of the ApoE gene variant have an increased risk of developing Alzheimer's.

The researchers concluded that adopting an active lifestyle in youth and midlife can have cognitive benefits later in life, and may have wide implications for preventive health care.

Physical and environmental factors associated with the risk of dementia remain largely undefined; however, equivocal evidence suggests that physical activity may have a relationship with the clinical expression of the disease.[2] In the Honolulu-Asia Aging

---

1 Stephenson, Joan, Ph.D. "Reducing Alzheimer Risk," JAMA 294: 2423, 2005.
2 Abbott, Robert D., Ph.D., et al. "Walking and Dementia in Physically Capable Elderly Men," JAMA 292(12): 1447-1453, 2004.

Study, the distance walked daily was assessed from 1991 to 1993 in 2,257 physically capable men ranging in age from 71 to 93. Follow-up for incident dementia was based on neurological assessment at 2 repeat examinations in 1994-1996 and 1997-1999. During the study, 158 cases of dementia were identified. After adjusting for age, the men who walked the least experienced a 1.8-fold excess risk of dementia when compared to the men who walked 2 miles/day. "Walking in this group of elderly men in Hawaii has also been associated with a lower risk of coronary heart disease, total mortality, and death due to cancer," the researchers added. "Although complex, this study and past evidence suggests that walking and active lifestyles in general are associated with a reduced risk of dementia."

The well-known Nurses' Health Study, headed by Jennifer Weuve, Sc.D., examined physical activity, including walking, and cognitive function in a large group of older women.[1] Participating in the study were 18,766 women, 70 to 81 years of age. Telephone assessments of cognition were evaluated twice about 2 years apart, from 1995 to 2001 and 1997 to 2003, including tests of general cognition, verbal memory, category fluency, and attention. On a global scale combining results of all 6 tests, women in the second through 50 quintiles of energy expenditure scored an average of 0.06, 0.06, 0.09, and 0.10 standard units higher than women in the lowest quintile.

"Compared with women in the lowest physical activity quintile, we found a 20% lower risk of cognitive impairment for those in the highest quintile," the researchers said. "Among women performing the equivalent of walking at an easy pace for at least 1.5 hours/week, mean global scores were 0.06 to 0.07 units higher when compared with those walking less than 40 minutes/week." The research team observed less cognitive decline among women who were more active, especially those in the 2 highest quintiles of energy expenditure.

In the famous Framingham Study, they continued, performance on tests of verbal memory predicted Alzheimer's disease up to 22 years later, and there was a 60% increase in the risk for each standard deviation difference in baseline (beginning of the study) performance. "Over 6 years of follow-up in the Kungsholmen Project, mean Mini-Mental State Beam scores were 0.84 points lower at baseline for those who subsequently developed Alzheimer's dis-

---

1 Weuve, Jennifer, Sc.D., et al. "Physical Activity, Including Walking, and Cognitive Function in Older Women," JAMA 292(12): 1454.-1461, 2004.

ease than those who did not, and those with poor performance on delayed verbal recall were 61% more likely to develop AD," the researchers said.

Several mechanisms may explain the relation between physical activity and cognitive function. Physical activity likely sustain the brain's vascular health by lowering blood pressure, improving lipoprotein profiles, and promoting endothelial nitric oxide production, adequate cerebral profusion.

As reported in Age and Ageing, 29 residents of a nursing home, ranging in age from 64 to 91, participated in a twice weekly exercise program or a twice weekly memory or recall session. The average attendance at the sessions was 91%, and 86% in the reminiscent (recall) session.[1] There was significant improvement between the exercise group and the reminiscent group in terms of grip strength, spinal flexion, chair-to-stand time, activities of daily living, and self-rating of depression. The researchers concluded that the elderly, while in a rest home, can improve their functional capacity by regular seated exercises. This 7-month, seated group exercise program improved physical and psychological improvements in frail, elderly patients in a nursing facility, reported Marion E. T. McMurdo and Lucy Rennie of the University of Dundee in Scotland.

Most of the research that has been done on the brain and exercise focuses on the influence of exercise on cerebral blood flow, neurotransmitter availability, and neural deficiency. Exercise's influence on mental health and cognitive ability has been the primary focus of research.[2] Researchers suggest that exercise has a direct impact on the brain, that is, it has a direct impact on cerebral blood flow, neurotransmitter availability, brain structure, and neural efficiency. The changes are related to improved mental health and cognitive function.

Exercisers have large increases in cerebral blood flow, increases in noradrenaline, and, in animal models, an increase in the number of synapses per Purkinje cells, increased central nervous system inhibitory abilities, faster reaction times and longer event-related potential latency, which is a measure of information processing in elderly fit people. (Noradrenaline/norepinephrine is a nerve transmitter. Purkinje cells are any number of nerve cells that are found in the middle layer of the cerebral cortex.)

---

1 McMurdo, Marion E. T., and Rennie, Lucy. "A Controlled Trial of Exercise by Residents of Old People's Homes," Age and Ageing 22: 11-15, 1993.

2 Etnier, Jennifer, and Landers, Daniel M., M.D. "Brain Function and Exercise: Current Perspectives," Sports Medicine 19(2): 81-85, 1995.

A conclusion from a report by the Centers for Disease Control and Prevention, and the American College of Sports Medicine, is that every adult American should participate in at least 30 minutes or more of moderate intensive physical activity on most — if not all — days of the week, reported Russell R. Pate, Ph.D., of the University of South Carolina School of Public Health in Columbia.[1] If those who lead a sedentary lifestyle developed a more active physical program, there would be tremendous health benefits to the public and to the individuals.

This does not have to be a vigorous exercise program, but small changes that increase daily physical activity will help to reduce the risk of chronic disease. For example, exercise training is known to improve coronary heart disease, risk factors such as cholesterol, blood pressure, body composition, glucose tolerance, insulin sensitivity, bone density, immune function, and psychologic function.

Skeletal muscle mass declines an average of 6% per decade after the age of 30. Exercise increases oxygen consumption by about 10-fold, which increases the rate of production of reactive oxygen species.[2] Aging is believed to be influenced by reactive oxygen species generation, and older people may be more susceptible to exercise-induced oxidative damage. In addition, aging is associated with increases in antioxidant enzymes. Researchers are still debating whether or not exercise training further upregulates the expression of these free radical scavenging enzymes.

Older people who participate in regular exercise may have higher requirements for antioxidant vitamins to compensate for a deficit in their intake of antioxidants from foods and supplements. Antioxidant vitamins include vitamin A, beta-carotene (provitamin A), vitamin C, and vitamin E.

Linda Teri, Ph.D. reported on a 12-week treatment period for 30 Alzheimer's disease patients. They were guided by their caregivers through individualized programs of endurance activities, such as walking, strength training, balance, and flexibility exercises.[3] One third completed all assigned exercises and 100% of the volunteers were compliant with the protocol with some exercise recommendations. Teri reported that exercise training in those with Alzheimer's disease is both needed and feasible.

1   Pate, Russell R., Ph.D., et al. "Physical Activity and Public Health: A Recommendation from the Centers for Disease Control and Prevention and the American College of Sports Medicine," JAMA 273(5): 402-407, 1995.

2   Fielding, R. A., and Meydani M. "Exercise, Free Radical Generation, and Aging," Aging, Clinical and Experimental Research 9: 12-18, 1997.

3   Teri, Linda, Ph.D., et al. "Exercise and Activity Level in Alzheimer's Disease: A Potential Treatment Focus," Journal of Rehabilitation, Res. Dev. 35(4): 411-419, October 1998.

Another study also showed that high levels of physical activity reduce the risk of cognitive impairment, Alzheimer's disease, and dementia of any type. As reported in Archives of Neurology, a research team evaluated 9,008 men and women 65 years of age or older, of which 4,615 completed a 5-year follow-up study. Of these, 3,894 were without cognitive impairment, 436 were diagnosed with cognitive impairment-no dementia, and 285 were said to have dementia.[1] Compared with those who did not exercise, physical activity was associated with a lower risk of cognitive impairment, that is, Alzheimer's disease and dementia of any type. There was a trend toward increased protection with greater physical activity.

Tai Chi Chuan exercise is said to have multiple cardiopulmonary, musculoskeletal, and postural benefits.[2] Tai Chi was devised over 300 years ago in the late Ming and early Qing dynasties in China. Tai Chi is translated as "supreme ultimate," and Chuan means "fist." It was originally conceived as shadow boxing, and it was subsequently transformed into a martial art in an effort to ward off foreign invaders or to suppress peasant insurrections. The unique characteristic of Tai Chi requires subduing the aggressive advances of an enemy through a soft flow of movement designed to dissipate force through or past one's own body. The technique is an important feature of the traditional Chinese approach to health, and it is associated with enhancing a sense of well-being and health. There are 108 forms of Tai Chi, many of which can be taught to an older person.

A research team at the Centers for Disease Control and Prevention in Atlanta, Georgia, evaluated sedentary adults — 60 women and 66 men — with a mean age of 50.6. They were assigned either to a control group, a moderate intensity walking group, low intensity walking group, low intensity walking plus relaxation group, or a Tai Chi program.[3] The women in the Tai Chi group experienced reductions in mood measurements and improvement in general mood. Women in the walking group reported greater satisfaction with physical attributes, and men in the walking group said they had an increased positive effect. No other differences were reported.

1   Laurin, D., et al. "Physical Activity and Risk of Cognitive Impairment and Dementia in Elderly Persons," Archives of Neurology 58: 498-504, March 2001.

2   Wolf, Steven L., Ph.D., et al. "Exploring the Basis for Tai Chi Chuan in a Therapeutic Exercise Approach," Archives of Physical Medicine and Rehabilitation 78: 886-892, 1997.

3   Brown, David R., Ph.D., et al. "Chronic Psychological Effects of Exercise in Exercise Plus Cognitive Strategies," Medical Science in Sports and Exercise 27(5): 765-775, 1995.

The research team added that there is equivocal support for the hypothesis that exercise plus positive strategy training are more effective than exercise programs lacking a structured cognitive component in promoting positive psychological benefits.[1]

In evaluating 2,216 men and women from 31 original studies that were published in Chinese and English journals, 9 studies showed that Tai Chi Chuan can be classified as moderate exercise, since it does not demand more than 55% of maximal oxygen uptake, reported the British Journal of Sports Medicine. When Tai Chi was compared with other forms of exercise of equal intensity, Tai Chi showed a significantly lower ventilator equivalent. Tai Chi has posture control, and it can help elderly reduce the likelihood of falls.

Exercise seems to improve mood and reduce symptoms of depression and anxiety in both healthy people and psychiatric patients, according to an article in Sports Medicine.[2] There are almost no contraindications for psychiatric patients to participate in exercise programs, except for cardiovascular disease and acute infections.

Heart rate is the best way to monitor exercise intensity, and psychiatric patients should be screened for cardiovascular disease before exercise is prescribed.

In a 12-week trial, 24 healthy men and women who were 65 years of age or older, showed that resistance training increased sub maximal walking endurance by 9 minutes (38%), whereas there was no change in the controls, according to Annals of Internal Medicine.[3]

Resistance training for 3 months improves both leg strength and walking endurance in healthy, community dwelling elderly people, according to Phillip A. Ades, M.D., of the Medical Center Hospital of Vermont in Burlington.

Although the brain shrinks with normal aging, the rate doubles with Alzheimer's disease, says Jeffrey Burns, M.D. Exercise may slow brain shrinkage in those with early Alzheimer's disease, according to a preliminary study by Dr. Burns and colleagues at the Alzheimer and Memory Program at the University of Kansas School of Medicine in Manhattan.[4]

---

1 Li, J. X., et al. "Tai Chi: Physiological Characteristics and Beneficial Effects on Health," British Journal of Sports Medicine 35: 148-156, 2001.

2 Mayer, T., and Broocks, A. "Therapeutic Impact of Exercise on Psychiatric Diseases: Guidelines for Exercise Training and Prescription," Sports Medicine 30(4): 269-279, 2000.

3 Ades, Phillip A., M.D., et al. "Weight Training Improves Walking Endurance in Healthy Elderly Persons," Annals of Internal Medicine 124(6): 568-572, 1996.

4 "Exercising May Slow Alzheimer's," New York Post, July 15, 2008, p. 18.

Regular physical exercise could represent an important and potent protective factor for cognitive decline and dementia in elderly people, according to Rene Verreault, M.D., of the Laval University Geriatric Research Unit in Quebec, Canada.[1] His study involved 9,008 randomly selected men and women, 65 and older, from a community sample. They were initially evaluated in the 1991-1992 Canadian Study of Health and Aging. Compared with no exercise, physical activity was associated with lower risks of cognitive impairment, Alzheimer disease, and dementia of any type.

Many observational studies have shown that physical activity reduces the risk of cognitive decline, but evidence thus far from randomized trials has been lacking. One research team conducted a randomized controlled trial of a 24-week physical activity intervention between 2004 and 2007 in Perth, Western Australia. They recruited volunteers who reported memory problems but did not meet criteria for dementia. In the process, 311 people, aged 50 and older, were screened for eligibility, while 89 were not eligible, 52 refused to participate. A total of 170 were randomized, and 138 completed the 18-month assessment. During the 18 months, participants were observed in changes in the Alzheimer Disease Assessment Scale-Cognitive Subscale scores, with a possible range of 0 to 70.

In the intent-to-treat analysis, those in the intervention group improved 0.26 points (95% confidence interval), while those in the usual care group deteriorated 1.04 points on the ADAS-Cog scores.

The researchers used the Community Healthy Activities Program for Seniors survey to assess physical activity. Physical activity measures included minutes per week spent on all exercise-related activities, minutes per week spent on all moderate-plus activities, and calories expended in all moderate-plus activities. Moderate-plus activities included moderate, hard, and very hard intensity activities (brisk walking, ballroom dancing, gym workouts, or swimming). Each person wore a pedometer to measure the total number of steps walked in a day.

Since 10,000 steps per day are associated with improved health outcomes, volunteers with a weekly step count greater than or equal to 70,000 were classified as active, and the others, non-active. "The results of this randomized trial indicate that a physical activity program of an additional 142 minutes of exercise per week on average moderately improved cognition relative to controls in

---

1 Verreault, Rene, et al. "Physical Activity and Risk of Cognitive Impairment and Dementia in Elderly Persons," *Archives of Neurology* 58: 498-504, 2001.

older adults with subjective and objective memory impairment," the researchers concluded.

Some Ways to Burn 100 Calories[1]
- Climbing stairs for 15 minutes
- Shoveling snow for 15 minutes (if your health permits)
- Running 1½ miles in 15 minutes
- Jumping rope for 15 minutes
- Bicycling 4 miles in 15 minutes
- Swimming laps for 20 minutes
- Performing water aerobics for 30 minutes
- Walking 2 miles in 30 minutes
- Raking leaves for 30 minutes
- Dancing fast for 30 minutes
- Bicycling 5 miles in 30 minutes
- Shooting baskets for 30 minutes
- Walking 1¾ miles in 35 minutes
- Gardening for 30-45 minutes
- Playing volleyball for 45 minutes
- Washing windows or floors for 45-60 minutes
- Washing and waxing a car for 45-60 minutes

Aerobic exercise can produce substantial improvement in mood in patients with major depressive disorders in a short time.[2] In a study at the Free University of Berlin, and the Benjamin Franklin Medical Center in the same city, researchers recruited 12 patients with a major depressive episode. Training consisted of walking on a treadmill following an interval training pattern, which was carried out for 30 minutes a day for 10 days. At the end of the training period, there was a clinically relevant and statistically significant reduction in depression scores, as recorded on the Hamilton Rating Scale for Depression.

Keeping active and remaining fit can help to prolong life, and it can help prevent or delay illnesses or disabilities as you grow older, according to Erin Brender, M.D.[3] "The benefits of physical activity extend throughout life and can improve many health conditions," Brender said.

---

1 Wallenfeldt, Jeff. "Mop That Floor, Tread That Mill. Medical and Health Annual. Chicago, IL: Encyclopaedia Britannica, Inc., 1997, pp. 344-345.
2 Dimeo, F., et al. "Benefits From Aerobic Exercise in Patients with Major Depression: A Pilot Study," British Journal of Sports Medicine 35: 114-117, 2001.
3 Brender, Erin, M.D., et al. "Fitness for Older Adults," JAMA 300(9): 1104, 2008.

In order to keep fit, follow these suggestions:

- Choose activities you enjoy.
- Make being fit part of your everyday life. Playing with children, gardening, walking, dancing, and housecleaning or a few activities that can improve your fitness.
- Combine a range of activities that include aerobic activity, such as, strengthening, flexibility, and balance.
- Start slowly and gradually build up to a total of at least 30 minutes of activity per day most days of the week. Activities can be broken up throughout the day.
- Keep safety in mind. Always wear comfortable, well-fitting shoes, and use appropriate safety gear. Avoid activities in extreme cold or heat. Drink plenty of fluids while engaging in physical activity.
- Aerobic exercises, which are exercises that increase oxygen use to improve heart and lung function, include walking, gardening, and swimming. They help to strengthen your heart, and lower blood pressure and cholesterol. They also improve your mood and sleep.

Strengthening activities include repetitive lifting of light weights or household items like canned foods. This improves your muscle and bone health. Strengthening leg and hip muscles with leg weight exercises can help to prevent falls.

Flexibility and balancing exercises include Tai chi, stretching, and yoga. They can help to prevent injuries and stiff joints.

Brender added that you should be aware of danger signs. Stop the activity and contact your doctor if you experience these symptoms:

- Pain or pressure in your chest, arms, neck, or jaw.
- Feeling lightheaded, nauseated, or weak.
- Becoming short of breath.
- Developing pain in your legs, calves, or back.
- Feeling an uncomfortable sensation of your heart beating too fast.

9. CARNITINE IS AN EXCEPTIONAL SUPPLEMENT

"The research on acetyl-L-carnitine is nothing short of extraordinary," according to Robert Crayhon, M.S.[1] "It prevents the deterioration of the brain during stress, and it helps the aging brain to function better. It also helps to prevent damage that can occur to nerve cells when there is a lack of oxygen in the brain. It is, therefore, no surprise that the nutrient is very helpful for stroke victims, who have been found to recover better on 1,500 mg/day of acetyl-L-carnitine." But what is carnitine?

Chemically, carnitine is a quaternary amine — the same chemical family that includes choline, which is related to the B Complex of vitamins — and it exists as two stereoisomers — structures that are mirror images of each other — called L-carnitine (the active form found in our tissues), and D-carnitine (biologically inactive form), according to Sheldon Saul Hendler, M.D., Ph.D.

L-carnitine is synthesized in the body, chiefly in the liver and kidneys, from 2 essential amino acids — lysine and methionine. Three vitamins — niacin (B3), B6, and vitamin C — as well as the mineral iron are also involved in the synthesis. "It is now established that L-carnitine is essential for the maintenance of good health in humans. L-carnitine is absolutely necessary for the transport of long-chain fatty acids into the mitochondria, which are the metabolic furnaces of the cells."[2]

1   Crayhon, Robert, M.S. The Carnitine Miracle. New York: M. Evans and Co., Inc., 1998, pp. 154ff.
2   Hendler, Sheldon Saul, M.D., Ph.D. The Doctors' Vitamin and Mineral Encyclopedia. New York: Simon & Schuster, 1990, pp. 348ff.

He went on to say that fatty acids are the major sources for pro-duction of energy in the heart and skeletal muscles, structures that are especially vulnerable to L-carnitine deficiency. A number of L-carnitine deficiency states have been identified, several of which are genetic in origin. Symptoms of these deficiencies include mus-cle weakness, severe confusion, and angina or heart pain.

Acetyl-L-carnitine is a special form of carnitine that has the ability to optimize brain function, adds Crayhon. It is able to cross the brain more effectively than regular carnitine, and, therefore, enhances brain-cell function better than regular carnitine. As we age acetyl-L-carnitine levels in our brains decline, and for optimal brain function, supplements of acetyl-L-carnitine become manda-tory. For those over 40, acetyl-L-carnitine is the preferred form of carnitine.

Acetyl-L-carnitine also acts to prevent the deterioration of brain cells that normally happen as we age, he said. It serves as a powerful antioxidant, increases levels of an important messenger molecule called acetylcholine, and it provides the brain with heal-ing energy. When a cell lacks energy, it dies. This is especially cru-cial for brain cells, since, when they die, they are almost impossi-ble to replace.

Acetyl-L-carnitine protects against the loss of receptors on brain cells that normally occurs with aging, Crayhon added. These receptors on brain cells permit the neurons in the brain to connect with each other. Within a nerve cell or neuron, information is sent with an electrical charge. However, when the message travels be-tween nerve cells, it is translated into a chemical — a neurotrans-mitter — that is sent from 1 neuron to another.

Since he wrote about so many nutritional supplements during his long career, you would not expect Robert C. Atkins, M.D., to have a favorite. But he did. It is carnitine, which he took in the greatest quantity every day.[1] "For a substance that is supposed-ly nonessential, carnitine is as necessary a nutrient as you'll ever find," he said. "While it is true that our bodies make this amino acid (protein), rarely do we have enough to keep us at our healthi-est." He added that suppose we had a simple treatment for slowing the downhill progression of Alzheimer's disease or for the speeding up the often lengthy recovery process following a stroke. Happily, we don't have to suppose, we already have it — acetyl-L-carnitine.

---

1   Atkins, Robert C, M.D. Dr. Atkins' Vita-Nutrient Solution, New York: Simon & Schuster, 1998, pp. 191ff.

"Acetyl-L-carnitine (ALC) is sort of a 'supercarnitine,' in many ways similar to the original amino acid, but in other ways it is far different," Atkins continued. "Better absorbed and probably more active than plain carnitine, it can refresh mental energy, improve mood, slow the aging of brain cells, and impede the advance of Alzheimer's. By energizing and balancing the central nervous system, it also strengthens our defenses against infections and immune problems."

For anyone older than 40, acetyl-L-carnitine is the preferred form of carnitine, Atkins said. A generally healthy person who wants to improve mental and physical performance should take about 500 to 1,000 mg/day of both carnitine and acetyl-L-carnitine. Since ALC invigorates the brain, don't take it in the evening, as it may interfere with sleep. Those with epilepsy should use it with caution, since their brains are already overly sensitive to neural stimulation.

In 12 Alzheimer's disease patients who were given a placebo, compared with 207 patients who received acetyl-L-carnitine hydrochloride at 3 g/day for 12 months, there was a trend for early-onset patients taking the supplement to decline more slowly than early-onset patients given a placebo, reported Neurology.[1]

However, early-onset patients tended to decline more rapidly than older patients given a placebo.

Acetyl-L-carnitine is able to reverse hippocampal and prefrontal neuronal loss and lipofuscin accumulation in aging animals, as well as improve learning and memory performance in the animals, according to the Annals of the New York Academy of Sciences. Lipofuscin is brown pigment granules that is considered one of the aging or wear-and-tear pigments. It is found in liver, kidney, heart muscle, adrenal, and ganglion (nerve) cells.[2]

The supplement helps to prevent lipid peroxidation in aged cells and increase levels of reduced glutathione and ubiquinol, which are antioxidants, the authors said. Lipid peroxidation is an interaction between fats and oxygen, which can lead to the destruction of cells. Acetyl-L-carnitine sustains electron transport, enhances oxidative phosphorylation, reverses the impairment of DNA/RNA transcriptase, and restores age-induced impaired turnover of mitochondrial inner membrane proteins. The supplement should be considered a neuroprotective agent, especially in dementia, due to

1 Thal, L. J., et al. "A 1-Year Multicenter Placebo-Controlled Study of Acetyl-L-Carnitine in Patients with Alzheimer's Disease," Neurology 47: 705-711, 1996.

2 Calvani, M., et al. "Action of Acetyl-L-Carnitine in Neurogeneration and Alzheimer's Disease," Annals of the New York Academy of Sciences 663: 483-486, 1992.

its antioxidant action, its ability to stabilize cell membrane function, and its ability to enhance cholinergic transmission. (Cholinergic refers to nerve cells or fibers that use acetylcholine as their
neurotransmitter.)

In a previous edition of the same publication, it was reported
that, in Alzheimer's disease, there appears to be membrane molecular alterations which affect phospholipid turnover, as well as
abnormalities of mitochondrial oxidative metabolism.[1] These biochemical defects, found in the brain tissue of AD patients, are possibly linked. Abnormalities in mitochondrial function, whether
primary or secondary dysfunction, may result in reduction in glu-
cose/sugar utilization and oxidative metabolism detected by positron emission temographic (PET) screening. These mitochondrial dysfunctions are thought to contribute to the accumulation of
the pathologic hallmark of AD, which are paired helical spiral filaments and amyloid plaques.

The authors added that acetyl-L-carnitine is an endogenous
(produced inside the body) substance that acts as an energy car-
rier at the mitochondrial level. The nutrient has pharmacologic
properties that are restorative, and even protect against processes that contribute to aging and neurogeneration.

A research team at the University of Modena in Italy evaluated
481 people from 44 geriatric and neurologic clinics who were treated with acetyl-L-carnitine at 1,500 mg/day for 3 months. The supplement has a structure similar to acetylcholine and may provide
protection against oxidative damage caused by free radicals, they
reported in Drugs, Experimental, and Clinical Research. The supplement brought improvement in mental, memory, emotional behavior, and depression, the research team said.[2]

Carnitine is especially needed for people who are malnourished,
those receiving dialysis or total parenteral nutrition (injection),
and those with liver disease.[3]

In a multicenter trial, giving acetyl-L-carnitine at 2 g/day for 1
year affected the progression of cognitive and functional impairment in Alzheimer's disease. The 2-gram dose was well tolerated,
except for some agitation, such as restlessness and motor over activity. There were 63 patients who received the supplement, and 67

1   Carta, A., and Calvani, M. "Acetyl-L-Carnitine: A Drug Able to Slow the Progress of
    Alzheimer's Disease," Annals of the New York Academy of Sciences 640: 228-232, 1991.

2   Salvioli, G., and Neri, M. "L-Acetylcarnitine Treatment of Mental Decline in Elderly," Drugs,
    Experimental, and Clinical Research 20(4): 169-176, 1994.

3   Bowman, Barbara A. B., Ph.D. "Acetyl-L-Carnitine and Alzheimer's Disease," Nutrition
    Reviews 50(5): 142-144, 1992.

others were given a placebo or look-alike pill. "While intraindividual variability was high, the treatment group showed a consistently reduced rate of progression, which was statistically significant for the Blessed Dementia Scale and for 3 neuropsychological tests."

The researchers added that acetyl-L-carnitine induces acetylcarnitine release in the striatum and hippocampus. The 2-gram dose of acetylcarnitine used in the study contained 1.6 grams of carnitine, which is about 5 to 10 times the average intake of the nutrient in the United States.

In a double-blind, placebo-controlled study at the University of Pittsburgh in Pennsylvania, acetyl-L-carnitine at 3 g/day was given to 7 probable Alzheimer's disease patients, compared to 5 placebo-treated probable Alzheimer's disease patients, and 21 age-matched healthy controls during a 1-year study.[1]

When compared to placebo, the Alzheimer's disease patients consuming carnitine showed significantly less deterioration in their Mini-Mental Status and Alzheimer's Disease Assessment Scale test scores, the researchers reported in Neurobiology of Aging.

A decrease in the phosphomonoesterase levels were seen in both carnitine groups, and the placebo Alzheimer's group, and was normalized in the carnitine group only. Phosphomonosterase is an enzyme that acts on monomers. It was also reported that there was a similar normalization of high-energy phosphate levels seen in the carnitine-treated group, but not in the placebo group. This was said to be the first direct in vivo demonstration of a beneficial effect of a drug on both clinical and central nervous system neurochemical parameters in Alzheimer's disease, according to Jay W. Pettegrew, M.D.

Carnitine acetyltransferase catalyzes (breaks down) the reaction between L-carnitine and acetyl-L-carnitine, and acetylcarnitine has been found to be of benefit in patients with Alzheimer's disease.[2] A research team evaluated 36 patients with AD, and 24 matched controls, upon autopsy in selected brain regions and in isolated cerebral micro vessels for carnitine acetyltransferase activity. They found a 25 to 50% decrease in carnitine acetyltransferase activity in those with AD. The findings provide a rationale for the use of acetyl-L-carnitine in the treatment of patients with Al-

1 Pettegrew, Jay W., M.D., et al. "Clinical and Neurological Effects of Acetyl-L-Carlnitine in Alzheimer's Disease," Neurobiology of Aging 16(l): 1-4, 1995.

2 Kalaria, Rajesh N., Ph.D., and Harik, Sami L., M.D. "Carnitine Acetyltransferase Activity in the Human Brain and Its Microvessels Is Decrease in Alzheimer's Diesease," annals of Neurology 32 (4): 583-586, 1992.

zheimer's disease, since the nutrient plays an important role in the oxidation of long-chain fatty acids by the mitochondria, and it may play a role in acetylcholine synthesis in the brain.

At Instituto Mario Negri in Milan, Italy, there was a placebo-controlled trial for one year, which involved 63 patients with Alzheimer's disease at 7 geriatric and 3 university centers. The men and women were over the age of 40.[1] The volunteers were given 2,500 mg tablets of acetyl-L-carnitine, or a placebo, orally after breakfast and lunch. Eighty-three percent of the patients completed the study. After 1 year of therapy, scores on virtually all of the tests had declined for both groups.

The tests included the Spontaneous Behavior Interview and the Blessed Dementia Scale. The treatment group showed less deterioration on all tests except word association. Mean scores for the treatment group were significantly better than for the controls on the Blessed Dementia Scale, the Raven Matrices, verbal judgment, mental calculation, memory, and concentration, as well as supraspan verbal learning.

The authors conclude that acetyl-L-carnitine therapy resulted in a "deceleration" of the decline in behavioral and cognitive function in patients with AD. It is believed that the supplement acts to enhance cholinergic and oxidative brain metabolism.

Mary Sano, Ph.D., and colleagues, conducted a double-blind, placebo-controlled study with 30 mild to moderately-demented patients with probable Alzheimer's disease. Each was assigned to receive either acetyl-levo-carnitine hydrochloride at 2.5 g/day for 3 months, followed by 3 g/day for 3 months, or a placebo.[2] Following 6 months of treatment, the treated group showed significantly less deterioration in timed cancellation tasks and Digit Span, and a trend towards less deterioration in time-verbal fluency tasks.

A subgroup with the lowest scores at the beginning of the study, who received acetyl-L-carnitine, had significantly less deterioration in verbal memory tests, and a significant increase in cerebrospinal fluid acetyl-L-carnitine levels, compared with the controls. The researchers concluded that acetyl-Levo-carnitine may retard the deterioration of some cognitive areas in patients with Alzheimer's disease.

---

1   Spagnoli, A., et al. "Long-Term Acetyl-L-Carnitine Treatment in Alzheimer's Disease," *Neurology* 41: 1725-1732, November 1991.
2   Sano, Mary, Ph.D., et al. "A Double-Blind Parallel design Pilot Study of Acetyl-Levo-Carnitine in Patients with Alzheimer's Disease," *Archives of Neurology* 49: 1137-1141, November 1992.

How Much Carnitine Should you Take?

Although the body makes its own carnitine, it doesn't make enough to give you optimal heart protection, according to Stephen L. DeFelice, M.D., in The Carnitine Defense.[1] Nor can you get enough from your diet.

Carnitine is available in small amounts in meat, chicken, fish, and dairy products. However, your body can only absorb about 25% of the carnitine that it gets through your diet. Regardless of what you eat and how much carnitine your body is able to make, you still need carnitine supplements, especially under high-stress conditions.

"Clinical studies suggest that you should take 1,500 to 3,000 milligrams of carnitine a day," DeFelice said. "I prefer the higher dose, but it is rather expensive." The liquid form may be preferred, since it enters the bloodstream more quickly, and more may be absorbed by the body, he added. But the liquid form tends to taste bitter. Most people prefer the capsules or tablets. "To make sure you don't forget your carnitine, take it with meals or just after meals," he continued. "Take your dose of carnitine at regular times each day, at least 8 to 12 hours between doses. If you miss a dose, it isn't necessary to double up your dosage."

Aging is characterized by a slow decline of the physiologic functions, with a progressive deterioration of various organs, and, consequently, of the organism until death, according to Mariano Malaguarnera and colleagues at the University of Catania in Italy. This appears to be associated with a substantial loss of the ability to regulate energy balance.[2]

In addition, mitochondria, because of their critical importance for energy production, have attracted the attention of scientists interested in unraveling the complex changes associated with aging and age-related diseases.

"L-carnitine is an endogenous (inside the body) molecule, and it is an important contributor to cellular energy metabolism, the Italian research team said. "It is present ubiquitously in the organism, and the main concentrations are found in the most active metabolic tissue, such as the myocardium and skeletal muscle."

They added that L-carnitine is indispensable for the transport of long-chain fatty acids across the inner mitochondrial mem-

1 DeFelice, Stephen L., M.D., and Kohl, Helen. The Carnitine Defense. Emmaus, PA: Rodale Press, Inc., 1999, pp. 108-109.
2 Malaguarnera, Mariano, et al. "L-Carnitine Treatment Reduces Severity of Physical and Mental Fatigue and Increases Cognitive Functions in Centenarians: A Randomized and Controlled Clinical Trial," American Journal of Clinical Nutrition 86: 1738-1744, 2007.

brane to their site of oxidation and the production of energy in the form of adenosine triphosphate (ATP), a phosphorylated nucleotide that supplies energy for many biochemical processes. "In our previous study, treatment with levocarnitine in elderly patients showed a progressive increase in total muscle mass and a significant reduction in muscle fatigue compared with placebo," the researchers added. "In the elderly, variations are found in the plasma concentration of L-carnitine, even if its causes are not known. In fact, the concentration of carnitine actually increases until about age 70, subsequently tending to diminish the parallel in the reduction in body mass index."

Their current study, which was reported in the American Journal of Clinical Nutrition in 2007, was aimed at evaluating the efficacy of L-carnitine in physical and mental fatigue, and on the cognitive functions of centenarians. The study involved 70 centenarians, ranging in age from 100 to 106, and it involved 24 men and 46 women. They were given L-carnitine for 6 months.

Sixty-six centenarians with onset of fatigue after slight physical activity completed the study, which consisted of a placebo-controlled, randomized, double-blind 2-phase study. The 2 groups were given 2 g/day of levocarnitine or a placebo. Efficacy measures included changes in total fat mass, total muscle mass, serum triglycerol, total cholesterol, HDL-cholesterol, LDL-cholesterol, Mini-Mental State Examination (MMSE), Activities of Daily Living survey, and a 6-minute walking test.

At the conclusion of the study, the researchers found that the levocarnitine-treated people, compared with the placebo group, showed significant improvement in: total fat mass, total muscle mass, plasma concentrations of total carnitine, plasma long-chain acylcarnitine, and plasma short-chain acylcarnitine. "Our study indicates that oral administration of L-carnitine produces a reduction in total fat mass, increases total muscular mass, and facilitates an increased capacity for physical and cognitive activity by reducing fatigue and improving cognitive functions," the researchers concluded.

L-carnitine readily penetrates the brain and exerts a number of metabolic and modulatory effects on the central nervous system tissue, according to Martin M. Zdanowicz, Ph.D., of Massachusetts College of Pharmacy and Health Sciences in Boston.[1]

---

1 Zdanowicz, Martin M., Ph.D. "Acetyl-L-Carnitine's Healing Potential," Nutrition Science News, October 2001, insert, pp. 1-7.

In a longitudinal study of 334 Alzheimer's patients[1], supplementation with the nutrient slowed disease progression in those younger than 61.

In another study involving 24 patients, carnitine supplements at 1 g/day for 1 month effectively treated symptoms of depression in those older than 70, who were hospitalized for the disease.[2]

In a study involving laboratory animals, researchers at the Tokyo Metropolitan Foundation for Research on Aging and Promotion in Japan, reported that treatment with acetyl-L-carnitine at 100 mg/kg of bodyweight, per ounce for three months, brought improved brain function.[3] Enhancements in choline parameters, high-affinity choline uptake, and acetylcholine synthesis were noted. The researchers added that their results indicate that acetyl-L-carnitine increases synaptic neurotransmitters in the brain and, therefore, improves learning capacity in the aging animals.

1 Brooks, J. O., et al. "Acetyl-L-Carnitine Slows Decline in Younger Patients with Alzheimer's Disease: A Reanalysis of a Double-Blind, Placebo-Controlled Study Using a Trilinear Approach," International Psychogeriatrics 10: 193-203, 1998.

2 Terapesta, E., et al. "L-acetylcarnitine in Depressed Elderly Subjects: A Cross-Over Study vs Placebo," Drugs, Experimental, and Clinical Research 20: 417-424, 1987.

3 Kobayashi, S., et al. "Acetyl-L-Carnitine Improves Aged Brain Function," Geriatrics & Gerontology International S599-S606, July 10, 2010.

10. Vitamins and Alzheimer's Disease

Since the brain is one of the most complex organs of the body, it requires a steady supply of vitamins and other nutrients. While all of the vitamins play significant roles, the most beneficial are vitamin C, vitamin D, vitamin E, vitamin A and the B Complex.

Vitamin Combinations

A number of studies have reported that Alzheimer's disease patients have high levels of free radicals, those harmful molecules that damage cells, as well as low levels of the protective antioxidants, which can neutralize the wayward chemicals. In fact, it can be shown that antioxidants can slow the progression of Alzheimer's disease.[1]

In one study, a research team measured levels of antioxidants and free radicals in 20 Alzheimer's patients who were adequately nourished, and 23 people without the disease. It was found that those with Alzheimer's had lower blood levels of vitamin E and vitamin A, and higher levels of malondialdehyde, a marker for free radicals. The study adds to the evidence which indicates a role for free radicals and antioxidants in Alzheimer's disease. It is theorized that abnormal amounts of free radicals drained the body of the essential antioxidants in these patients.

In 2,200 male and female patients, 65 years of age or older, men and Hispanics had lower blood levels of vitamin B12 and vitamin

---

1 Bourdel-Marchasson, I., et al. "Antioxidant Defenses and Oxidative Stress Markers in Erythrocytes and Plasma from Normally Nourished Elderly Alzheimer's Patients," Age and Ageing 30: 235-241, 2001.

C, and folic acid (the B vitamin) concentrations than women and non-Hispanic white men, respectively, according to the Journal of the American College of Nutrition.[1] Those who were taking a multivitamin supplement had higher serum vitamin concentrations than those who did not take a supplement. There were significant associations between blood levels of folic acid and measures of cognitive function.

In a prospective study of 633 volunteers, 65 years of age or older, after an average follow-up of 4.3 years, 91 of the people with vitamin information met the criteria for the clinical diagnosis of Alzheimer's disease, reported Martha Clare Morris, M.D., of Rush Institute on Aging in Chicago, Illinois.[2]

None of the vitamin E-supplemented users had Alzheimer's disease, compared with 3.9 predicted, based on the crude observed incidence among nonusers, and 2.5 predicted based on age, sex, years of education, and health at follow-intervals.

None of the 23 vitamin C users had Alzheimer's disease, compared with 3.3 predicted, based on the crude observed incidence among nonusers, and 3.2 predicted when adjusted for age, sex, education, and follow-up intervals. However, there was no relation between AD and the use of multivitamins.

At St. Mary's Hospital in London, England, a research team evaluated 38 patients, 74 to 90 years of age, for blood levels of vitamin A, vitamin C, and carotenoids. Ten of the patients had Alzheimer's disease, and 10 others were diagnosed with multi-infarct dementia. Twenty were nondemented controls.[3] Both Alzheimer's disease patients and those with multi-infarct dementia had significantly lower levels of vitamin E and beta-carotene (provitamin A) than the controls. Vitamin A levels were significantly lower in only the AD patients.

Since vitamin A, vitamin E, and beta-carotene act as antioxidants, reduced levels could result in increased degeneration of the nervous system, thereby exacerbating the dementia, the researchers added.

The brain is highly susceptible to free radical damage because of low levels of endogenous antioxidants. Low levels of vitamin C have been associated with cognitive impairment, low vitamin E

1 Lindeman, R. D., et al. "Serum Vitamin B12, C and Folate Concentrations in the New Mexico Elder Health Survey: Correlations with Cognitive and Affective Functions," Journal of American College of Nutrition 19(1): 68-76, 2000.

2 Morris, Martha Clare, M.D., et al. "Vitamin E and Vitamin C Supplement Use and Risk of Incident Alzheimer Disease," Alzheimer's Disease Association Disord. 12(3): 121-126, 1998.

3 Zaman, C, et al. "Plasma Concentrations of Vitamins A and E and Carotenoids in Alzheimer's Disease," Age and Ageing 21: 91-94, 1992.

levels are associated with dementia and Down's syndrome, and oxidative processes have been associated with both vascular dementia and Alzheimer's disease.[1] Increasing fruit and vegetable intake may increase antioxidant protection.

Vitamin E

A study in 1997 found that 2,000 IU/day of vitamin E delayed the admission to a nursing home by an average of 230 days over placebo for Alzheimer's disease patients.[2]

A neurologist at the Mayo Clinic in Jacksonville, Florida, recommended giving vitamin E in the early stages of Alzheimer's disease. Patients on warfarin and high-dose vitamin E are at risk for hemorrhage, the researcher added. Estrogen replacement therapy and anti-inflammatory medications may also be protective.

Nutrition Week reports that a group of Alzheimer's disease patients that was given 2,000 IU/day of vitamin E showed a significant delay in the progression to 1 of 4 major milestone symptoms, namely, inability to perform basic daily admission to a nursing home; progression to severe dementia; or death.[3]

A pathogenesis of Alzheimer's disease seems to have an oxidative stress component, according to an article in the American Journal of Clinical Nutrition. Beta-amyloid is found abundantly in AD patients, and this substance is toxic to neuronal cell cultures through a mechanism which involves free radicals.[4]

Vitamin E prevents oxidative damage caused by beta-amyloid in cell cultures, and it delays memory deficits in animal models.

In the Alzheimer's Disease Cooperative Study, 2,000 IU/day of vitamin E slowed functional deterioration leading to nursing home placement.

The amyloid B protein (ABP) is a 40 to 42 chain amino acid peptide which accumulates in Alzheimer's disease plaques, according to Christian Behl and colleagues at the Salk Institute for Biological Studies in San Diego, California.[5] It was found that vitamin E inhibits ABP-induced cell death, and it can prevent some types of cell deaths, which includes those caused by glutamate and cys-

1 Latham, Rosemary, and Orrell, Martin. "Antioxidants and Dementia," The Lancet 349: 1189, April 26, 1997.

2 Zwillich, T. "Vitamin E High on List of Alzheimer's Therapies," Family Practice News, August 15, 1999, p. 27.

3 "Alzheimer's and Vitamin E," Nutrition Week 27(1): 7, May 2, 1997.

4 Grundman, M. "Vitamin E and Alzheimer Disease: The Basis for Additional Clinical Trials," American Journal of Clinical Nutrition 71: 630S-636S, 2000.

5 Behl, Christian, et al. "Vitamin E Protects Nerve Cells from Amyloid B Protein Toxicity," Biochemical and Biophysical Research Communication 186(2): 944-950, July 31, 1992.

teine starvation, 2 amino acids. The data revealed that amyloid B protein associated with AD plaques and the internal B25-35 fragment are toxic to the sympathetic nerve precursor cell line PC12, and that this toxicity can be blocked with vitamin E. The researchers suggest that reduced levels of vitamin E and other antioxidants may occur in malnourished Alzheimer's disease patients, and that there is evidence for a deficiency of the vitamin in Alzheimer's diseased brains.

If glutamate and ABP toxicity, as observed in cultured neuronal cells, play a role in Alzheimer's disease, then the ingestion of antioxidants such as vitamin E may alleviate some of the damage and slow the clinical progression of the disease, the research team reported in Biochemical and Biophysical Research Communication.

The body's major natural defense against free radicals and the damage they can do to the body is the antioxidant vitamins A, C, and E, and the selenium-containing enzyme glutathione peroxidase. Of these, fat-soluble vitamin E is considered the primary defense against cell membrane damage that is linked to a range of degenerative diseases.[1]

In nature, 8 substances have been found to have vitamin E activity, namely, d-alpha, d-beta, d-gamma, and d-delta tocopherol, and d-alpha, d-beta, d-gamma, and d-delta tocotrienol. Of these, d-alpha tocopherol has the highest biopotency, and its activity is the standard against which the others are compared.

In selecting an over-the-counter vitamin E supplement, considerable research recommends that you buy the natural form of the vitamin (d-alpha tocopherol). The synthetic form is dl-alpha tocopherol.[2]

Natural vitamin E is retained by the body twice as efficiently as the synthetic form, according to the American Journal of Clinical Nutrition. The human body seems to select the natural form of the molecule over the synthetic form. In other words, 400 IU of natural vitamin E and. 800 IU of the synthetic form would be roughly equal.

---

1 The Vitamin E Fact Book. LaGrange, IL: Research and Information Service, 1989.
2 Burton, G. W., et al. "Human Plasma and Tissue Aipha-Tocopherol Concentrations in Response to Supplementation with Deuterated Natural and Synthetic Vitamin E," American Journal of Clinical Nutrition 67: 669-684, 1998.

Vitamin C

At the Debrecen Medical School in Hungary, vitamin C and de-hydroascorbic acid levels in the blood and cerebrospinal (CSF) flu-id of 12 patients with senile dementia of moderate-grade Alzheim-er's type were found to be significantly lower than in 15 young, healthy volunteers. (Dehydroascorbic acid is the reversibly oxidat-ed form of ascorbic acid or vitamin C.)[1] An intravenous infusion of 2 g of vitamin C in 5 of the patients showed an active transport process for vitamin C from the blood through the blood-CSF bar-rier. The study confirmed that the free radical scavenging function of vitamin C in the central nervous system, which consists of the brain and spinal cord. Therefore, the monitoring of ascorbate lev-els in the blood of demented patients is recommended because of its protective role in the free radical process that occurs in demen-tia. The beta-amyloid precursor proteins cluster only in the pres-ence of free radicals, and vitamin C may reduce the harmful effects of free radicals in the brain.

Beta-Carotene

In studying 5,182 patients ranging in age from 55 to 95, over a 3-year period, after adjusting for various variables, a low dietary intake of beta-carotene (provitamin A) was associated with im-paired cognitive function, according to researchers at Erasmus University Medical School in Rotterdam, the Netherlands.[2]

Vitamin E

Vitamin E Content of Selected Foods[3]

Food/100 g or 1 serving	IU of Vitamin E
Oils and Fats	
Wheat germ oil	177.07
Safflower oil	97.00
Sunflower oil	72.56
Peanut oil	26.15
Mayonnaise	19.17
Soybean oil	7.92
Butter	3.20

1 Barabas, Judit, et al. "Ascorbic Acid in Cerebrospinal Fluid: A Possible Protection Against Free Radicals in the Brain," Archives of Gerontology and Geriatrics 21: 43-48, 1995.
2 Warsama, Jema J., et al. "Dietary antioxidants and Cognitive Function in a Population-Based Sample of Older Persons: The Rotterdam Study," American Journal of Epidemiology 144: 275-280, 1996.
3 The Vitamin E Fact Book, Vitamin E Research and Information Service, LaGrange, Illinois, 1989, p. 18-19.

Grains	
Wheat germ, stabilized	17.00
Brown rice, boiled	3.00
Oatmeal, rolled, cereal	2.00
Nuts	
Sunflower seeds, raw	73.76
Almonds	37.50
Peanuts, dry roasted	11.47
Peanut butter	9 24
Vegetables	
Asparagus, fresh	2.68
Spinach	10.00

THE B COMPLEX

Independence and self-esteem are strongly determined by physical and mental capacities, and there is growing evidence to support the view that continued physical activity and good nutritional status are important determinates of physical and cognitive function, explain Irwin H. Rosenberg and Joshua W. Miller of Tufts University in Boston, Massachusetts.[1] They added that it is possible that some of the decline in cognitive function associated with aging is preventable or reversible with improved vitamin use.

With regards to neurocognitive function, vitamin B1 (thiamine) deficiency can result in beriberi or Wernicke-Korsakoff psychosis; vitamin B3 (niacin, niacinamide and nicotinic acid) deficiency causes pellagra and dementia; pantothenic acid (a B vitamin) results in a deficiency in myelin degeneration; vitamin B6 (pyridoxine) results in a deficiency in peripheral neuropathy and convulsions; folic acid (a B vitamin) deficiency causes irritability, depression, or paranoia; a vitamin B12 deficiency is found in peripheral neuropathy, subacute combined system degeneration, and dementia.

They reported that volunteers who had lower levels of vitamins, such as folic acid, vitamin B12, vitamin B2 (riboflavin), and vitamin C, all scored poorly on tests of memory and nonverbal abstract thinking. In 28 healthy people over the age of 60, cognitive performance and electroencephalographic indices of neuropsychological function found relationships between vitamins B1 and B2, and iron status and ECG patterns.

---

1 Rosenberg, Irwin H., and Miller, Joshua W. "Nutritional Factors and Physical and Cognitive Functions of Elderly People," *American Journal of Clinical Nutrition* 55: 1237-1243, 1992.

Other researchers have shown low or low-normal vitamin B12 and folic acid levels associated with neuropsychiatric disorders in elderly people, especially depression. In one study, 17% of geriatric inpatients with major depression had elevated homocysteine levels without other evidence of folic acid and/or B12 deficiency. The authors focused on 3 measures of homocysteine levels, since the relationship of this circulating amino acid with folic acid, B6, and B12 as a model for approaching the concept of subclinical vitamin deficiency and neurocognitive function in elderly people. Homocysteine is normally a benign substance, but it can build up to toxic levels and cause considerable damage.

Elderly patients have been found to have the loss of ability to make stomach acid, which occurs in about 30% of those over 65 years of age, primarily as a function of the development of atrophic gastritis, the researchers continued. Low pH values enhance the absorption of B12 and folic acid. Also, elderly people have been found to have a reduced ability to absorb both folic acid and protein-bound B12, compared with healthy young controls.

The effect of B12 deficiency is well known, they added, and it can result in paresthesia (a tingling sensation), ataxis (difficulty with coordination), mood disturbances, delusions, and paranoia. Vitamin B6 is important in the synthesis of several neurotransmitters, including epinephrine, norepinephrine, serotonin, and gamma-amino butyrate.

A folic acid deficiency can result in irritability, forgetfulness, and paranoia, and a deficiency in the vitamin has been observed in patients with psychiatric disorders, including depression, dementia, schizophrenia, and epilepsy. It has been suggested that one can have a normal vitamin concentration in the blood, but still have physiologic impairment due to a vitamin deficiency. Homocysteine is a perfect model, since it can indicate deficiencies without blood levels of the vitamin being normal.

The authors believe that the tools are now available to evaluate the hypothesis that subtle defects in vitamin status may explain some of the neurocognitive impairment associated with the aging process. As reported in Gerontology, 19 men and 30 women, with a mean age of 73.8, were given intramuscular injections of 1 mg of vitamin B12; 1.1 mg of folic acid; and 5 mg of vitamin B6 for 8 times over a 21-day period. The volunteers were evaluated over 269 days.[1] From the beginning of the study to day 21, blood lev-

---

1 Henning, B. F., et al. "Long-Term Effects of Vitamin B12, Folate, and Vitamin B6 Supplements in Elderly People with Normal Serum Vitamin B12 Concentrations," Gerontology 47: 30-35, 2001.

els of the B vitamins increased significantly, but returned to origi-nal levels after the vitamins were withdrawn. Total homocysteine, methylmalonic acid, and 2-methyleitrie acid levels decreased dur-ing the treatment period. Cystathionine levels did not differ signif-icantly from those at the start of the therapy. Evaluating methyl-malonic acid and 2-methylcitric acid in elderly patients with men-tal disturbances may be a cost-effective way to improve or main-tain mental functioning, the researchers said.

Cystathioniuria is the inability to metabolize cystathionine — involved in the conversion of the amino acid methionine to cyste-ine — and high levels in the blood are associated with mental re-tardation. Methylmalonic acid is involved in fatty acid metabolism, and elevated levels are due to a vitamin B12 deficiency.

In evaluating cognition in 70 men, 54 to 81 years of age, lower concentrations of vitamin B12 and folic acid, and higher concen-trations of homocysteine, were associated with poor spatial cop-ing skills, according to researchers at Tufts University in Boston, Massachusetts.[1]

They reported that blood levels of homocysteine were a strong predictor of spatial copying performance than either B12 or folic acid concentrations. Higher amounts of vitamin B6 were related to better performance on 2 measures of memory. Adequate levels of B12, B6, and folic acid are said to inactivate toxic levels of the ami-no acid, according to the American Journal of Clinical Nutrition.

Vitamin B1 (Thiamine)

In their studies at the University of South Florida in Tampa, Michael Gold, M.D., and colleagues, found that patients with Al-zheimer's disease had significantly lower blood levels of vitamin B1 than did patients with other forms of dementia. They also found a disproportionally higher number of patients with Alzheimer's dis-ease that had deficiencies in plasma thiamine.[2]

Gold added that blood levels of the vitamin and red blood cell count levels did not correlate. That is, a number of patients with deficient plasma B1 had normal red blood counts of the vitamin. If substantiated, this finding has serious implications for the treat-ment of Alzheimer's disease, since there may be a large subset of patients with the disease who are deficient in vitamin B1. Since

1 Riggs, Karen M., et al. "Relation of Vitamin B12, Vitamin B6, Folate, and Homocysteine to Cognitive Performance in the Normative Aging Study," American Journal of Clinical Nutrition 63: 306-314, 1996.

2 Gold, Michael, M.D. "Plasma and Red Blood Cell Thiamin Deficiency in Patients with Dementia of the Alzheimer's Type," Archives of Neurology 52: 1081-1085, November 1995.

these patients have not been studied in a clinical setting, it is not known whether these patients have a unique cognitive profile, or have a unique natural history. "However, he has had a few patients who improved with 3 to 5 g/day of the vitamin." There is conflicting data on the nutritional status of Alzheimer's patients, and there may be a degree of malabsorption involved. Gold suggests that the metabolic derangement in the central nervous system may cause a more rapid shuttling of B1 from the blood into the central nervous system so that the vitamin is then rapidly absorbed.

Seven women and 4 men, 59 to 83 years of age, with Alzheimer's disease, participated in a double-blind crossover study evaluating 3 g/day of oral thiamine hydrochloride for 3 months, compared with a niacinamide (B3) placebo at 250 mg 3 times daily.[1] Results showed that the Mini-Mental State Exam was higher during the 3 months with 3 g/day of thiamine than with the B3 placebo. The patients were not B1 deficient in the conventional sense, they were not malnourished, and they were not alcoholics.

At the Clarke Institute of Psychiatry in Toronto, Canada, the activities of 3 thiamine diphosphate metabolizing enzymes were measured in autopsied cerebral cortex of 18 patients with Alzheimer's disease and 20 matched controls, reported Archives of Neurology.[2] The researchers found levels of thiamine diphosphate were significantly reduced by 18 to 215 in all 3 cortical brain areas. The B1 constituents were normal in the Alzheimer's disease group. The B1 substance decrease may be explained by a cerebral or cortical deficiency in Alzheimer's disease of adenosine 5'-triphosphate (ATP), which is needed for thiamine diphosphate synthesis.

A chronic subclinical thiamine diphosphate deficiency could result in impaired brain function in Alzheimer's disease, and there might be modest improvement with vitamin B1 supplementation in cognitive status of some of the AD patients. ATP is a phosphorylated enzyme that supplies energy for many cellular processes in the body.

In comparing patients with Alzheimer's disease, and 15 controls without the disease, for the intake and functional levels of B1, B6, and vitamin C, there were similar levels of the vitamins in both groups, except for vitamin B1, which had lower functional values

1 Blass, J. P., et al. "Thiamine and Alzheimer's Disease: A Pilot Study," Archives of Neurology 45: 833-835, August 1998.

2 Mastrogiacomo, Frank, B.Sc, et al. "Brain Thiamine, Its Phosphate Esters, and Its Metabolizing Enzymes in Alzheimer's Disease," Annals of Neurology 39: 585-591, 1996.

for those with Alzheimer's, according to the Canadian Journal of Psychiatry.[1]

Assessment techniques included blood pyridoxal phosphate, B6 blood levels of vitamin C, and thiamine pyrophosphate activity (B1).

Thiamine is important in the metabolism of acetylcholine and in its release from presynaptic neurons. In giving Alzheimer's patients between 3 and 8 g/day of B1 orally, there may have been a mild beneficial effect on dementia of the Alzheimer's type, reported the Journal of Geriatrics, Psychiatry and Neurology.[2]

Vitamin B3 (Niacin)

It was Richard P. Huemer, M.D., who pointed out that the concept of subclinical deficiency has, for the most part, been rejected by the scientific community. Glen Green, M.D., who published a paper on subclinical pellagra, described mental symptoms in patients with frank deficiency of vitamin B3, but who responded to treatment with niacin supplements.[3] "It was only in 1983 that the medical establishment acknowledged the existence of subclinical deficiency in a report summarized in the Journal of the American Medical Association," Huemer said. "Gingival dysplasia was identified as a symptom of marginal vitamin C depletion, a subclinical deficiency."

Vitamin B12 (Cyanocobalamin)

A vitamin B12 deficiency is present in up to 15% of the elderly population, as documented by high levels of methylmalonic acid with or without elevated total homocysteine concentrations with low or low-normal vitamin B12 concentrations, according to Sally P. Stabler of the University of Colorado Health Sciences Center in Denver, and colleagues there and at the Columbia University College of Physicians and Surgeons in New York. Methylmalonic acid is an intermediate in fatty acid metabolism, and it is found in elevated levels of a B12 deficiency, they reported in the American Journal of Clinical Nutrition.[4] "Clinical signs and symptoms

1 Agbayewa, M. O., et al. "Pyridoxine, Ascorbic Acid and Thiamine in Alzheimer and Comparison Subjects," Canadian Journal of Psychiatry 37(9): 661-662, September 1992.

2 Meador, K., et al, "Preliminary Findings of High-Dose Thiamine in Dementia of Alzheimer's Type," Journal of Geriatrics, Psychiatry and Neurology 6(4): 222-229, October-December 1993.

3 Huemer, Richard P., M.D. The Roots of Molecular Medicine. New York: W. H. Freeman and Co., 1986, p. 206.

4 Stabler, Sally P., et al. "Vitamin B12 Deficiency in the Elderly: Current Dilemmas," American Journal of Clinical Nutrition 66: 741-749, 1997.

of a B12 deficiency are insensitive in elderly people and comorbidity in these people makes response to therapy difficult to interpret," the researchers said.

Many elderly people with high levels of homocysteine have undiagnosed vitamin B12 deficiency with elevated blood levels of methylmalonic acid concentrations, they continued. Therefore, these patients should not be given folic acid supplements — the B vitamin that works with B12 — before their B12 status is determined.

"Oral B12 supplementation may be effective in lowering blood levels of methylmalonic acid values in the elderly, but the dose of B12 in most common multivitamin preparations is too low for this purpose," they added.

Since a B12 deficiency and Alzheimer's disease and other dementias are common in elderly patients, it seems likely that many of them will have combinations of disorders. Since it would take an astute clinician to determine what percentage of cognitive dysfunction in a specific individual could be attributed to only a B12 deficiency, it seems prudent to aggressively diagnose and treat a vitamin B12 deficiency.

To determine whether the increased prevalence of low blood levels of vitamin B12 in elderly people represents a true deficiency, blood concentrations of B12 and folic acid, and metabolites that are sensitive indicators of a B12 deficiency, were measured in 548 surviving members of the original Framingham Study cohort.[1] John Lindenbaum and colleagues found that the prevalence of a B12 deficiency was about 12% in a large sample of free-living elderly Americans. However, many elderly people with "normal" blood vitamin concentrations are metabolically deficient in both B12 and folic acid.

When a research team evaluated 6 patients with Alzheimer's disease, they found that 4 of them had low levels of B12. Many elderly people do have low B12 status.[2]

At West Penn Hospital in Pittsburgh, Pennsylvania, David C. Martin, M.D., and colleagues, evaluated 22 people (18 completed the study) with low blood levels of vitamin B12 and evidence of cognitive dysfunction during an 8-month period.[3] The participants

1 Lindenbaum, John, et al. "Prevalence of Cobalamin Deficiency in the Framingham Elderly Population," American Journal of Clinical Nutrition 60: 2-11, 1994.

2 McCaddon, A., and Kelly, C. "Familial Alzheimer's Disease and Vitamin B12 Deficiency," Age and Ageing 23: 334-337, July 1994.

3 Martin, David C, M.D., et al. "Time Dependency of Cognitive Recovery with Cobalamin Replacement: Report of a Pilot Study," Journal of the American Geriatric Society 40(2): 168-172, 1992.

were given 1,000 mcg of vitamin B12 via muscular injection daily for 1 week, then weekly for 1 month, and finally monthly thereafter for 6 months. The Mattis Dementia Rating Scale was administered before the study began, and at least 8 months afterward. Following 8 months of B12 therapy, 11 of the 18 patients showed cognitive improvement. Patients symptomatic for less than 12 months gained an average of 20 points on the just-mentioned scale, whereas those symptomatic for greater than 10 months lost an average of 3 points. Two patients symptomatic for only 3 months normalized their testing, gaining 31 and 28 points, respectively.

Martin said that early therapy is necessary for full cognitive recovery. Only the patients who are symptomatic for less than 1 year showed improvement with therapy, and the most progressive responders had been symptomatic for less than 6 months. With longer duration of illness, Martin continued, there may be a loss of the ability for neuronal repair at the stage of widespread myelinolysis (dissolution of the myelin sheath of nerve fibers).

He went on to say that an elevated red blood cell volume was poorly correlated with low blood levels of B12, suggesting that an abnormal complete blood count is an inadequate screen for B12 deficiency. He said that a study by Lindenbaum, et al., found that 40 patients with B12 deficiency and without anemia or macrocytosis (large numbers of macrocytes in blood) responded to vitamin therapy. Of these, 13 patients had memory loss; 8 were reported to have complete recovery; and 3 exhibited partial recovery.

The study revealed that B12 therapy may lead to improved cognitive recovery in some patients if therapy is started early after the onset of cognitive symptoms. The window of opportunity of effective intervention may be as short as 1 year, and Martin encourages physicians to screen for B12 deficiency, especially in those patients with mental changes.

In the United States, fortification of cereals with folic acid began on January 1, 1998. Fortification with the vitamin was made mandatory by the FDA at a level of 140 mcg/100 grams of food, which was intended to increase the dietary intake of folic acid in people by 70 to 130 mcg/day, reported Kelly F. Wyckoff and Vijay Ganji of Rash University Medical Center in Chicago, Illinois and Georgia State University in Atlanta.[1]

---

1 Wyckoff, Kelly F., and Ganji, Vijay. "Proportion of Individuals with Low Serum Vitamin B12 Concentrations Without Macrocytosis Is Higher in the Post-Folic Acid Fortification Period Than in the Pre-Folic Acid Fortification Period," *American Journal of Clinical Nutrition* 86: 1187-1192, 2007.

The fortification program was designed to reduce the risk of a woman having a child with neural tube defects, which was reduced by 19% following the fortification of cereals with the vitamin. In this condition, the spinal cord is pushed through the wall of the spinal canal between the vertebrae. The incomplete development of the spinal cord can increase the chances of the child dying.

Folic acid fortification has also lowered circulating homocysteine, which was said to reduce the risk of cardiovascular disease, the researchers said. However, high levels of the vitamin may lead to the correction of hematologic abnormalities associated with a vitamin B12 deficiency. This may delay the patient seeing a doctor, since the patient may be feeling tired or exhausted because of a vitamin B12 deficiency, resulting in irreversible neurologic damage.

The amount of folic acid needed to correct the macrocytosis of vitamin B12 deficiency has not been defined because, knowingly, patients are not given folic acid to treat a vitamin B12 deficiency, the researchers continued. However, the Upper Intake Level for folic acid was set by the Food and Drug Administration at 1,000 mcg/day.

"In the post-folic acid fortification period, those with low blood levels of vitamin B12 are 3 times as likely to be without macrocytosis (large numbers of macrocytes in the blood as seen in pernicious anemia), than are those in the pre-folic acid fortification period," the researchers added.

Commenting on the just-named study in the same issue of the American Journal of Clinical Nutrition, Ingeborg Brouwer and Petra Verhoef of Universiteit in Amsterdam, the Netherlands, and Unilever Food and Health Research Institute in Vlaardingen, the Netherlands, said that it is uncertain as to what extent the masking of a vitamin B12 deficiency by folic acid is a concern.[1] "Doctor's delay appears to be a nonissue if appropriate markers of vitamin B12 are measured, but the patient's delay should be considered," the authors said. "Considering the ongoing discussion of what the best markers and cutoff values for vitamin B12 deficiency are, it is also hard to say how many people would be at risk." They added that other possible negative effects of folic acid fortification should be further investigated. Cofortification with vitamin B12 may solve some, but not all, of the possible adverse effects.

---

1 Brouwer, Ingeborg, and Verhoef, Petra. "Folic Acid Fortification: Is Masking of Vitamin B12 Deficiency. What We Should Really Worry About?" ibid, pp. 897-898.

In 8 male and 10 female patients — 75 and 69 years of age, respectively — those who were healthy but had cognitive impairment suggestive of Alzheimer's disease, were compared with 9 men and 9 women volunteers — 74 and 75 years of age, respectively — who acted as controls.[1] Those with Alzheimer's disease had low blood levels of vitamin B12 and haptocorrin saturated when compared to the controls. The disparate mechanisms seem to inhibit the assimilation of active B12 and the elimination of its inactive analogs, thus contributing to the development of B12 tissue deficiency in Alzheimer's patients, the researchers said.

At the Institute of Psychiatry in Toronto, Canada, a research team evaluated 40 patients with either possible or probable Alzheimer's disease, 31 with dementia, and 26 with mild cognitive impairment to determine the relationship between vitamin B12 and folic acid, according to Acta Psychiatrica Scandinavia.[2]

It was found that only in the AD group that vitamin B12 was significantly correlated with the Mini-Mental State Examination evaluation. Using regression analysis, vitamin B12 contributed significantly to the variance in the exam. There was no correlation between the test and blood or red blood cell folic acid, or B12 in the other dementias, or in the cognitively nondementia group.

However, the research team concluded that there may be a specific relationship between vitamin B12 levels and the severity of cognitive impairment in patients with Alzheimer's disease.

At Clinica Universitaria de Navarra in Pamplona, Spain, researchers studied a 64-year-old man, who was taken to a psychiatry department with progressive impairment of cerebral functions, including dementia, diarrhea, and fecal incontinence for the previous several months.[3]

The patient was vitamin B12 deficient without megaloblastic anemia, and he had an abnormal Schilling test that was not due to intrinsic factor deficiency. Intrinsic factor is a substance produced by gastrointestinal mucosa that helps to absorb vitamin B12. A Schilling blood count test determines the number and arrangement of certain cells. (It was named after Victor Schilling (1883–1960), a German hematologist.) Treatment with the B vitamins and longer-term oral antibiotic therapy resulted in the complete

1 McCaddon, A., M.D., et al. "Analogues, Ageing and Aberrant Assimilation of Vitamin B12 in Alzheimer's Disease," Dement. Geriatr. Cogn. Disord. 12: 133-137, 2001.

2 Levitt, A. J., et al. "Folate, Vitamin B12, and Cognitive Impairment in Patients with Alzheimer's Disease," Acta Psychiatrica Scandinavia 86: 301-305, 1992.

3 Subtil, J. C, et al. "Dementia Due to Bacterial Overgrowth in a Patient with Billroth II Anastomosis," Rev. Esp. Enf. Digest 88(6): 431-433, 1996.

and permanent resolution of the neurologic and digestive symptoms, the researchers added. When evaluating for dementias that are curable, it is necessary to take into account bacterial overgrowth, which is a problem that can produce a variety of disorders.

Alzheimer's type dementia patients are more likely to have lower blood vitamin B12 concentrations than nondemented older counterparts, reported Carol S. Johnston, Ph.D., R.D., and Julia A. Thomas, M.S., R.D., of Arizona State University in Tempe.[1] They added that risk factors for vitamin B12 deficiency in the elderly include lack of intrinsic factor, atrophic gastritis, which reduces gastric acid and pepsin secretion that impairs B12 release from food, therefore, inhibiting absorption, and Helicobacter pylori infection of the stomach. The latter is a bacterium that is associated with several gastroduodenal diseases.

Folic Acid (B9)

A research team at the Sanders-Brown Center on Aging at the University of Kentucky at Lexington, evaluated 30 nuns at a convent, who later died when they were 78 to 101 years of age. A negative correlation was found between blood levels of folic acid and the severity of atrophy of the neocortex, reported the American Journal of Clinical Nutrition.[2]

Atrophy may be specific to low folic acid levels, because none of the other 18 nutrients, lipoproteins, or nutritional markers measured in the blood had significant negative correlations with atrophy. In this group of nuns, low blood levels of folic acid were strongly associated with atrophy of the cerebral cortex, the surface layer of gray matter of the cerebrum that functions mostly in coordination of sensory and motor information, the researchers added. Atrophy is the wasting of tissues, organs or the entire body.

INOSITOL

Inositol (myoinositol) is an essential building block of cell membrane fats, reported Robert A. Ronzio, Ph.D.

Inositol is available in citrus fruits (except lemons), cantaloupe, whole grain bread, cooked beans, green beans, and nuts.

---

1 Johnston, Carol S., Ph.D., R.D., and Thomas, Julia A., M.S., R.D. "Holotranscobalamin II Levels in Plasma Are Related to dementia in Older People," Journal of the American Geriatric Society 45(6): 779-780, June 1997.

2 Snowdon, D. A., et al. "Serum Folate and the Severity of Atrophy of the Neocortex in Alzheimer's Disease: Findings from the Nun Study," American Journal of Clinical Nutrition 71: 993-998, 2000.

It is a constituent of the inositol-containing phospholipid, phosphatidylinositol, a component of inner-cell membranes. Derivatives of inositol function as a hormone relay signal to cells.[1] Diverse hormones such as vasopressin (from the pituitary gland), epinephrine (from the adrenal gland), and releasing factors from the hypothalamus stimulate the release of inositol triphosphate from phosphatidylinositol.

In a double-blind crossover study at Beersheva Mental Health Center in Israel, inositol — not a vitamin but associated with the B Complex — at 6 g/day versus glucose for 1 month involved 11 Alzheimer's patients. It was found that there was an overall improvement in the Cognitive Subscale of the Cambridge Mental Disorder of the Elderly Examination (CAMDEX) with inositol, although it was not significant, according to Yoram Barak. However, language and orientation improved significantly more with the inositol than with the placebo.[2]

There were no serious side effects, and the research team suggests that higher doses of inositol should be studied in Alzheimer's disease patients for longer periods.

Vitamin D

In a 6-year population-based study involving 858 patients 65 years of age and older, a research team at the University of Exeter in England said that the levels of vitamin D were associated with an increased risk of substantial cognitive decline.[3] The cognitive decline was determined using the Mini-Mental State Examination (MMSE) and the Trail-Making Tests A and B. After adjusting for cofounders, patients with severe vitamin D deficiency showed a 60% increased risk of substantial cognitive decline when compared to those with sufficient levels of the vitamin.

In addition, a severe vitamin D deficiency was associated with a 31% increased risk of substantial decline on the Trail-Making Test A, when compared with sufficient levels of the vitamin.

1   Ronzio, Robert A., Ph.D. The Encyclopedia of Nutrition and Good Health. New York: Facts On File, Inc., 1997, p. 247.

2   Barak, Yoram, et al. "Inositol Treatment of Alzheimer's Disease: A Double-Blind, Crossover Placebo Controlled Trial," Prog. Neuro-Psychopharmacol and Biological Psychiatry 20: 729-735, 1996.

3   Llewellyn, D. J., et al. "Vitamin D and Risk of Cognitive Decline in Elderly Persons," Archives of Internal Medicine 170(13): 1135-1141, 2010.

Vitamin E to the Rescue

A research team at Rush Institute for Healthy Aging in Chicago evaluated 2,889 community residents, aged 65 to 102, as to whether or not antioxidant nutrients — including vitamin E, vitamin C, and beta-carotene-are associated with reduced cognitive decline with age.[1] They reported a 36% reduction in the rate of decline among those in the highest quintile of total vitamin E intake, when compared with those in the lowest quintile. They also observed a reduced decline with higher vitamin E intake from foods. "Vitamin E intake from foods or supplements is associated with less cognitive decline with age," the researchers said.

Research also suggests that oxidative stress is important in the pathogenesis of Alzheimer's disease. Beta-amyloid, which is found in abundance in the brains of AD patients, is toxic to neuronal cell cultures, through the development of free radicals. Vitamin E prevents the oxidative damage induced by beta-amyloid in cell culture, and delays memory deficits in animal models.

One clinical trial using vitamin E reported that the vitamin may slow functional deterioration leading to nursing home placement. In this study conducted by the Alzheimer's Disease Cooperative Study, patients with moderately advanced Alzheimer's disease were given 2,000 IU/day of vitamin E.[2]

1 Morris, Martha Clare, M.D., et al. "Vitamin E and Cognitive Decline in Older Persons," Archives of Neurology 59: 1125-1132, 2002.
2 Grundman, Michael. "Vitamin E and Alzheimer Disease: The Basis for Additional Clinical Trials," American Journal of Clinical Nutrition 71(Suppl.): 630S-636S, 2000.

11. Minerals and Alzheimer's Disease

Although minerals have not been studied as extensively as vitamins in relation to Alzheimer's disease, they do play important roles in the development of the disease. As we learn in Chapter 15, they are especially valuable in deactivating potentially dangerous levels of aluminum.

Calcium

In evaluating 18 non-demented patients, 22 with Alzheimer's type dementia and 20 with vascular type senile dementia, the Alzheimer-type group showed significant decreases in blood levels of calcium as well as increases in serum parathyroid hormone, urinary calcium, and a tendency of reduced vitamin D when compared with the non-demented group.[1] The researchers added that calcium and calcium regulating hormones may play a role in senile dementia.

Aluminum silicates in the plaques of Alzheimer's disease patients may be secondary to calcium deficiency because: 1) the level of calcium is a major influence on microtubules assembly/disassembly; 2) the neurofibrillary tangles in senile dementia of the Alzheimer's disease type seem to represent disordered assemblies of microtubules; 3) microtubules are closely related to structure, development and functioning of postsynaptic densities that are involved in senile plaques; 4) a calcium deficiency occurs in

---

1 Ogihara, T., et al. "Possible Participation of Calcium-Regulating Factors in Senile Dementia in Elderly Female Subjects," Gerontology 35(Supp. 1): 25-30, 1990.

a range of neurological diseases in which neurofibrillary tangles and plaques are neuropathological features of the disease. Microtubules are important components of the cytoskeleton, a network of protein filaments in the cytoplasm that control cell shape.[1] The researchers suggest that calcium supplements or a maintenance of calcium levels may provide some protection against cognitive decline in Alzheimer's disease.

IRON

Free radical damage to neurons has been documented in Alzheimer's disease patients, according to the Proceedings of the National Academy of Sciences (USA). The study reported that redox-active iron was associated with senile plaques and neurofibrillary tangles, which are pathological hallmark lesions of Alzheimer's disease.[2]

Iron binding appears to be dependent on available histidine residues and on protein metabolism. Iron accumulation could be an important contributor to the oxidative damage that is found in Alzheimer's disease.

There is a significant ferritin (iron) immunoreaction which accompanies senile plaques and many blood vessels in Alzheimer's brain tissue. The iron reaction is observed both diffusely (spread) in the proximity of plaques and in cells associated with the plaques.[3] Data suggest a disruption of brain iron homeostasis (balance) in Alzheimer's disease by alterations in the normal cellular distribution of the mineral and the proteins responsible for iron regulation. This might lead to oxidative damage and the potential for metal neurotoxicity in Alzheimer's disease, they said.

MAGNESIUM

In 20 Alzheimer's disease patients with a mean age of 70, whose brains were removed at autopsy within 48 to 72 hours after death, results showed a non-homogenous distribution of magnesium in the normal human brain, according to Magnesium Research.[4] In

---

1 Deary, I. J., and Hendrickson, A. E. "Calcium and Alzheimer's Disease," Lancet, May 24, 1986, p. 1219.

2 Smith, M. A., et al. "Iron Accumulation in Alzheimer Disease Is a Source of Redox-Generated Free Radicals," Proceedings of the National Academy of Sciences (USA) 94:9866-9868, September 1997.

3 Connor, J. R., et al. "A Histochemical Study of Iron, Transferrin, and Ferritin in Alzheimer's Diseased Brains," Neuroscience Research 31: 78-83, 1992.

4 Andrasi, E., et al. "Distribution of Magnesium Concentrations in Various Brain Areas in Alzheimer's Disease," Magnesium Research 13(3): 189-196, 2000.

9 patients with the disease, magnesium levels were found to be significantly decreased in brain regions of the deceased patients when compared with controls.

ZINC

A number of studies have shown that zinc enhances aggregation of beta-amyloid protein, a main component of senile plaques found in Alzheimer's disease brains, according to researchers at the University of Auckland School of Medicine in New Zealand. Chelatable zinc has been shown to accumulate in the cytoplasm of neurons in other neurological disorders, where neurons appear to be dying of apoptosis (programmed cell death).[1]

Although there is debate, some studies show that total zinc is significantly reduced in several brain regions of Alzheimer's disease patients, which creates a paradox of zinc being reduced in several areas of the brain, while there are higher quantities of zinc in senile plaques consistent with Alzheimer's disease.

As noted earlier, it is unknown whether there is a causal link between zinc and Alzheimer's. In Trace Elements and Electrolytes, a research team studied the role of zinc in the pathogenesis of Alzheimer's disease, and reported that an excess of the mineral may enhance aggregation and deposition of amyloid in the brain, whereas a zinc deficiency may enhance neurofibrillary tangle formation.[2] Zinc levels in the tissue of Alzheimer's disease patients have produced various results, however, zinc supplementation or chelation is not warranted, they said. Zinc supplementation in those with severe cognitive impairment and evidence of a zinc deficiency should be considered, the researchers suggested.

In 9 adults with Alzheimer's disease, compared with 8 controls, postmortem blood levels of zinc showed a statistically significant elevation in Alzheimer's patients at 136.4 mcg/dl, compared with age-matched controls at 71.1 mcg/dl, according to Biological Trace Element Research.[3] A beta-amyloid formation is involved in the pathogenesis of Alzheimer's disease, according to Science. Concentrations of zinc above 300 nM (nanomolar) rapidly destabilize A-netal-40 solutions, including amyloid formation.[4] Alterations in

1   Cuajungoo, Math P., et al. "Zinc and Alzheimer's Disease: Is There a Link?" Journal of Brain Research Reviews 23: 219-236, 1997.

2   Nachev, P. C, and Larner, A. J. "Zinc and Alzheimer's Disease," Trace Elements and Electrolytes 13(2): 55-59, 1996.

3   Rulon, L. L., et al. "Serum Zinc Levels and Alzheimer's Disease," Biological Trace Element Research 75: 79-85, 2000.

4   Bush, A. I., et al. "Rapid Induction of Alzheimer Amyloid Formation by Zinc," Science 265: 1464-1467, September 2, 1994.

zinc cerebral metabolism may be involved in the pathogenesis of Alzheimer's disease, the researchers added.

In 6 Alzheimer's disease patients, oral zinc at 30 mg/day — which did not increase blood levels of the mineral significantly — showed modest improvement on psychometric testing and the cognitive portion of the Alzheimer's Disease Association scale scores in 4 patients, according to the South African Medical Journal.[1]

The addition of zinc in the diet may prevent or delay the onset of dementia in those at risk, since the mineral is important in enzymes dealing with DNA replication, repair, and transcription, as well as in neuronal DNA polymerases, according to Lancet.[2]

The best dietary sources of zinc include meat, poultry, seafoods, bran and whole grains, brewer's yeast, vegetables, and others. Zinc supplements are available over-the-counter.

Pneumonia is a major public health problem in the elderly, especially as they are more at risk of infections due to the age-associated decline in immune function.[3] These changes in immune response, in addition to malnutrition, contribute to the increased frequency and severity of pneumonia and to the morbidity due to pneumonia in the elderly.

"Our study suggests that elderly with low blood levels of zinc might benefit from zinc supplementation," the researchers added. "Such a measure has the potential to reduce not only the number of episodes and duration of pneumonia and the number of new antibiotic prescriptions and days of antibiotic use due to pneumonia, but also all-cause mortality in the elderly." Zinc has been shown to play an important role in the regulation of the T-cell-mediated function, and a deficiency in the mineral has been shown to cause thymus involution (returning an enlarged organ to its original size), and to depress lymphocyte proliferation, interleukin-2 production, delayed-hypersensitivity skin responses, and antibody response to T-cell-dependent antigens.

---

1   Potpcnik, F. C., et al. "Zinc and Platelet Membrane Microviscosity in Alzheimer's Disease: The In Vivo Effect of Zinc on Platelet Membranes and Cognition," South African Medical Journal 87(9): 1116-1119, September 1997.

2   Burnet, F. M. "A Possible Role of Zinc in the Pathology of Dementia," Lancet, January 24, 1981, pp. 186-188.

3   Meydani, Simin K., et al. "Serum Zinc and Pneumonia in Nursing Home Elderly," American Journal of Clinical Nutrition 86: 1167-1173, 2007.

COPPER

Progressive cognitive impairments are characteristic in the dementia of Alzheimer's disease,[1] and "an increased concentration of copper in cerebrospinal fluid with normal plasma copper concentrations has been noted in some patients with Alzheimer's disease." Copper interacts with amyloid precursor protein and beta-amyloid peptide in the self-aggregating plaques and neurofibrillary tangles characteristic of Alzheimer's disease, and may contribute to the pathogenesis of this disorder via cellular oxidative stress.

SELENIUM

Blood levels of selenium may be inversely associated with performance in neurological tests, according to a study involving 1,024 patients who were 65 years of age or older (the InCHIANTI population-based study).[2]

1 Desai, Vishal, and Kaler, Stephen G. "Role of Copper in Human Neurological Disorders," American Journal of Clinical Nutrition 88(Suppl.): 855S-858S, 2008.
2 Shahar, A., et al. "Plasma Selenium Is Positively Related to Performance in Neurological Tasks Assessing Coordination and Motor Speed," Movement Disorders 25(12): 1909-1915, 2010.

12. Herbs and Alzheimer's Disease

Although a number of herbs are associated with Alzheimer's disease, the crown jewel of the plants in this regard is Ginkgo biloba, since it has been researched extensively for improving memory loss and cognitive function.

Ginkgo Biloba

Ginkgo biloba is the oldest living tree species in the world, having survived unchanged in China for over 300 million years, according to Harold H. Bloomfield, M.D.. Also known as the maidenhair tree, Ginkgo was the only plant to survive the atomic bomb dropped on Hiroshima. Charles Darwin called the tree a living fossil.[1]

The Ginkgo is a popular ornamental tree that is found in parks and along the streets in the United States, its distinctive leaves often found on sidewalks. Just as this hardy tree can live to a ripe old age, it can also help baby boomers to overcome their angst and die young — as late as possible, Bloomfield commented.

The October 22, 1997 issue of the Journal of the American Medical Association published research showing that Ginkgo biloba extracts appear to slow Alzheimer's disease. The double-blind study lasted for 1 year and was conducted by Pierre L. LeBars, M.D., and colleagues at the New York Institute for Medical Research.

---

1   Bloomfield, Harold H., M.D. Healing Anxiety With Herbs. New York: HarperCollins Publishers, 1998, pp. 16ff.

The research team reported that 27% of patients who took 120 mg/day of Ginkgo extract for 6 months or longer improved their mental functioning, including memory, reasoning, and the ability to learn, compared with only 14% of those given a placebo.

The study began with 309 patients, 45 or older, with the most suffering from Alzheimer's disease but also some of the dementia caused by strokes, Bloomfield added. The study found that Ginkgo can stabilize or even improve mental performance in one-third of those who are mildly impaired by Alzheimer's.

"The form of Ginkgo biloba extract used in the study is called EGb 761, and it is widely used in Europe for the treatment of Alzheimer's," Bloomfield continued. "German studies have demonstrated that 240 mg of EGb 761 a day is perhaps more effective than the 120 mg daily dose that was used in the just-named study."

The most potent Ginkgo formulations use a strictly controlled process that was developed in Germany. The extract is sold in the United States under the trade names GinkgoId and Dinkgo-D.

Bloomfield added that Ginkgo increases blood flow to the brain and has excellent restorative effects on the nervous system. The active components of the supplement have a profound tonic effect on the mind and body, and EGb 761 has been shown to inhibit the reuptake of norepinephrine, serotonin, dopamine, and acetylcholine, which are important neurotransmitters in the brain.

The extract acts as an antioxidant and a nerve cell membrane stabilizer, Bloomfield continued. It also enhances oxygen and glucose utilization and increases blood flow in arteries, veins, and capillaries.

Experiments involving learned helplessness, and behavioral despair in lab animals demonstrated that the supplement exhibited some antianxiety and antidepressant activities.

Ginkgo is also reportedly of benefit in many symptoms of aging:

1. Anxiety and depression.
2. Memory impairment.
3. Poor concentration and decreased alertness.
4. Diminished intellectual capacity.
5. Vertigo and headache.
6. Tinnitus (ringing in the ears).
7. Macular degeneration (the most common form of blindness in adults).
8. Inner ear disturbances, which can cause partial deafness.
9. Poor circulation in the extremities.
10. Impotence due to impaired blood flow to the penis.

In a data review, researchers found intake of Ginkgo to show promise in patients with dementia, normal aging, and cerebrovascular disorders, as well as low levels of drug interactions, according to an article in Archives of Physical Medicine and Rehabilitation.[1]

Clinical indications for the use of Ginkgo include memory, information processing, and activities of daily living. Conditions in which the herb shows promise are Alzheimer's disease, stroke, aging, edema (swelling), tinnitus, and macular degeneration, the research team added.

Most Ginkgo products contain a ratio of 50:1 by weight — 50 pounds of leaf for each pound of extract — and are standardized to include 24% to 26% Ginkgo flavonol glycosides. Doses range from 80 to 480 mg/day, the research team said.

At the Freie Universitat Berlin in Germany, S. Kanowski, M.D., reported that there is evidence from extensive research that the Ginkgo special extract, EGb 761, showed a beneficial influence on some systems and mechanisms involved in the pathology of Alzheimer's disease. The nutrient exerts a protective effect on energy metabolism and neuronal cells under conditions of impaired oxidative phosphorylation, and serves as a potent free-radical scavenger, thus preventing peroxidation of membrane lipids by oxygen free radicals. Lipid peroxidation is an interaction between fats and oxygen, which can lead to the destruction of ceils.[2] It has been demonstrated that free radicals play a key role in B-amyloid neurotoxicity, and it is well known that oxidative energy metabolism is impaired in Alzheimer's disease, Kanowski said.

In experimental studies, the supplement has proven to enhance the density of cortical muscarinic receptors in aged animals, as well as the high-affinity choline uptake into acetylcholine producing hippocampal neurons. Muscarine is a toxin with neurologic effects. It is a cholinergic substance whose effects resemble acetylcholine, Ginkgo also enhances global and regional cerebral blood flow by reducing blood viscosity and probably vascular resistance, Kanowski continued.

In their study, patients were given an oral daily dose of 240 mg of Ginkgo biloba extract (EGb) to those suffering from dementia or Alzheimer's type of vascular dementia. Following 24 weeks of

---

1   Diamond, B. J., et al. "Ginkgo Biloba Extract: Mechanisms and Clinical Indications," Archives of Physical Medicine and Rehabilitation 81: 668-678, May 2000.

2   Kanowski, S., M.D. "Proof of Efficacy of the Ginkgo Biloba Extract EGb 761 in Outpatients Suffering from Mild to Moderate Primary Degenerative Dementia of the Alzheimer's Type or Multi-Infarct Dementia," Pharmacopsychiatry 29: 47-56, 1996.

therapy, the proportion of multiple responders was significantly higher in the treated group than in the controls, that is, 28 to 10%.

In 2 other studies, there is considerable evidence that doses of the supplement between 120 and 240 mg/day are affected in age-related cognitive impairment in those not yet diagnosed with dementia, Kanowski added.

Based on his studies and the information available, Kanowski said that Ginkgo biloba extract (EGb 761), should be considered in the treatment of dementia patients, since its excellent tolerability is especially advantageous.

Researchers evaluated 36 patients with classical symptoms of organic brain syndrome, who participated in a placebo-controlled trial of 40 mg — 3 times daily — of a Ginkgo biloba extract (EGb 761) for 8 weeks.[1] The results showed a highly significant difference after 4 weeks of therapy, and also after 8 weeks in both the saccadic (jerky) test and the psychometric evaluation.

In a double-blind controlled trial of Alzheimer's-type dementia, patients were given 240 mg/day of a special extract of Ginkgo biloba (EGb 761) over a 3-month period, and there was an improvement in the SKT-test from 19.67 to 16.78 in the treated group, versus a deterioration from 18.11 to 18.89 points in the placebo group, the German researchers reported in the Journal of Psychiatric Research.[2]

If you suffer from any deficiency of circulation, consider using Ginkgo, which is widely used in Germany to increase blood flow throughout the body.[3] "Ginkgo is a nontoxic and not an anticoagulation, and it works by increasing the elasticity of the membranes of the red blood cells, making it easier for them to squeeze through small arteries and capillaries," says Andrew Weil, M.D. Many people report both physical and mental improvement after using the herbal remedy for at least 2 months, he added. Standard extracts are available over-the-counter in health food stores and other outlets. The recommended dose is 40 mg 3 times daily with meals.

In 1975, French researchers evaluated the potential benefits of Ginkgo biloba extract in a group of 60 patients — 55 women and 5 men — who had been diagnosed with cerebrovascular insufficiency, and 30 women who served as controls and who were given ar-

1   Hofferberth, B. "The Effect of Ginkgo Biloba Extract on Neurophysiological and Psychometric Measurement Results in Patients with Psychotic Organic Brain Syndrome," Arzeimittelforschung 39(8): 918-922, August 1989.

2   Maurer, K., et al. "Clinical Efficacy of Ginkgo Biloba Special Extract EGb 761 in Dementia of the Alzheimer Type," Journal of Psychiatric Research 31(6): 645-655, 1997.

3   Weil, Andrew, M.D. 8 Weeks to Optimum Health. New York: Alfred A. Knopf, 1997, pp. 199-200.

got alkaloid derivatives.[1] Pretrial examination recorded the extent of dizziness, headaches, movability, sensory manifestations, and other parameters. The volunteers were also given typical psychometric tests. Following the study, the research team determined that there was a 79% improvement in those given the Ginkgo extract, compared with only 21% in the placebo group. The treatment group received 120 mg/day of the herbal extract for 3 months.

At the Whittington Hospital in London, England, researchers examined the benefits of Ginkgo extract on 31 patients over the age of 50 with signs of memory impairment, reported Donald J. Brown, N.D.[2] For the double-blind study, half of the participants were given 40 mg of Ginkgo extract 3 times daily, while the others received a look-alike pill. Psychometric tests were evaluated at the beginning of the study and after 12 and 24 weeks of therapy.

The patients who received the Ginkgo supplement showed significantly superior improvement when compared to those given a placebo, Brown said. Besides demonstrating that the extract had a beneficial effect on mild to moderate memory loss of organic origin, the study also revealed that electroencephalogram (EEG) measurements in the Ginkgo group indicated improved brain function. The extract is said to increase the rate of information transmitted to nerve cells.

In a study reported in the Proceedings of the National Academy of Sciences, a research team gave Ginkgo supplements or a placebo to laboratory mice.[3] Following Ginkgo supplementation, 1 gene in the brain's hippocampus and 9 in the cortex increased in activity by more than 3 times. The hippocampus is the center of learning and memory, while the cerebral cortex controls memory, speech, logical and emotional responses, as well as voluntary movement. All of the activated genes are involved in promoting normal brain activities and protecting brain cells from serious damage. The researchers found that the Ginkgo supplement significantly increased the activity of 10 genes involved in normal brain function, and the study suggested that the use of the herbal supplement in many brain disorders has a clear and genetic basis.

As reported Nouveau Presse Medica, in experimental models of ischemia, edema, and hypoxia (lack of oxygen), Ginkgo biloba extract reduced vascular, tissue, and metabolic disturbances, along

1 Moreau, P. "Un Noveau Stimulant Circulatoire Cerebral," *Nouveau Presse Medica* 4: 2401-2402, 1975.

2 Murray, Frank. *Ginkgo Biloba*. McGraw-Hill, 1996, p. 13.

3 Watanabe, C. M. H., et al. "The In Vivo Neuromodulatory Effect of the Herbal Medicine Ginkgo Biloba," *Proceedings of the National Academy of Sciences* 98: 6577-6580, 2001.

with neurological and behavioral consequences.[1] It is suggested that Ginkgo biloba may protect the membrane ultra structure against free radical damage, and modulate some enzymatic systems and ionic pumps to have the vascular, rheological, and metabolic effects. The researchers added that the herb increases resistance and diminishes hyperpermeability in the capillaries, and, in the veins, it reinforces vascular tension and restores to the return circulation its efficacy in cleansing the metabolic waste products from hypoxia and acidosis.

In a double-blind trial involving 202 patients, they were given 120 mg/day of EGb 761, or a look-alike pill, according to the Journal of the American Medical Association. The supplemented group had an Alzheimer's Disease Assessment Scale-Cognitive subscale score of 1.4 points, better than the placebo group, and a Geriatric Evaluation by Relative's Rating Instrument (GERRI) score of 0.14 points better than the controls.[2]

The research team headed by Pierre L. Le Bars, M.D., of the New York Institute for Medical Research in Tarrytown, said that the supplement was safe and appeared to be capable of stabilizing and, in a substantial number of cases, improving the cognitive performance and social functioning of demented patients for 6 months to 1 year. The patients in this study were 45 years of age or older, and they had a diagnosis of uncomplicated dementia of either the Alzheimer's type or multi-infarct dementia.

The research team added that the extract contains a variety of compounds that may act synergistically on diverse processes involved in the homeostasis of inflammation and oxidative stress, providing membrane protection and neurotransmitter modulation, which may be the basis for the herb's effect on the central nervous system.

ST. JOHN'S WORT

Some evidence indicates that St. John's wort can raise levels of some neurotransmitters, such as serotonin and dopamine, helping to treat mild to moderate depression.[3]

In a study using human vascular cells and a cell-free medium, low levels of the herb had a pronounced antioxidant effect. The

---

1 Clostre, F. "From the Body to the Cellular Membranes: The Different Levels of Pharmacological Action of Ginkgo Biloba Extract," Nouveau Presse Medica 15: 1529-1538, 1986.

2 Le Bars, Pierre L., M.D., Ph.D., et al. "A Placebo-Controlled, Doable-Blind, Randomized Trial of an Extract of Ginkgo Biloba for Dementia," JAMA 278(16): 1327-1332, 1997.

3 Hunt, E. J., et al. "Effect of St. John's Wort on Free Radical Production," Life Sciences 69: 181-190, 2001.

ability of the herb to quench free radicals could explain some of its benefits, since antioxidant levels are often compromised when people have a disease condition.

In an article in the British Medical Journal, 324 outpatients with mild to moderate depression, 157 — 17% women with a mean age of 46.5) — received 250 mg of St. John's wort (Hypericum perforatum L.) extract twice daily for 6 weeks. The controls were 167 volunteers — 71% women with a mean age of 45.4 — who took 75 mg of Norfanil imipramine, a drug prescribed for depression, twice daily for 6 weeks.[1]

The mean score on the anxiety-somatization subscale of the Hamilton Scale was 3.79 in the hypericum group and 4.26 in the controls, suggesting a significant benefit of the herb over the drug, according to Helmut Woelk of the University of Giessen in Germany.

In addition, the tolerability scores were better for the herb at 1.67, compared with 2.35 for the drug. Adverse events occurred in 39% of those taking the herb, compared with 63% given the drug.

Herbal Remedies

Galanthamine (Galanthus nivalis) is derived from the bulbs of a spring flower called common snowdrop. For Alzheimer's disease, some experts have recommended 5 mg 3 times daily, then increased to 30 to 40 mg/day. It is available in 5 to 10 mg coated tablets and 5 mg ampoules.[2] A 1983 report suggested that Odysseus (in Homer's poem The Odyssey) used the herb as an antidote to Circe's poisonous drugs. If this is true, this would have been the first recorded use of galanthamine to reverse drug intoxication.

"Combining herbs with certain drugs may alter their action or produce unwanted side effects," the publication said. "Don't use galanthamine while taking drugs to relieve depression (MAO inhibitors such as Marplan and Nardil), or if you have been exposed to organophosphate fertilizers that are used in gardens and on farms." In addition, don't use this herb if you have a slow pulse, poor muscle tone, recent heart attack, epilepsy, Parkinson's disease, diabetes, or a blockage of the respiratory, digestive, or urinary tract. And consult a health care practitioner before taking the herb, the publication added.

---

1 Woelk, Helmut. "Comparison of St. John's Wort and Imipramine for Treating depression: Randomized Controlled Trial," British Medical Journal, September 2, 2000, pp. 536-539.

2 Petrow, Charles W., Pharm. D., and Avila, Juan R., Pharm. D. The Complete Guide to Herbal Medicines. New York: Pocket Books, 2000, pp. 220-221.

Experts are not yet sure what causes the memory loss and personality changes characteristic of Alzheimer's disease, but they do know that acetylcholine plays a major role, reported James A. Duke, Ph.D. This is a neurotransmitter that enables nerve impulses to pass from one nerve cell to another.[1] "Scientists have observed that people with AD run low on acetylcholine, which seems to explain why their mental function declines," Duke said. "This observation also directed researchers to 2 treatment options: Either help AD patients to make more acetylcholine or inhibit the action of cholinesterase, so that the acetylcholine that the patients have might last longer and let more nerve impulses through. Drugs currently approved to treat AD are cholinesterase inhibitors, namely tacrine (Cognex) and donepezil (Aricept). While they slow the progress on AD, they can't reverse it."

Duke added that Nicolette Perry, a British pharmacy researcher, has studied herbal cholinesterase inhibition and has come up with the herbs that do the best job: balm or lemon balm, lime, sage, hyssop, and rosemary. "Now I don't know of any research that proves these herbs to be as powerful as the AD drugs, or that shows they have any effect on AD patients, but I think that's because the herbs haven't been studied. There are intriguing signs that they may help," Duke said.

A HERBAL PROGRAM FOR ALZHEIMER'S

The following herbs have well-known positive effects on brain function:[2]

- Ginkgo biloba, 40 mg., 1 capsule twice daily.
- Gotu kola, 500 mg, 1 capsule twice daily.
- Siberian ginseng, 100 mg, 1 capsule twice daily.

MUSHROOMS

Treatments for reducing neuronal (nerve) cell death are important for preventing as well as treating neurodegenerative diseases, including dementia and motor dysfunction.[3]

Since neuronal cell death is caused by endoplastic reticulum (ER) stress in many neurodegenerative diseases — Alzheimer's

---

1 Duke, James A., Ph.D., and Castleman, Michael. Anti-Aging Prescriptions. Emmaus, PA: Rodale Press, Inc., 2001, pp. 213ff.

2 Golan, Ralph, M.D. Optimal Wellness. New York: Ballantine Books, 1995, p. 328.

3 Kagai, Kaouri, et al. "Dilinoleoyl-phosphatidylethanolamine From Hericum Erinaceum Protects Against ER Stress-Dependent Neuro2a Cell Death via Protein Kinase C Pathway," Journal of Nutritional Biochemistry 17: 525-530, 2006.

disease, Parkinson's, Huntington's, etc. — it is reasonable to sus-pect that molecules able to weaken ER stress might reduce both the risk for and the extent of damage in neurodegenerative diseas-es, the researchers said. "Since neurodegenerative diseases have a rather long incubation period prior to diagnosis, reducing the risk before the identification of quite advanced disease is important," they continued. "Therefore, reducing the risk of neurodegenera-tion by the consumption of food products might be a viable and important option for target populations."

This led the research team to screen ER stress-attenuating mol-ecules, which might reduce the risk of neurodegenerative disease from an edible mushroom, Hericium erinaceum, which is known in Japan as Yamabushitake, in China as Hou Tou Gu, and in the United States and Europe as Lion's Mane.

As a result of their screening, they determined that Dilinoleo-yl-phosphatidylethanolamine (DLPE) was one of the molecules that was effective in reducing ER stress-dependent cell death, in both human and animal trials. A purified form of DLPE, now com-mercially available as Amylobam 3399, was found to reduce the ER stress-dependent cell death, thus protecting neuronal cells.

Lion's Mane is available over-the-counter in 180 vegetable tab-lets. Recommended dosage is 2 to 3 times daily with meals, or as prescribed by a health-care provider.

At Shizuoka University in Japan, Hirokazu Kawagishi and Cun Zhuang conducted a study involving 50 patients with an average age of 75.0 years and 50 controls with an average age of 77.2. They were evaluated for the efficacy of H. erinaceum at a rehabilitation hospital in the Gunma prefecture of Japan.[1] The patients were suf-fering from cerebrovascular disease, Parkinson's disease, diabetic neuropathy, and 7 patients in the treatment group were diagnosed with dementia. Those in the treatment group received 5 g/day of the mushroom in their soup for 6 months. Patients were evaluated before and after treatment based on the Functional Independence Measure (FIM), which is an international standard for evaluating eating, dressing, evacuating, walking, bathing, etc., as well as per-ceptive capabilities — understanding, expression, communication, problem solving, memory, etc. Following 6 months of the mush-room therapy, 6 of 7 dementia patients demonstrated improve-ment in their perceptual capacities, and all 7 had improvements in

---

1   Kawagishi, Hirokazu, and Zhuang, Cun. "Bioactive Compounds from Mushrooms," Heterocycles 72: 45-52, 2007.

their overall FIM scores. Of special interest, 3 bedridden patients were able to get up to eat meals following the therapy.

"Our review introduces some bioactive substances, including toxins, from mushrooms, and it is clear that there is only a fine line between medicinal compounds and toxins," the researchers concluded. "It is said that there are over 140,000 species of mushrooms on earth, but less than 1% have been studied. Nevertheless, we believe that unknown mushrooms are a vast source of new bioactive substances."

Several compounds — hericenones, erinacines, and DLPF, isolated from H. erinaceum, have shown significant efficacy in protecting neuronal cells against ER stress or oxidative stress-induced cell death, both in vitro and in vivo. Results to date indicate that the mushroom compound appears to be effective in treating dementia, especially the Alzheimer's-type dementia.[1] "Overall, it appears that H. erinaceum may have great potential as a medicine or dietary supplement for Alzheimer's-type dementia," the researchers added.

GREEN TEA

Environmental factors associated with the risk of Alzheimer's disease, a common cause of dementia, remain largely undefined, although several risk factors for vascular dementia have been identified.[2] "The present results suggest that higher consumption of green tea is associated with lower prevalence of cognitive impairment in humans," researchers say.[3] "The results might partly explain the relative low prevalence of dementia, especially Alzheimer's disease, in Japan than in Europe and North America."

Of those in the study, 16.9% consumed less than 3 cups of green tea/week; 10.8% consumed 4 to 6 cups/week or 1 cup/day; and 72.3% consumed over 2 cups/day.

Higher green tea consumption was significantly associated with a lower prevalence of depressive symptoms in community-dwelling elderly people.[4] A more frequent consumption of green

---

1 Kawagishi, Hirokazu, and Zhuang, Cun. "Compounds for Dementia from Hericum Erinaceum," Drugs of the Future 33(2): 149-155, 2008.

2 Kuriyama, Shinichi, et al. "Green Tea Consumption and Cognitive Function: A Cross-Sectional Study from the Tsurugaya Project," American Journal of Clinical Nutrition 83: 355-361, 2006.

3 Nourhashemi, F., et al. "Alzheimer Disease: Protective Factors," American Journal of Clinical Nutrition 71(Suppl.): S643-S649, 2000.

4 Niu, Kaijun, et al. "Green Tea Consumption Is Associated with Depressive Symptoms in the Elderly," American Journal of Clinical Nutrition 90: 1615-1622, 2009.

tea was associated with a lower prevalence of depressive symptoms in the community-dwelling older population.[1]

At the just-named university, a research team, headed by Atsushi Hozawa, reported that green tea consumption was inversely associated with psychological stress in a cross-sectional study of 42,093 Japanese people, over 40 years of age, even after adjustment for possible confounding factors.[2][3]

BACOPA MONNIERI

A study involving 81 healthy patients over 55 years of age found that supplementation with an extract of Bacopa monnieri may improve memory performance.[4] The patients were randomized to receive 300 mg/day of the extract or a placebo for 12 weeks. The researchers reported that supplementation with the herbal extract was associated with a significant improvement in verbal learning, memory acquisition, and delayed recall. However, some patients experienced gastrointestinal tract side-effects.

The study concurs with previous findings with the traditional use of the herb.

GREEN TEA AND BODY WEIGHT

Studies have related obesity to a variety of illnesses, including Alzheimer's disease.

At Oklahoma State University in Stillwater, a research team determined that green tea supplementation may reduce body weight and body mass index (BMI), improve lipid profile, and decrease oxidative stress.[5] The study involved 35 obese volunteers with metabolic syndrome, who were randomized selected to be given 4 cups/day of water (the controls), 4 cups/day of green tea, or 2 capsules/day of green tea extract for 8 weeks. At the end of the study,

1 Shimbo, M., et al. "Green Tea Consumption in Everyday Life and Mental Health," Public Health Nutrition 8: 1300-1306, 2005.

2 Hozawa, Atsushi, et al. "Green Tea Consumption Is Associated with Lower Psychological Distress in a General Population: The Ohsaki Cohort 2006 Study," American Journal of Clinical Nutrition 90: 1390-1396, 2009.

3 Hintikka, J., et al. "Daily Tea Drinking Is Associated with a Low Level of Depressive Symptoms in the Finnish General Population," European Journal of Epidemiology 20: 359-363, 2005.

4 Morgan, A., et al. "Does Bacoba Monnieri Improve Memory Performance in Older Persons? Results of a Randomized, Placebo-Controlled, Double-Blind Trial," Journal of Alternative and Complimentary Medicine 16(7): 753-759, 2010.

5 Basu, A., et al. "Green Tea Supplementation Affects Body Weight, Lipids, and Lipid Peroxidation in Obese Subjects with Metabolic Syndrome," Journal of the American College of Nutrition 29(1): 31-40, 2010.

a significant decrease in body weight and BMI were reported in the green tea group when compared with the controls.

In addition, the green tea users reported a decrease in LDL-cholesterol, the bad kind, the LDL/HDL ratio, and malondialdehyde. Malondialdehyde is a marker for fatty acid oxidation. The falavonoids in both the green tea extract and the capsules were equally beneficial.

13. Combination Nutrients

A research team in Germany reported that dementias of the Alzheimer's type and Parkinson's disease are characterized by a transmitter-specific loss of neurons which progress to several neuronal systems over the course of the illness.[1] Oxidative stress has been proposed as a means of neurodegeneration in dementia of the Alzheimer's type and Parkinson's disease, and there is evidence of increased free radical oxygen activity and impaired defenses in dementia of the Alzheimer's type, although less true in Parkinson's disease. Several antioxidant vitamins — including vitamins A, C, and E — may have beneficial free radical scavenging mechanisms for dementia of the Alzheimer's type. The effects of selegiline, a MAO-B inhibitor, has shown a slowing of the progression of Parkinson's disease, and it has been used in dementia of the Alzheimer's type, together with a small improvement on selective remaining tests was also observed.

The use of desferrioxanine, a chelating agent for the removal of iron and aluminum, when given intramuscularly over a 2-year period to 48 patients with dementia of the Alzheimer's type, showed a significant slowing of the rate of decline, but there were some concerns about the study.

Alphalipoic acid is a cofactor for mitochondrial dehydrogenase and can enhance energy metabolism, the researchers continued, and this substance has potential as a therapeutic agent in dementia of the Alzheimer's type.

---

1 Frolich, L., and Riederer, P. "Free Radical Mechanisms in Dementia of the Alzheimer's Type and the Potential for Antioxidative Treatment," Drug Research 45(1): 443-446, 1995.

The researchers added that Ginkgo biloba extract has a strong free radical action, and it could possibly be of benefit. Pharmacologic drugs that show effects on oxygen free radical mediated mechanisms also have other pharmacologic properties which might be beneficial in the treatment of dementia of the Alzheimer's type.

Selegiline hydrochloride (L-Deprenyl) is available as Alzene, Deprenyl, Eldeoryl, and other formulations. Used to treat Parkinson's disease and Parkinson's-like syndromes, the drug issued in conjunction with Levodopa/carbidopa Atamet and Sinemet is recommended following infection of an injury to the central nervous system, due to damage to blood vessels in the brain, or after exposure to certain toxins. The drug inhibits a nervous system enzyme — monoamine oxidase (MAO), which is found in the brain and intestinal tract, and it acts to break down various chemicals that play a role in the initiation and control of voluntary muscle movements.[1]

Alzheimer's disease has not responded well to orthomolecular treatment, reported Abram Hoffer, M.D., Ph.D., one of the world's leading researchers in this type of treatment. He treated 5 patients with large doses of vitamin B3, vitamin C, and other vitamins, and the treatment was effective in the senile state not caused by Alzheimer's.[2] "Nevertheless," he continued, "I still consider it to be a disease of malnutrition, brought on by chronic malnutrition or other factors. F. Abalan[3] suggested it is caused by malabsorption. Thus, in his experience, normal serum albumin levels are achieved only with massive protein feeding. The usual neurological, psychiatric, and biochemical findings can be accounted for if there is massive malabsorption. This explains why large doses of vitamins are often ineffective."

In a study that was consistent with Abalan's hypothesis, Alzheimer's brains were unable to make enough tetrahydrobiopterin (Bh4), which is a cofactor in the synthesis of the neurotransmitters dopamine, noradrenalin, and serotonin, Hoffer added. A deficiency in Bh4 causes several neurological and mental abnormalities. For example, in Alzheimer's there is a decrease in synthesis of Bh4 from dihydroneopterin triphosphate because of a defect in the

1 Visaili, Gayla, project editor. Prescription & Over-the-Counter Drugs. Pleasantvi-lle, NY: The Reader's Digest Association, Inc., 1998, p. 668.

2 Hoffer, Abram, M.D., Ph.D. Orthomolecular Medicine for Physicians. New Canaan, CT: Keats Publishing, Inc., 1989, pp. 165-166.

3 Abalan, F. "Alzheimer's Disease and Malnutrition: A New Etiological Hypothesis," Medical Hypothesis 15: 385-393, 1984.

enzyme that eliminates phosphate. It was found that Alzheimer's brains have more neopterin and less Bh4 than the controls.

Another possibility is to use Warfarin (coumadin), a blood thinner, Hoffer said. Arthur C. Walsh, M.D.,[1] pioneered the use of Warfarin for treating senile dementia, and with good results. Walsh described a 56-year-old lawyer/engineer who could not be cared for at home since he was extremely confused and could not walk because he was so weak. Following 1 week on the anticoagulant, he was physically much better, could walk alone, and was cooperative. In preparation for sending him to a state hospital, the medication was stopped and, within a few days, he had regressed to his earlier condition. In the state hospital the Warfarin was stopped, and he soon became bedridden and died in 3 months. An autopsy confirmed that he had Alzheimer's disease.

"I believe the heavy metal toxicity hypothesis by Carl C. Pfeiffer, M.D.[2] should be investigated," Hoffer continued. "One should look not just for aluminum but also for excess copper, lead, mercury, cadmium, and silver. If they are present in excess amounts, methods can be developed to remove them. Chelation therapy can be used to find these metals and remove them.

An article in The Nutrition Report discussed 20 patients with long-term sporadic Alzheimer's disease, who were given supplements of vitamin B6, iron, and coenzyme Q10. It was found that there was a significant improvement in a variety of mental and functional tests after 1 year of therapy.[3]

It is thought that coenzyme Q10 reduces the free radicals formed by iron, and that vitamin B6 plays a role in neurotransmitter synthesis. The combination of these nutrients have a positive effect on reducing the signs and symptoms of Alzheimer's disease, the researchers said.

A Japanese research team evaluated 27 Alzheimer's disease patients supplementing them with coenzyme Q10 at 60 mg/day; sodium ferrous citrate (iron) at 150 mg/day; and vitamin B6 at 180 mg/day; which demonstrated considerable effectiveness of mito-

---

1 Walsh, Arthur C. M.D. "Treatment of Senile Dementia of the Alzheimer's Type by a Psychiatric-Anticoagulant Regimen," Journal of Orthomolecular Medicine, 1987. (Entire article)

2 Pfeiffer, Carl C., M.D. Mental and Elemental Nutrients. New Canaan, CT: Keats Publishing, Inc., 1975. (Entire book)

3 "Iron, B6 and Coenzyme Q10 in Alzheimer's," The Nutrition Report 12(10): 75, October 1994.

chondrial activation with this therapy, according to an article in The Lancet.[1]

The patients in the same family, who were found to have missense mutation of the amyloid beta-protein precursor gene at Codon 717, were given the just-named therapeutic regimen. Codon is a set of consecutive nucleotides in a strand of DNA or RNA. Missense, as used in genetics, is a mutation that causes a sequence in which there is a substitution of one amino acid (protein) residue for another.

For Patient 1, a 49-year-old woman with a 1-year history of progressive memory loss, her mental state improved to almost normal after 6 months of therapy. Her daily activity improved from FAST Stage 5 (moderate AD disease) to 1 (normal), and she had increased blood flow to the cerebral cortex, decreased symptoms of clinical dementia, and faster alpha wave activity in the power spectra of the electroencephalogram. She was able to ride a motorcycle and take care of Patient 2. When she stopped the therapy, her symptoms returned, but improved with the resumption of the regimen.

Patient 2 was her 58-year-old sister, who had had progressive dementia for 4 years. Her mental state and daily activity improved gradually with the above-named protocol. This patient also had adult T-cell leukemia, and, at 18 months of therapy, her mental and physical condition deteriorated because of her high fever and hypercalcemia (excessive calcium in the blood).

The researchers believe that this natural treatment prevented the progression of dementia for 1½ to 2 years in both patients.

In evaluating 341 patients with Alzheimer's disease of moderate severity, who received selegiline at 10 mg/day; vitamin E at 2,000 IU/day; both of these agents or a placebo for 2 years, it was found that in the adjusted analysis there was no statistically significant difference in the outcomes among the 4 groups, reported Mary Sano, Ph.D., and colleagues, in the New England Journal of Medicine.[2]

However, in an analysis that indicated the beginning scores on the Mini-Mental State Examination, there was significant delays in the time to primary outcome for patients treated with selegiline, vitamin E, or combination therapy, compared with placebo.

---

1 Imagawa, Masaki, et al, "Coenzyme Q10, Iron, and Vitamin B6 in Genetically Confirmed Alzheimer's Disease," The Lancet 340: 671, September 12, 1992.

2 Sano, Mary, Ph.D., et al. "A Controlled Trial of Selegiline, Alpha-Tocopherol, or Both, As Treatment for Alzheimer's Disease," The New England Journal of Medicine 336(17): 1216-1222, April 24, 1997.

Both supplements delayed functional deterioration, especially as reflected by the need for institutionalization, therefore, both should be considered for use in patients with moderate dementia. In those with moderately severe impairment from Alzheimer's disease, treatment with either of the agents slows its progression, Sano said.

In an article in Age, Denham Barman, M.D., of Omaha, Nebraska, assessed the role of free radicals in the etiology of senile dementia of the Alzheimer's type (SDAT), and the potential benefit of antioxidant therapy. It is suggested that SDAT results from a mutation in a mitochondrial DNA molecule early in the development of Alzheimer's disease.[1]

It is suggested that this may impair oxidative phosphorylation, while increasing the production of singlet oxygen and hydrogen peroxide. Phosphorylation is the addition of phosphorus to an organic compound, such as glucose, to produce glucose monophosphate. Like oxygen, glucose has 2 sides, good and bad. For example, specialized nerve cells in the brain can only run on sugar/glucose. Hydrogen peroxide is naturally produced in the body, and it is involved in cellular processes such as hormone regulation and the metabolism of protein, carbohydrates, fats, vitamins, and minerals. It is used for microbial infections, but intravenous or oral injections should be monitored by a physician.

Singlet oxygen can react with atmospheric pollutants to cause fog formation, and it may have harmful biological effects.

The mutated mitochondrial DNA is distributed to the cells of the developing organisms that, with advancing age, cellular dysfunction occurs in areas associated with Alzheimer's disease in the brain, Harman said. Cell damage and death are attributed to free radical damage secondary to reduced adenosine 5-triphosphate (ATP) production, thereby increasing the formation of hydrogen peroxide and a hydroxyl radical. This happens due to the aging of normal and defective mitochondria.

SDAT is best described as accelerated normal neuronal aging, and it is theoretically possible that reduction of maternal free radical reactions by dietary manipulation or supplementation with antioxidants — such as coenzyme Q10 — may be of benefit, Harman continued. Supplementation of antioxidants in the general population may also decrease the incidence of this syndrome by slow-

---

1 Harman, Denham, M.D. "Free Radical Therapy of Ageing: A Hypothesis on Pathogenesis of Senile Dementia of the Alzheimer's Type," Age 16: 23-30, 1993.

ing the rate of free radical damage to the abnormal mitochondria in those who are predisposed to SDAT.

By improving mitochondrial function with vitamin B2 (riboflavin), vitamin E, and coenzyme Q10, the function of SDAT patients may be temporarily improved by enhancing some impaired neurons, and slowing mitochondrial decline. Sodium ferrous citrate (iron), and vitamin B6 (pyridoxine) have also shown a benefit in improving mental function, Harman concluded.

Evidence suggests that oxidative stress plays an important role in the development of Alzheimer's disease. Ginkgo biloba, vitamins A, C, and E, and estrogen may act as free radical scavengers, and may be of pharmacological benefit.[1] Antioxidants which can prevent or reduce the production of free radicals include selegiline; MAO-B inhibitor; tenilsetam, which is believed to be an ACE inhibitor.

As reported elsewhere in this book, the standardized extract from the leaves of Ginkgo biloba contains 24% ginkgo flavone glycosides and 6% terpene lactones. In 8 of 11 studies evaluating EGb 761 extract in cerebrovascular insufficiency and organic psychosyndrome, there were 7 studies with evidence of a positive effect and 1 negative study. However, only 2 of the studies dealt with dementia of the Alzheimer's type.

In 13 studies using selegiline, beneficial effects were seen for at least symptoms of Alzheimer's dementia. There is considerable evidence that selegiline may act as an antidementive agent, the researchers added. Dementia is the loss of cognitive function.

The research team is convinced that vitamin E, selegiline. Ginkgo biloba, and idebenone may slow the progression of Alzheimer's disease.

The dual action of a cholinesterase inhibitor provides a new way of treating or delaying the symptoms of Alzheimer's disease, according to John Schiezer in Medical Tribune. Galantamine/galanthamine, a derivative of the daffodil plant, in addition to inhibiting acetylcholine, also stimulates nicotine receptors.[2] He reported that Paul R. Solomon, Ph.D., of Williams College in Williamstown, Massachusetts, said that there are data to suggest that stimulating nicotine receptors produces improvement in learning, memory, attention, and concentration. "All these things are very provocative, and it raises the issue that if you are able to stimulate nicotine re-

---

1 Rosler, M. et al. "Free Radicals in Alzheimer's Dementia: Currently Available Therapeutic Strategies," Journal of Neural Transmission 54(Suppl.): 211-219, 1998.

2 Schiezer, John. "Galantamine Found to Improve Cognition in Alzheimer's," Medical Tribune 40(16): 2, September 23, 1999.

ceptors, not through smoking, but with a drug, it could have a beneficial effect."

In an initial double-blind study involving 636 patients with mild to moderate Alzheimer's disease, 423 people were given galantamine twice daily for 6 months, while 213 received placebos. Sixty-two percent of the patients were women, with a mean age of 75. The volunteers were tested using the cognitive portion of the Alzheimer's Disease Assessment Scale, and the cognitive scores of those who took the drug were an average of 3.7 to 3.8 points higher than scores of those given a placebo.

Poor cognition recently joined the list of ills associated with hyperhomocysteinemia or high levels of homocysteine in the blood, reported Sally P. Stabler of the University of Colorado Health Sciences Center in Denver.[1] She noted that, in the same issue of the magazine, J. W. Miller, et al.[2] in a study at the University of California at Davis, found a large Mexican-American group that confirms the association of hyperhomocysteinemia and impaired cognitive performance that was previously found in other larger studies.

"There are plausible reasons for a causal relation because elevated homocysteine is a marker indicating deficiency of vitamin B12, folic acid (the B vitamin), or both, and it is a well documented risk factor for vascular disease, which is related to both vascular dementia and Alzheimer's disease," Stabler added.

Vitamin B12 is required for a healthy central nervous system — brain and spinal cord — and up to 10% of patients with pernicious anemia (due to a B12 deficiency) have prominent mental symptoms, including memory loss. In addition, the 2 vitamins are necessary to ensure adequate methylation by S-adenosylmethionine in the synthesis of neurotransmitters, myelin, and phosphatidylcholine, as well as other compounds important to the nervous system.

She added that a small but intriguing study showed that vitamin B12 replacement improved cognitive performance and abnormalities on EGG (electroencephalogram) in B12-deficient seniors. Vascular dementia and the plaques and neurofibrillary tangles in Alzheimer's disease would seem to be irreversible, however, and lowering homocysteine before the onset of the disease would be necessary to show a treatment benefit.

"Because folic acid status has improved in the United States during the past 5 years — food fortification, etc. — with the re-

1 Stabler, Sally P. "Vitamins, Homocysteine, and Cognition," American Journal of Clinical Nutrition 78: 359-360, 2003.
2 Miller, J. W., et al. "Homocysteine and Cognitive Function in the Sacramento Area Latino Study on Aging," ibid, pp. 441-447.

sult that total homocysteine values decreased, it may be possible to show a decline in the incidence of vascular dementia, strokes, and other cardiovascular events, or even Alzheimer's disease over the next decade," she continued.

The 10 to 20% of seniors who have metabolic evidence of a vitamin B12 deficiency may benefit from replacement supplementation, Stabler continued. If a B12 deficiency is suspected in someone with hyperhomocysteinemia, it would be prudent to treat them with a high dose of oral or parenteral (injection) B12, because a B12 deficiency is known to cause central nervous system demyelination. While over-the-counter vitamin therapy clearly improves folic acid and vitamin B12 status — also known to lower homocysteine levels — higher doses of oral B12 supplements may not be available in the usual multivitamin supplements.

In a study at the University of Paris XIII in France, which involved 1,743 men and women, ranging in age from 45 to 80, with a history of myocardial infarction, unstable angina, or ischemic stroke, those with prior stroke who were given B vitamins plus omega-3 fatty acids, were significantly less likely to have a decreased score on the temporal orientation task, compared to those given a placebo.[1] The treatment included 3 mg of vitamin B6; 0.02 mg of vitamin B12; 0.56 mg of folic acid; and 600 mg of EPA plus DHA omega-3 fatty acids. Although no other significant effects on cognitive function were found, some disease history-specific and age-specific beneficial effects were reported. These results could be useful in interventions aimed at preventing cognitive decline in high-risk patients, the researchers concluded.

---

1 Andreeva, V. A., et al. "Cognitive Function After Supplementation with B vitamins and Long-Chain Omega-3 Fatty Acids; Ancillary Findings from the SU.FOL.OM3 Randomized Trial," *American Journal of Clinical Nutrition* 94(1): 278-286, May 18, 2011.

14. OTHER SUPPLEMENTS AND THERAPIES

Elsewhere in this book, I discuss a variety of vitamins, minerals, and herbs that are useful in dealing with dementia and Alzheimer's disease. Here are other supplements that may be beneficial.

MELATONIN

Lying in the center of the brain is the pineal gland, which is about the size and shape of a kernel of corn. It produces the hormone melatonin, however, the hormone declines with age. Of all the ills that accompany aging, perhaps the most feared is the loss of mental function. You can fight cancer and heart disease, but when you become senile, there is no "you" left to wage a good fight, explained Russel J. Reiter, Ph.D. and Jo Robinson.

But dementia is not the inevitable consequence of advanced years.[1] "In 1993, Italian gerontologists studied the mental functioning of 22 elderly people and 13 younger adults. They found a clear correlation between melatonin production and mental acuity. The better the patient performed on a test known as the Mini-Mental State Exam, the higher their levels of melatonin. A year later, Japanese researchers produced a similar finding. The elderly were producing more than twice as much melatonin as Alzheimer's patients of a similar age."

They go on to say that free radicals are believed to be a significant factor in the neuronal damage characteristic of Alzheimer's-

---

1 Reiter, Russel J., Ph.D., and Robinson, Jo. Your Body's Natural Wonder Drug: Melatonin. New York: Bantam Books, 1995, pp. 146ff.

type dementia. An indication that this is true is that tissue taken from the brains of Alzheimer's patients at autopsy contains higher levels of a by-product of lipid peroxidation. Since melatonin may be the body's most potent antioxidant, and it is one of the few antioxidants to penetrate the blood-brain barrier, a person with a deficiency in this protective hormone is likely to suffer a greater amount of free radical damage to the brain.

The blood-brain barrier is a barrier created by the modification of brain capillaries that prevents many substances from leaving the blood and crossing the capillary walls into brain tissues. "As we have shown..., melatonin causes a significant increase in glutathione peroxidase, another antioxidant for the protection of the brain," Reiter added.

Can melatonin extend human life? Reiter said that these are some of the possible mechanisms:
- Reducing free-radical damage.
- Stimulating an aging immune system.
- Protecting the cardiovascular system.
- Stabilizing the body's biological rhythms to help you sleep.
- Restoring the nightly cycle of rest and repair.
- Stimulating the production of growth hormone.

What are free radicals, which are mentioned often in this book? Because of stress, aging, infection, and other factors, chemical bonds become split to such an extent that a molecule is left with an unpaired electron, making it reactive and unstable, explained J. E. Williams, O.M.D. This is called a free radical.[1]

"Free radical molecules react with the first compatible molecule to restore their stability, altering the structure of both in the process," Williams added. "Normally the body has adaptive mechanism that automatically restore metabolic stability by providing extra molecules to neutralize free radicals. This neutralization process, the adding of electrons by taking one from another molecule, is called reduction, and it is the natural opposite pole of oxidation. The process is referred to as the oxidation-reduction cycle."

He added that free radical accumulation can be caused by exposure to pollution, radiation, smoke, stress, lack of exercise, or repetitively over exercising.

Even though tissue damage has begun, no specific disease is manifest, he continued. The person with active free radical pathology may only feel tired or vaguely not well, but the stage is set

---

1 Williams, J. E., O.M.D. Viral Immunity. Charlottesville, VA: Hampton Roads Publishing Co., Inc., 2002, p. 202.

for illness as a wide range of diseases, such as Alzheimer's disease, cancer, heart disease, allergies, cataracts, diabetes, macular degeneration, mental impairment, and most of the other chronic degenerative diseases.

In studying 11 nursing home residents suffering from dementia — mean age of 85 — most of them were given 3 mg of melatonin each evening. There were minimal side effects, but with a significant reduction in agitated behavior, and a significant decrease in daytime sleepiness. Improving sleep may help to reduce fatigue, and, therefore, reduce the symptoms of agitation, according to an article in Archives of Gerontology and Geriatrics.[1]

PHOSPHATIDYLSERINE (PS)

In evaluating elderly patients, 65 to 93 years of age, with cognitive decline, results showed that 300 mg/day of phosphatidylserine versus placebo brought improvements in both behavioral and cognitive parameters, according to Aging (Milano).[2]

In an article in Psychopharmacological Bulletin, 51 patients with Alzheimer's disease were treated for 12 weeks with bovine cortex phosphatidylserine at 100 mg 3 times daily, or a placebo. There were significant improvements in several cognitive measures in those treated with the supplement when compared with placebo, the researchers said.[3]

Derived from phospholipids, PS is thought to play a key role in the function of brain cells, thereby helping them to maintain or improve cognitive functions.[4]

T. H. Crook, who was involved with the just-named study, who, with the Memory Assessment Clinics in Bethesda, Maryland, in conjunction with researchers from Vanderbilt University School of Medicine in Nashville, Tennessee; Stanford University School of Medicine in Palo Alto, California; and a pharmaceutical company in Italy conducted a study involving 149 volunteers ranging in age from 50 to 75.

The volunteers were given 300 mg/day of PS (100 mg in 3 equal doses), versus a placebo group, for 12 weeks. Assessments were

---

1 Cohen-Mansfield, J., et al. "Melatonin for Treatment of Sundowning in Elderly Persons with Dementia: A Preliminary Study," Archives of Gerontology and Geriatrics 31: 65-76, 2000.

2 Cenacchi, T., et al. "Cognitive Decline in the Elderly: A Double-Blind, "Placebo-Controlled, Multicenter Study on Efficacy of Phosphatidylserine Administration," Aging (Milano) 5(2): 123-133, 1993.

3 Crook, T. H., et al. "Effects of Phosphatidylserine in Alzheimer's Disease," Psychopharmacological Bulletin 28(1): 61-66, 1992.

4 Murray, Frank. 100 Super Supplements for a Longer Life. (English and Chinese). New York: McGraw-Hill, 2000, pp. 282ff.

tabulated periodically during the study, as well as during a 4-week follow-up after the study ended. The researchers reported that PS was well tolerated, and, after 3 weeks of therapy, improvements had been recorded in learning names and faces, recalling names and faces, and recognizing faces.

Since this progress was not maintained throughout the 12 weeks of the study, the researchers segregated 57 people into a subgroup, who were considered more memory impaired. Average age was 64.3 years. While improving in the just-mentioned categories, the participants also exhibited a significant improvement with PS therapy in recalling telephone numbers, misplaced objects recall, paragraph recall (Wechsler Memory Scale-Logical Memory Subtest), and ability to concentrate while reading, conversing and performing tasks.

The researchers reported that the PS therapy had improved the subgroup's performance by an average of 2 points in their ability to learn names and faces, essentially "turning back the clock" roughly 12 years. In other words, from being a cognitive-age equivalent of a person of 64, these volunteers were restored, on average, to a cognitive age of 52.

HUPERZINE A (HUPA)

This is an extract from the moss Huperzia serrata, which grows at high elevations and in cold climates, according to Debasis Bagchi, Ph.D., and Jean Barilla, M.S. Known as Qian Ceng Ta, it has been used in Chinese folk medicine for centuries. In China, it was used to treat fever and inflammation, and, in recent years, it has been a prescription medication for treating dementia.[1]

Researchers claim that it helps to alleviate memory problems in the elderly, as well as those with Alzheimer's disease, the authors said. HupA, a lycopodium alkaloid, was first isolated from Huperzia serrata (also known as Lycopodium serratum) at the Zheijiang Academy of Medicine and Shanghai Institute of Materia Medica, Chinese Academy of Sciences, and by Dr. Alan Kozikowski at Georgetown University in Washington. D. C.

HupA, a selective cholinesterase inhibitor, has proven superior to other acetylcholinesterase inhibitors recommended for Alzheimer's disease, the authors continued. Cholinesterase is a family of enzymes that catalyzes (brings about) the hydrolysis of acylcholines.

---

1 Bagchi, Debasis, Ph.D., and Barilla, Jean, M.S. Huperzine A: Boost Your Brain Power. New Canaan, CT: Keats Publishing, Inc., 1998, pp. 29ff.

"Cholinergic mechanisms play a role in controlling cerebral blood circulation and blood flow," the authors said. "These mechanisms depend on adequate amounts of acetylcholine, which can act to dilate or constrict blood vessels, depending on where in the brain it is released. A deficiency of acetylcholine will prevent proper regulation of blood vessel size and result in impairment in brain function. As the loss of cholinergic function progresses, memory becomes increasingly impaired."

Huperzine A has gained considerable notice because of its unique anti-acetylcholinesterase activity, as well as memory-enhancing effects in a broad range of behavioral models, the authors added. It exhibits significant inhibition of acetylcholinesterase activity in all brain regions tested, including hippocampus, striatum, hypothalamus, and frontal cortex.

In a study published in Pharmacologica Sinica (12: 250-253, 1991), R. W. Zhang, et al., evaluated the therapeutic effects of HupA in 56 patients with multi-infarct dementia, which resulted from small strokes. The patients — 52 men and 4 women — were about 64 years of age. Also studied were 104 patients with senile and presenile memory disorders (58 men and 46 women).

The volunteers were divided into 2 smaller groups, with 1 group given HupA and the other serving as controls. The controls were treated intramuscularly with only a salt solution.

The intramuscularly dose of HupA for multi-infarct dementia was 50 mcg twice daily for 4 weeks. For senile and presenile simple memory disorders, the dosage was 30 mcg twice a day for 2 weeks. The supplement is also available in tablet form.

"The Weschler memory scale was used to determine whether there was improvement of memory function in the patients," the authors said. "Hup-A treatment significantly improved the memory of patients in both the Hup-A treatment groups, with minimal observed side effects."

The Chinese tea Huperizia serrata, which is grown in the mountains of China, has been reported to improve memory in the elderly, according to Medical Tribune. Huperzine A is a synthetic compound derived from the plant, and it may be beneficial for Alzheimer's disease and more effective than tacrine. Cognex, an anticholinesterase agent with nonspecific central nervous system stimulatory effects, and used in the early stages of Alzheimer's disease.[1] A pure form of the compound was tested in a Chinese study of about

---

1 Chinese Herbal Brew May Yield New Alzheimer's Drug," Medical Tribune, September 23, 1993, p. 6.

300 patients, and it was found to be effective, safe, and a promising candidate for the treatment of Alzheimer's disease.

Huperzine A increases acetylcholine levels in the brain and thus improves cognitive function, the publication said. Acetylcholine is a neurotransmitter which transfers nerve impulses across a synapse/juncture.

Fifty patients with Alzheimer's disease were given 4 tablets of HupA, and 53 others received 4 placebo tablets twice daily for 8 weeks, reported Chung Kao Yao Li Hsueh Pao, a Chinese publication.[1] Of those treated with the supplement, 58% showed improvement in memory, cognitive and behavioral functions.

As reported in Acta Pharmacologica Sinica, Xi-Can Tang of the Shanghai Institute of Materia Medica in China, found that HupA is a potent selective inhibitor of AchE (acetylcholinesterase), with rapid absorption and penetration into the brains of lab animals. In addition, HupA exhibited a broad range of memory-enhancing activities in the animals.[2]

At Mercy Medical Center in Rockville Center, New York, Alan A. Mazurck, M.D., conducted a study involving HupA patients with dementia and memory loss. In the trial, 22 patients were given 50 mcg of the supplement twice a day, 2 patients received 100 mcg twice a day, and 5 patients were increased to 100 mcg twice daily.[3]

Over half of the patients showed an improvement or an arrest of progression of their dementia, which represents a significant result, Mazurck said. While more studies are needed to determine the exact dosage, this therapy is clearly a major advancement in the treatment of dementia and memory loss, he said.

HupA has been used as a prescription drug in China since the 1990s, and it has reportedly been used by over 100,000 with no serious side effects, according to Natural Medicine Journal.[4]

When given at 200 mcg twice daily, HupA produced measurable improvements in memory, cognitive function, and behavioral factors in 58% of the Alzheimer's patients, which contrasted with only 36% showing improvement in the controls, the publication continued.

---

1 Xu, S. S., et al. "Efficacy of Tablet Huperzine A on Memory, Cognition, and Behavior in Alzheimer's Disease," Chung Kao Yao Li Hsueh Pao 16(5): 391-395. September 1995.

2 Tang, Xi-Can. "Huperzine A: A Promising Drug for Alzheimer's Disease," Acta Pharmacologica Sinica 17(6): 481-484, November 1996.

3 Mazurck, Alan A. "An Open Label Trial of Huperzine A in the Treatment of Alzheimer's Disease," unpublished, 1997.

4 "Huperzine A: A New Treatment for Alzheimer's Disease in China," Natural Medicine Journal, March 1999, p. 22.

PYCNOGENOL

As often reported, free radicals can damage cells and promote the aging process. However, Pycnogenol, a supplement made from French maritime pine bark extract, contains a natural complex of antioxidants that quenches these wayward chemicals.[1]

A research team used laboratory mice that age at an accelerated rate. Typically, these animals develop premature learning and memory problems, immune deficits, and abnormalities in blood-cell formation. The researchers compared aspects of aging in the mice who were given the supplement with those not given the therapy. Those given Pcynogenol for 2 months showed increases in antibody-forming cells, white blood cells, and blood-cell-forming activity in bone marrow. Those not given the supplement showed declines in these markers of aging. The supplement may slow the age-related declines in immunity and blood-cell formation, as well as restore these functions to more youthful levels, the researchers added.

Pcynogenols, from grapeseed skin or pine bark, are potent free radical scavengers, according to Julian Whitaker, M.D. The standard dosage of the extract should be 150 to 300 mg/day. This assumes that the extract has a procyanidin content of 85 to 95%.[2]

SAMe

Four patients with Alzheimer's disease participated in an open trial using S-adenosyl-L-methionine (SAMe), reported an article in the Journal of Clinical Psychopharmacology. The patients had been ill for 2 to 10 years, and they were randomly selected to alternately receive either 200 mg by intravenous bolus or 400 mg by intravenous infusion of SAMe between 10 and 11 a.m., daily, for 14 days.[3] The SAMe solution was prepared fresh daily, and. the therapy led to marked increases in membrane fluidity, the researchers said.

A study from Neurology found that cerebrospinal fluid (CSF) levels of SAMe in dementia and especially Alzheimer's disease patients were very low compared with neurologic controls.[4]

---

1 Lin, F. J., et al. "Pycnogenol Enhances Immune and Kaemopoietic Functions in Senescence-Accelerated Mice," Cellular and Molecular Life Sciences 54: 1168-1172, 1998.

2 Whitaker, Julian, M.D. Dr. Whitaker's Guide to Natural Healing. Rocklin, CA: Prima Publishing, 1995, pp. 356-357.

3 Cohen, B. M., et al. "S-Adenosyl-L-Methionine in the Treatment of Alzheimer's disease," Journal of Clinical Psychopharmacology 8(1): 43-47, February 1988.

4 Reynolds, E. H., et al. "S-Adenosylmethionine and Alzheimer's Disease," Neurology 39(Suppl. 1):397, March 1989.

Using 1,200 mg of SAMe daily for 3 months in 2 patients, and a double-blind crossover study using 1,200 mg of SAMe or a placebo for 3 months in 5 patients with AD, showed that SAMe improved measures of cognitive function as well as mood and speed of mental processing.

Oral SAMe was associated with a rise in CSF-SAM and monoamine metabolites, as well as an increase in red blood cell levels of folic acid, the B vitamin. Impaired methylation in the central nervous system may be a contributing factor in some forms of dementia, the researchers added. Methylation is the addition of methyl groups.

NADH

NADH is an enzyme helper that functions in oxidation/reduction actions in cells. NADH, which contains the B vitamin niacin (B3), assists dehydrogenase, a family of enzymes that removes hydrogen atoms from substances (oxidation).[1]

In a trial of 17 patients suffering from dementia of the Alzheimer's type in Vienna, Austria, 10 mg of nicotinamide adenine dinucleotide (NADH) was given daily in 5 mg tablets in the morning, 30 minutes before the first meal.[2] Based on the Mini-Mental Exam, the mean improvement was 8.35 points, according to Jorg G. D. Birkmayer, M.D., Ph.D. The improvement on the global deterioration scale had a mean value of 1.82. The therapy lasted from 8 to 12 weeks, and there were no side effects reported.

NADH plays a vital role in energy production, especially in the brain and nervous system, according to Earl Mindell, R.Ph., Ph.D. The more NADH, the greater the capacity of cells to produce energy.[3] He went on to say that many researchers believe that the loss of NADH as we age may promote diseases normally associated with brain aging, such as Alzheimer's disease and Parkinson's disease. Levels of NADH are 20 to 50% lower in Alzheimer's disease patients than in those of the same age who remain free of Alzheimer's.

In one study, Alzheimer's patients who received 10 mg of NADH daily showed a noticeable improvement in cognitive function and

---

1 Ronzio, Robert A., Ph.D. The Encyclopedia of Nutrition and Good Health. New York: Facts On File, Inc., 1997, p. 312.

2 Birkmayer, Jorg G. D., M.D., Ph.D. "Coenzyme Nicotinamide Adenine Dinucleotide: New Therapeutic Approach for Improving Dementia of the Alzheimer Type," Annals of Clinical and Laboratory Science 26(1): 1-9, 1996.

3 Mindell, Earl, R.Ph., Ph.D. Earl Mindell's Supplement Bible. New York: Simon & Schuster, 1998, pp. 108ff.

memory. The usually recommended dosage is two 5-mg tablets daily on an empty stomach.

For Alzheimer's disease, Robert C. Atkins, M.D., prescribed NADH with all degrees of memory loss, and he reported that a surprisingly high percentage of the patients regained at least some of their short-term memory.[1]

DHA

In evaluating 20 elderly people — average age of 83 — living in a home for the elderly, with mild to moderate dementia of cerebrovascular origin, 10 of the patients were given 6 capsules of docosahexaenoic acid (DHA) capsules containing 0.76 g/day of DHA for 1 year. Another 10 patients acted as controls, reported an article in Lipids.[2] In the DHA group, different mental assessment scores improved, but there was no change in the controls. There were significant differences in the dementia scores 3 to 6 months after DHA supplementation. Also, in the DHA patients, the content of DHA and eicosapentaenoic (EPA) acid increased without altering other fatty acid concentrations, including arachidonic acid. Red blood cell deformability significantly improved with DHA supplements, however, there was a positive correlation between blood levels of DHA/arachidonic acid ratios and dementia scores.

Arachidonic acid is a polyunsaturated fatty acid that is related to the hormone-like substances called prostaglandins and leukotrienes. It belongs to the omega-6 family of unsaturated fatty acids and they are derived from linoleic acid, an essential fatty acid.

DHA is a polyunsaturated fatty acid that is found in cold-water fish and fish oils. DHA belongs to the omega-3 family of fatty acids, and, together with EPA, reduce blood clot formation, among other things.

L-Arginine

At the Health Administration Center in Sapporo, Japan, Yoshinori Ohtsuka, M.D., Ph.D., evaluated 16 elderly patients (13 women and 3 men), with a mean age of 79, with cerebrovascular disease, who had been living in a nursing home for 2 to 4 years, according to an article in the American Journal of Medicine.[3]

---

1   Atkins, Robert C., M.D. *Dr. Atkins' Vita-Nutrient Solution*. New York: Simon & Schuster, 1998, p. 268.

2   Terano, T., et al. "Docosahexaenoic Acid Supplementation Improves the Moderately Severe Dementia from Thrombotic Cerebrovascular Disease," *Lipids* 34: 345S-346S, 1999.

3   Ohtsuka, Toshinori, M.D., Ph.D. "Effect of Oral Administration of L-Arginine on Senile Dementia," *American Journal of Medicine* 108: 439, April 1, 2000.

The patients were given the amino acid L-arginine at a dose of 1.6 g/day for 3 months. Results showed that lipid peroxide levels declined from 4.3 to 4.1 nmol/ml. Months later the mean level had increased to 4.9 nmol/ml.

Cognitive function increased in all the patients following the amino acid therapy from a score of 16 to 23, and returned to 17 by 3 months after the therapy ended. In general, the patients showed more expressive faces and quicker responses, and there were no side effects reported.

Low doses of L-arginine, a form of protein, at 2 g/day were effective in lowering lipid peroxidation. The author suggested that L-arginine increases nitric oxide as a neurotransmitter, increases brain blood flow due to increased nitric oxide levels, and reduces oxidative stress.

Ashwagandha

Ashwagandha root (Withania somnifera), an Ayurvedic medicine herb that grows in southern India, is used to treat dementia, asthma, bronchitis, psoriasis, arthritis, insomnia, and nervous exhaustion, reported Earl L. Mindell, R.Ph., Ph.D, and Donald. R. Yance, Jr.[1] The medication is used as a restorative tonic for those weakened by stress or long illness. It has long been recommended to promote growth, anti-anemic and anti-aging activity, and a general tonic to prevent disease.

Testosterone

Older men with lower levels of free testosterone, the male hormone, may be more likely to develop depression than are men with higher levels, according to Joan Stephenson, Ph.D.[2] An Australian study involved 4,000 men, ranging in age from 71 to 89, of whom 203 were diagnosed with depression. After controlling for such factors as education level and cognitive scores, the research team found that the odds of depression in men with free testosterone concentrations in the lowest quintile (less than 6 ng/dl) was almost 3 times higher than that of men with a free testosterone concentration of at least 10 ng/dl.

If the link between testosterone levels and depression is causal, older men with depression may benefit from systematic screening

1 Mindell, Earl, R.Ph., Ph.D., and Yance, Donald R., Jr., C.N. Dr. Earl Mindell's Russian Energy Secret. Laguna Beach, CA: Basic Health Publications, Inc., 2001, p. 17.

2 Stephenson, Joan, Ph.D. "Testosterone and depression," JAMA 299: 1764, 2008. (The Australian study originally appeared in Archives of General Psychiatry.)

of free testosterone concentrations and testosterone supplementation, the researchers said.

LIGHT THERAPY

There are studies that show that light therapy can help mitigate sleep problems. As reported in Family Practice News, in another study 27 women and 5 men — 65 to 90 years of age — with Alzheimer's disease, 15 received 1 hour of exposure to bright natural light each morning for 12 weeks, and 17 were exposed to only natural low-light conditions.[1] It was reported that there was a clear trend toward increased sleep efficiency, reduced nighttime wakefulness, and reduced nighttime activity in those receiving the light therapy, when compared to the controls.

In an article in the American Journal of Psychiatry, 10 Alzheimer's disease patients with sundowning behavior (delirium during the day or evening), and sleep disturbances were given 2 hours per day of exposure to bright light between 7 and 9 p.m., for 1 week.[2] Sleep-wakefulness on the evening nursing shift improved with light treatment in 8 of 10 patients, and there was a reduction in total daily activity occurring at nighttime during the light treatment week. The researchers agreed that the relative amplitude of the circadian locomotor activity rhythm increased during the light treatment week. Those with more severe sundowning at the beginning of the treatment had a greater clinical improvement. They added that evening bright light pulses may help to reduce sleep-wake cycle disturbances in some Alzheimer's disease patients. (Circadian refers to biologic variations or rhythms within a cycle of about 24 hours.)

---

1 Moon, M. A. "Light Therapy Aids Alzheimer's Sleep Disorders," Family Practice News, September 1, 2000, p. 16.

2 Satlin, Andrew, M.D., et al. "Bright Light Treatment of Behavioral and Sleep Disturbances in Patients with Alzheimer's Disease," American Journal of Psychiatry 49(8): 1028-1032, August 1992.

15. Avoid Toxic Metals and Pollutants

The jury is still sequestered as to whether or not aluminum contributes to Alzheimer's disease. However, data seems to suggest that it and other metals and pollutants are viable candidates.

Aluminum

Aluminum — alum, aluminum silicate, and sodium potassium aluminate — is a metallic ion that is widely distributed in water and soil, explained Robert A. Ronzio, Ph.D. Drinking water often contains aluminum in excess of levels leached from soil and clay, since aluminum hydroxide is often added to municipal water supplies to clarify drinking water.[1]

"Aluminum seems to accumulate in the brain with age, and high levels of the metal are found in the brains of those with Alzheimer's disease," Ronzio said. "Whether this is a cause or an effect of senility is not known, but a controversial report from Great Britain correlated the occurrence of Alzheimer's with the increased levels of aluminum in drinking water." Aluminum is widely found in foods and drugs, he continued. As an example, aluminum compounds make processed foods more creamy and pourable. They are found in infant formulas, pickles, relishes, beer, cream of tartar, grated cheese, canned foods, baking powder, self-rising flour, antacids (Maalox), over-the-counter analgesics (buffered aspirin).

---

1 Ronzio, Robert A., Ph.D. The Encyclopedia of Nutrition and Good Health. New York: Facts on File, Inc., 1997, p. 17.

The average daily intake from all sources ranges from 10 to 100 mg. Most of this is not absorbed but is excreted. "Accumulating evidence suggests that aluminum may be harmful," Ronzio continued. "It causes dialysis dementia, senility and brain damage in those undergoing hemodialysis for kidney failure. Excessive aluminum also impairs the body's immunity."

As reported in Mineral and Metal Neurotoxicology, the evidence for the association of Alzheimer's disease and aluminum includes:[1]

1. Cellular and biochemical changes occurring both in vitro (in the body) and in vivo (in lab glassware) tests at aluminum concentrations equivalent to those found in various subcompartments of the Alzheimer's diseased brain.

2. The slowing of clinical progression of Alzheimer's disease by desferrioxamine, a chelator drug which removes aluminum from the brain.

3. Epidemiological data which show an increased incidence of Alzheimer's disease in relation to the aluminum content of drinking water.

4. Neurotoxicologic studies and laboratory investigations utilizing experimental aluminum encephalopathy, on the learning and memory performance in test animals.

5. Similarities in the pathoclisis, the sites of toxic action of aluminum and the neocortical regions selectively affected by the Alzheimer's disease process.

Walter J. Lukiw, Ph.D., of Louisiana State University Medical Center in New Orleans, adds that aluminum has a wide array of adverse effects on the structural, biochemical, and genetic integrity of the central nervous system in mammals and humans. He said that our aging population at genetic risk for Alzheimer's disease may be prudent to limit their exposure to the metal.

While the role of aluminum toxicity in promoting Alzheimer's disease has been debated, there is a great deal of evidence that there is a connection, according to Robert M. Giller, M.D. and Kathy Mathews. Autopsies of those with Alzheimer's have revealed increased levels of aluminum as well as silicon.[2] "An extremely convincing argument for the role of aluminum in Alzheimer's is that patients who are undergoing kidney dialysis often develop 'dialysis dementia' as a combined result of using antacids contain-

---

1   Lukiw, Walter J., Ph.D. "Alzheimer's Disease and Aluminum," Mineral and Metal Neurotoxicology, Chapter 12: 113-126, 1997.

2   Giller, Robert M., M.D., and Matthews, Kathy. Natural Prescriptions. New York: Carol Southern Books, 1994, p. 10.

ing aluminum and elevated levels in the water used for dialysis," noted Giller. "While it is difficult to completely eliminate aluminum from your life, it is prudent to make an effort to avoid as many sources of the metal as possible."

Aluminum Products to Avoid

1. Aluminum cookware.

2. Antacids. Many antacids contain aluminum hydroxide, which is an aluminum salt. Di-Gel, Gelusil, Maalox, Mylanta, Riopan, and Rolaids have been reported to contain the metal. Dr. Giller does not recommend that you take antacids containing aluminum for your calcium supplementation. Read the labels, as there are many antacids that do not contain aluminum.

3. Buffered aspirin can contain up to 88 mg of aluminum per dose. Read the labels.

4. Douches can contain aluminum salts, and we do not know how much of these salts the body absorbs.

5. Medicines for diarrhea can contain up to 600 mg of aluminum salts. Check labels before you buy.

Aluminum is the most modern of common metals that is widely used in building materials and wrappings, food additives, aluminum-containing antacids, cooking utensils and other applications, reported an article in Epidemiology.[1]

A research team at Southampton General Hospital in the United Kingdom evaluated 106 men with Alzheimer's disease; 59 men with other dementing illnesses; 226 men with brain cancer; and 441 men with other diseases of the nervous system. The volunteers were between the ages of 42 and 75. The researchers reported that there was little association between Alzheimer's disease and higher aluminum or lower silicon concentrations in the drinking water when compared with controls. They added that the risk of Alzheimer's from aluminum in the drinking water at concentrations below 0.2 mg/liter is small.

The suggestion that aluminum is a cause in the development of amyloid plaques and neurofibrillary tangles and dementia in Alzheimer's disease originated in 1965, when animals were injected with aluminum compounds, which induced the formation of neurofibrillary tangles, according to H. M. Wisniewski and G. Y. Wen,

---

1 Martyn, Christopher N., et al. "Aluminum Concentrations in Drinking Water and Risk of Alzheimer's Disease," Epidemiology 8(3): 281-286, May 1997.

at the New York State Institute for Basic Research in Developmental Disabilities in Staten Island, New York.[1]

Some studies have suggested a relationship between amyotrophic lateral sclerosis (Lou Gehrig's disease), Guam Parkinsonian-dementia complex, and aluminum in the environment, the researchers said. They added that desferrioxamine has been used to slow the rate of cognitive decline in Alzheimer's patients, but this evidence is countered by studies of the pathology of AD and aluminum-induced encephalopathy, which indicates that the metal does not cause Alzheimer's neuropathology. However, they suggest that in cases of kidney failure, those undergoing dialysis, or those with a damaged blood-brain barrier, should control their intake of aluminum.

A research team at Argyll and Bute Hospital in Argyll, Scotland, evaluated 22 patients with alcoholic dementia, 20 with senile dementia of the Alzheimer's type, and 7 controls for blood levels of minerals.[2] They found that blood levels of cesium, which is used in photoelectric cells, were elevated in the alcoholic dementia patients when compared with the controls and those with Alzheimer's. Both blood and red-cell aluminum concentrations were higher in the alcoholic dementia patients compared with the controls.

In an article in the Journal of Clinical Epidemiology, a research team evaluated 130 Alzheimer's disease patients with matched controls concerning the aluminum content of antiperspirants and deodorants. They found no connection with Alzheimer's disease.[3] For aluminum-containing antiperspirants, the overall adjusted odds ratio was 1.6, with a trend toward a higher risk with increasing frequency of use. For antacids, regardless of their aluminum content, the overall adjusted odds ratio was 3.1. The researchers added that their study did not show consistent findings regarding the relationship between aluminum and Alzheimer's disease in the products they tested.

Researchers at Erasmus University Medical School in Rotterdam, The Netherlands, reported that for many decades aluminum has been a controversial potential risk factor for Alzheimer's disease. Epidemiologic data suggest that exposure to the metal from

---

1 Wisniewski, H. M., and Wen, G. Y. "Aluminum and Alzheimer's Disease," Aluminum in Biology and Medicine/CIBA Foundation Symposium 169, 1992, pp. 142-146.

2 Gibb, R. C, et al. "Elevation of Serum Cesium in Alcoholic Dementia," Trace Elements and Electrolytes 13(4): 205-208, 1996.

3 Graves, A. B., et al. "The Association Between Aluminum-Containing Products and Alzheimer's Disease," Journal of Clinical Epidemiology 43(1): 35-44, 1990.

drinking water is associated with an increased risk for the disease.[1] At first glance, they added, this is surprising since drinking water represents only a small percentage of one's total possible exposure to aluminum. At best, these investigations demonstrate an association, but do not establish cause and effect. However, it has been observed that the rate of decline of an untreated control group of Alzheimer's disease patients was twice as rapid as a control group treated with the drug desferrioxamine.

Many questions remain, they continued, but there is a strong indication that aluminum may be just one of several factors involved in the pathogenesis of Alzheimer's. Perhaps genetic or environmental factors, or a combination of both, are involved.

Tau is 1 of 6 isoforms of a family of proteins that are abundant in neural tissue, they continued. In Alzheimer's disease, there is a high concentration of the insoluble, highly-phosphorylated form of this protein that makes up the hydrophobic neurofibrillary tangles found in AD patients.

High concentrations of aluminum from poorly-treated drinking water can increase the risk of Alzheimer's disease by 2.6 times, according to the American Academy of Neurology.[2] Aluminum levels should not exceed 100 mcg/liter. However, there was no association found between AD and aluminum water levels less than 100 mcg/liter.

In a French study, 3,777 volunteers, 65 years of age or older, there was an inverse relationship between calcium levels in drinking water and cognitive impairment.[3] However, high levels of aluminum had an adverse effect when silica concentrations were low, but there was a protective effect when the pH and the silica levels were high. Aluminum concentrations in drinking water may be associated with a high risk of cognitive impairment only when the concentration of silica is low, they said.

Although the early chemists considered silica an elementary element, Antoine Lavoisier, in 1787, suspected that it was an oxide of an undiscovered element. In 1823, Jons J. Berzelius, the Swedish chemist, discovered the element, which he called silicon (from the Latin silex or silicis, meaning flint or hardness).[4]

1 Savory, John, Ph.D., et al. "Aluminum Tau Protein, and Alzheimer's Disease: An Important Link?" Nutrition 14(3): 313-314, 1998.
2 "Aluminum in Water and Alzheimer's Disease," American Academy of Neurology. Press release, March 5, 1996.
3 Jacquin-Gedda, Helene, et al. "Silica and Aluminum in Drinking Water and Cognitive Impairment in the Elderly," Epidemiology 7(3): 281-285, 1996.
4 Ensminger, A., et al. Foods and Nutrition Encyclopedia. Clovis, CA: Pegasus Press, 1983, p. 1994.

Human intake of silicon is said to be about 1 g/day. It is found in the fibrous parts of whole grains, liver, kidney, etc. However, much of silicon is lost in the refining of grains. It is rapidly excreted in urine and feces.

Silicon is most commonly found in the mineral silica, and silicon may have an important biological role in helping to prevent aluminum accumulation in organisms, according to The Lancet. Beer is a rich source of bioavailable silicon.[1] Drinking beer affected silicon status in 6 male volunteers, where it was found that 42 to 75% of the silicon was excreted within 8 hours of drinking 2 pints of beer. The authors suggest that beer drinking must be taken into consideration in the epidemiology of disease in which aluminum is thought to be a potential etiologic factor.

Using laboratory animals, a research team gave 450 mg/kg/day of aluminum nitrate nonahydrate by gavage (feeding tube) 5 days a week for 5 weeks. Animals were also given silicon in their drinking water. Aluminum levels for all tissues were significantly lower in the groups exposed to silica then in the positive control group. There were also significant reductions in urinary aluminum levels of these same groups.[2]

The study suggests that silicon effectively prevents gastrointestinal aluminum absorption, which may help protect against the neurotoxic effects of aluminum.

In one test, 3 healthy volunteers ingested aluminum alone (the controls), aluminum with oligomeric silica (17 mg), and aluminum with monomeric silica (17 mg). In a second study, 5 healthy volunteers consumed both forms of silica for a total of 34 g.[3] It was found that oligomeric silica reduced the availability of aluminum by 67%, compared with the control. Monomeric silica had no effect, since it was readily taken up from the gastrointestinal tract and rapidly excreted in the urine. On the other hand, oligomeric silica was not detectably absorbed or excreted. The researchers added that oligomeric silica has a soluble high-aluminum affinity and can reduce the aluminum availability from the human gastrointestinal tract. An oligomeric polymer contains only a few repeating units (less than 20). A monomeric polymer consists of a single component.

As reported in the New England Journal of Medicine, a 45-year-old man who was in rehabilitation for intravenous substance

---

1 Bellia, J. P., et al. "Beer: A Dietary Source of Silicon," The Lancet, January 22, 1994, p. 235.

2 Belles, M., et al. "Aluminum Accumulation in Rats: Relevance to the Aluminum Hypothesis of Alzheimer Disease," Alzheimer Disease Association Disord. 12(2): 83-87, 1998.

3 Jugdaohsingh, R., et al. "Oligomeric But Not Monomeric Silica Prevents Aluminum Absorption in Humans," American Journal of Clinical Nutrition 71: 944-949, 2000.

abuse was found with a 3-month history of seizures, incoordination, dysarthia (slurred speech), myoclonic jerks, postural tremor, emotional lability, and short-term memory loss.[1] He admitted that for 4 years he had been concentrating his methadone preparation, which was diluted with a grape-flavored drink, by heating it in an uncoated aluminum pot. He would then reconstitute the residue for intravenous injection.

Raymond L. Yong, M.D., and colleagues at the University of British Columbia in Vancouver, Canada, prescribed chelation therapy with a continuous intravenous infusion of desferrioxamine at a rate of 50 mg/hour. The procedure was stopped several times because of kidney dysfunction, but the condition improved with supportive measures and an adjustment in the infusion rate. "Our patient demonstrated the characteristic encephalopathy of aluminum toxicity, first described by A.C. Alfrey, et al.,"[2] the researchers said. "Other manifestations include microcytic anemia, adynamic bone disease, and osteomalacia (weakened bones). "Desferrioxamine is the only aluminum-chelating agent used routinely in patients undergoing dialysis. Desferrioxamine should be considered for the treatment of chronic aluminum toxicity in patients who are not undergoing hemodialysis.

Regarding Alzheimer's disease, aluminum may activate some processes, inhibit some enzymes, and cross-link macromolecules, reported Accounts of Chemical Research. The illness involves the formation of neurofibrillary tangles composed of paired heliofilaments, and these proteins involved in filament formation are perhaps hyperphosphorylated. It is well known that aluminum binds strongly with phosphates.[3]

Therefore, aluminum is an excellent candidate to promote the formation of the characteristic paired filaments that is seen in Alzheimer's disease, reported R. Bruce Martin, Ph.D., of the University of Virginia in Charlottesville.

LEAD

A research team at the University of Rhode Island at Kingston exposed Macaca fascicularis monkeys, from birth to age 400 days, to lead levels that produced no obvious signs of toxicity, according

---

1 Yong, Raymund L., M.D., et al. "Aluminum Toxicity Due to Intravenous Injection of Boiled Methadone," New England Journal of Medicine 354(11): 1210-1211, 2006.

2 Alfrey, A. C., et al. "The Dialysis Encephalopathy Syndrome Possible Aluminum Intoxication," New England Journal of Medicine 294: 184-188, 1976.

3 Martin, R. Bruce. "Abundance of Neurotoxic Products in Acid Rain," Accounts of Chemical Research 27: 204-210, 1994.

to the February 6, 2008 issue of the Journal of the American Medical Association.[1]

After about 23 years, examination of the brains of the lead-exposed monkeys showed many hallmarks of Alzheimer's disease, in spite of undetectable levels of lead in their blood. Brains of the animals contained neuronal plaques and neurofibrillary tangles, and exhibited increased expression of AD-related genes. This study suggests that lead exposure early in life may predispose animals to later neurodegenerative disease, possibly through alterations in DNA methylation and oxidation," reported Tracy Hampton, Ph.D.

MERCURY

At the University of Basel In Switzerland, blood mercury concentrations were measured in 33 Alzheimer's disease patients, and 45 age-matched controls with major depression, as well as a control group of 65 people with various nonpsychiatric disorders, reported the Journal of Neural Transmission.[2]

It was found that blood levels of mercury were over 2-fold higher in the AD patients, compared with both groups serving as controls. In early onset Alzheimer's disease, the mercury levels were almost 3-fold higher when compared with the controls. The increases were unrelated to the mercury in amalgam fillings and those with and without dentures.

These results indicated elevated blood levels of mercury in the Alzheimer's patients, and suggest that the increase in mercury is associated with high cerebral fluid levels of amyloid beta-peptide, the researchers added. The sources of the elevated blood levels of mercury may be an unidentified environmental source, or mercury may be released from brain tissue with advanced neuronal death.

According to researchers at the University of Calgary in Canada, it is well known that mercury vapor is continuously released from silver amalgam tooth fillings, and that it is absorbed into the brain.[3] Using laboratory rats, the animals were exposed to mercury vapor at concentrations present in the mouth and air of some humans with many amalgam fillings. During the exposure, average rat brain concentrations increased significantly 11- to 47-fold during the mercury vapor exposure. It was found that a neurochem-

---

1   Hampton, Tracy, Ph.D. "Alzheimer Disease Trigger," JAMA 299(5): 513, 2008.
2   Hock, C., et al. "Increased Blood Mercury Levels in Patients with Alzheimer's Disease," Journal of Neural Transmission 105: 59-68, 1998.
3   Pendergrass, James C, et al. "Mercury Vapor Inhalation Inhibits Binding of GTP to Tubulin in Rat Brain Similarly to a Molecular Lesion in Alzheimer Diseased Brains," Neurotoxicology 18(2): 315-324, 1997.

ical lesion occurred that was similar to that seen in Alzheimer's brain homogenates (mixtures).

TRACE MINERALS

In an article in Neurotoxicology, a research team evaluated the hair and nails of 180 Alzheimer's patients and compared them with controls. Alzheimer's patients had significant imbalances in bromine, calcium, cobalt, mercury, potassium, and zinc, and bromine was elevated in hair, nails, and brain of the AD patients.[1] Levels of calcium and cobalt in hair were decreased in the Alzheimer's patients, while mercury was decreased in these patients when compared to controls. It was also found that potassium levels were elevated in the nails of AD patients compared with controls, while zinc levels were raised in the hair and nails of the patients compared with controls.

In studying subcellular fractions of Alzheimer's disease brains, elevated bromine and mercury, and reduced rubidium, selenium, and zinc, were found in the brains of AD patients compared with controls, according to an article in Brain Research.[2] It was also reported that there were increased ratios of mercury/selenium, mercury/zinc, and zinc/selenium in the brains of AD patients. Selenium and zinc may play a protective role against mercury toxicity, and they may be used to detoxify mercury in AD brains. Mercury could well be an important toxic element in AD disease, they said.

Chronic poisoning from occupational inhalation or skin absorption of mercury (paints, household items, pesticides, etc.) can cause a metallic taste, oral inflammation, blue gum line, extremity pain and tremor, weight loss, and mental changes (depression and withdrawal).[3] In studying 7 brain regions from 58 Alzheimer's disease patients and 21 controls, there were statistically significant elevations of iron and zinc in multiple regions of the AD brain compared to controls, according to Neurotoxicology.[4] Mercury elevation in Alzheimer's disease brains was found in most regions that were studied, but the high variability of mercury levels in both AD and the controls prevented the AD-control difference from reaching statistical significance.

1 Vance, D. E., et al. "Trace Element Imbalance in Hair and Nails of Alzheimer's Disease Patients," Neurotoxicology 19(2): 197-208, 1998.
2 Wenstrap, D., et al. "Trace Element Imbalances in Isolated Subcellular Fractions of Alzheimer's Disease Brains," Brain Research 533: 125-131, 1990.
3 Stevens, Mark A., editor. Merriam-Webster's Collegiate Encyclopedia. Springfield, MA: Merriam-Webster, Inc., 2000, p. 1052.
4 Cornett, C. R., et al. "Imbalances of Trace Elements Related to Oxidative Damage in Alzheimer's Disease Brains," Neurotoxicology 19(3): 339-346, 1998.

Selenium, which is a protective agent against mercury toxicity, was considerably elevated in only the AD amygdala, the researchers added. Increased amounts of iron and zinc in AD brains may enhance neurodegeneration through free-radical damage. Amygdala is an almond-shaped mass of gray matter in the anterior extremity of the temporal lobe.

Environmental Pollutants

In evaluating data from 3 independent studies on the association between occupations with probable medium to high exposure to extremely low frequency (less than 300 Hz), electromagnetic fields, and sporadic Alzheimer's disease, Eugene Sobel, M.D., and colleagues at the University of Southern California Medical School in Los Angeles, found the odds ratio for women was 3.8.[1]

The predominant occupations with this type of exposure were seamstresses, dressmakers, and tailors. The researchers said that these electromagnetic fields may adversely influence calcium homeostasis (balance) and/or inappropriately activate the immune system cells, such as microglial cells (cellular elements in the central nervous system), which initiate events that result in neuronal degeneration.

Alzheimer's may be, in part, an autoimmune disorder initiated by chronic inflammatory processes because the plaques have been found to contain monocytes and macrophages. In an autoimmune disease (arthritis, lupus, etc.) the body simply attacks its own tissues.

As reported in Occupational Environment and Medicine, there is no support for the hypothesis that occupational exposure to solvents is a cause of dementia.[2] Researchers evaluated 204 cases of dementia, 225 controls with brain cancer, and 441 other controls. Those with dementia had less often worked as a painter or printer, and they were less likely to have worked for more than 1 year as a printer, painter, launderer, or at a dry cleaning establishment.

A research team from the University of Washington at Seattle, headed by Walter A. Kukull, evaluated 23,000 people, 60 years of age or older, and found 193 cases of Alzheimer's disease. There were 243 controls who were free of dementia or neurological dis-

---

1 Sobel, Eugene, M.D., et al. "Occupation with Exposure to Electromagnetic Fields: A Possible Risk Factor for Alzheimer's Disease," American Journal of Epidemiology 142(5): 515-524, 1995.

2 Palmer, K., et al. "Dementia and Occupational Exposure to Organic Solvents," Occupational Environment and Medicine 55(10): 712-715, 1998.

ease.[1] They reported a history of exposure to 1 or more solvents yielded an Alzheimer's disease odds ratio of 2.3. This ratio went up to 6.0 only in men. They concluded that past exposure to organic solvents may be associated with the onset of Alzheimer's disease.

Commenting on the study, Olav Axelson of University Hospital in Linkoping, Sweden, said that, while Kukull's study is potentially important, there is room for doubt regarding the validity of the AD-solvent connection.[2] The author is concerned about selection bias in their recruitment of both participants and controls. This does not necessarily mean lack of validity in that the results are misleading, but perhaps further studies may be needed, he said.

Also commenting on the Kukull study, Margrit L. Bleecker, M.D., of Children's Hospital in Baltimore, Maryland, said that heavy alcohol consumption seemed to have a strong effect on solvent-related mental disorders.[3] High cumulative exposure to organic solvents can result in adverse signs and symptoms in the central nervous system, but it is controversial as to whether or not low-level occupational solvent exposure is associated with definitive central nervous system disorders. (The central nervous system consists of the brain and spinal cord.)

Neurobehavioral changes associated with solvent exposure are primarily due to membrane alterations to contrast to Alzheimer's disease, where the cognitive decline is related to synaptic and neuronal loss that produce a depletion in cholinergic markers, she added. However, intracellular neurofibrilliary tangles and amyloid deposits in the brain that are required for the definitive diagnosis of AD are not found in the brain after chronic solvent exposure.

The numerous risk factors associated with Alzheimer's disease suggest a combination of genetic factors and environmental exposures as the most likely etiologies. Since solvents are used in adhesives, glues, coatings, degreasing and cleaning agents, and some paints that are in most households, she suggests the Kukull findings are premature. However, these findings are noteworthy, but, until replicated, they are not a cause for alarm, she said.

More than 9 million workers are exposed to solvents in the workplace, so the potential for the development of significant psychiatric disorders is significant, according to Psychosomatic Med-

---

1 Kukull, Walter A., et al. "Solvent Exposure As a Risk Factor for Alzheimer's Disease: A Case-Control Study," American Journal of Epidemiology 141(11): 1059-1071, 1995.

2 Axelson, Olav. "Invited Commentary: Possibility That Solvent Exposure Is A Risk Factor for Alzheimer's Disease," ibid, pp. 1075-1079.

3 Bleecker, Margit L. "Invited Commentary: Solvent Exposure As a Risk Factor for Alzheimer's Disease: A Multiple Insult Hypothesis," ibid, pp. 1072-1074.

icine.[1] The study involved 33 men and 5 women (mean age of 43.8 years and 12.2 years of education), who were exposed to solvents, compared with 23 men and 16 women without a history of chemical exposure (mean age of 40.1 years and 13.4 years of education). It was found that 71% of those exposed to solvents met the criteria for Diagnostic and Statistical Manual of Mental Disorders, 4th Edition, Axis 1 disorder, compared with 10% of the controls.

Anxiety and mood clusters were the most prominent diagnosis in the exposed individuals, according to Lisa Morrow, Ph.D. Also, 36% of the exposed volunteers met the criteria for a dual diagnosis of mood and anxiety disorder.

As reported in Quarterly Journal of Medicine, there are some studies suggesting that patients with organic brain disease all had a history of prolonged heavy exposure to commonly used organic solvents.[2] People in industries such as carpet layers and painters are exposed to levels of solvent vapor throughout their working lives. These organic solvents include carbon tetrachloride, trichloroethylene, and methylbutylketone, which have known nervous system toxicity.

A Swedish study found that those with previous neuropsychiatric diagnosis were at a greater risk to solvent exposure. In another study, those with organic brain disease were found to have greater risk from past solvent exposure than controls with psychiatric disease. An excess of motor neuron disease deaths has been recorded in leather workers and their wives.

While the author is not suggesting that organic solvents are responsible for all unexplained neurologic disease, the evidence is accumulating that long-term exposure may play a part. The author, who is with the University Medical School in Aberdeen, United Kingdom, encourages physicians and neurologists to take an occupational history of their patients, and take seriously any occupational exposure to organic chemicals in those with neurologic disease.

---

1 Morrow, Lisa, Ph.D., et al. "Increased Incidence of Anxiety and Depressive Disorders in Persons with Organic Solvent Exposure," Psychosomatic Medicine 62: 746-750, 2000.
2 Seaton, A. "Organic Solvents and the Nervous System: Time for a Reappraisal?" Quarterly Journal of Medicine 84(305): 637-639, September 1992.

16. DRUGS: THE GOOD, THE BAD AND THE UGLY

Even medications approved by the Food and Drug Administration for the treatment of dementia may produce little, if any, clinically meaningful benefit. The most recent FDA review shows that these drugs pass muster statistically, on scales that measure patients' cognitive function, but that is not the whole story.[1]

Results of the review, originally published in the Annals of Internal Medicine, point to an urgent need for more thorough, independent research on the pharmacologic treatment of dementia. Guidelines based on the review advise physicians that because evidence is scant, the drugs should not be used routinely for patients with dementia. "The decision to initiate therapy should be based on individual assessment," said Amir Qaseem, M.D., Ph.D., senior medical associate in clinical programs and quality of care at the American College of Physicians. "The benefits of treatment may be very modest, or there may be none at all." Qaseem added that there are public health concerns about dementia, as the leading edge of the baby-boom generation approaches 65, since the prevalence of Alzheimer's disease is expected to quadruple in the next 50 years, to 1 in 45 Americans. Drugs can often alleviate symptoms, but there is no cure.

The guidelines focus on the 5 medications that are approved for the treatment of dementia, Voelker continued. Four are cholinesterase inhibitors (donepezil, galantamine, rivastigmine, and tacrine). The fifth is the neuropeptide-modifying agent memantine.

---

1 Voelker, Rebecca. "Guideline: Dementia Drugs' Benefits Uncertain," JAMA 299(15): 1763, 2008.

Sales of the 5 drugs were just shy of $3 billion in 1997. Donepezil and memantine accounted for 85% of the sales, while tacrine Cognex has fell out of favor because of its damaging side-effects, Voelker said.

Kenneth Schellhase, M.D., of the Medical College of Wisconsin at Milwaukee, advised physicians to weigh potential benefits against adverse side-effects and. the cost of the medications. Depending on the patient's insurance, a 1-month supply of donepezil or memantine costs between $150 and $160. Qaseem and Schellhase added that current studies do not address how long the medications should be taken or which patients may derive more benefit from a specific drug. Unfortunately, there are no head-to-head trials that compare the drugs with one another.

Ronald Petersen, M.D., Ph.D., of the Alzheimer's Association Medical and Scientific Advisory board, said that, "we have the choice of a few drugs that are modestly effective. We need not only to learn more about existing drugs, but also to develop new ones that prevent neuronal (nerve) damage from deposits of amyloid protein in the brain....This is almost reaching a crisis proportion," added Petersen, who is also director of the Mayo Clinic Alzheimer's Disease Research Center in Rochester, Minnesota. "If nothing is done to delay the onset and slow the progression of dementia, it alone will bankrupt the health-care system."

Medications for high blood pressure may also reduce the risk of Alzheimer's disease.[1] A research team, headed by Peter P. Zandi, M.D., of Johns Hopkins University in Baltimore, Maryland, followed over 3,300 people, over 65 years of age, for 6 years, obtaining information on mental status and the use of drugs for high blood pressure. Of the group, 104 developed Alzheimer's. "Taking any drug to reduce blood pressure — enzyme inhibitors, beta blockers, calcium channel blockers, and diuretics — was associated with a 36% decrease in the risk of Alzheimer's," said Bakalar.

Diuretics (water pills) were associated with a greater risk reduction at 43%. One drug, potassium-sparing diuretics, was associated with the greatest risk reduction — 74% — compared with those who took no blood pressure medication. Analysis showed that the results were independent of the medicines' ability to control blood pressure, and the researchers were uncertain why the water pills proved so effective.

---

1 Bakalar, Nicholas. "For Blood Pressure, and Maybe Alzheimer's, Too, New York Times, March 21, 2006, p. F6.

In the study, originally appearing in Archives of Neurology in May 2007, the researchers acknowledge that the study has limits, especially because it is observational in nature, which studied patients over time, as opposed to a controlled experiment.

"Our findings raise an interesting hypothesis that needs to be investigated further before we can make conclusive recommendations as to what people should or should not be taking," Zandi added. "But the study raises the possibility that taking potassium-sparing diuretics may reduce the risk of Alzheimer's."

The introduction of the first antipsychotic drug, chlorpromazine (Thorazine), into clinical practice over 50 years ago revolutionized psychiatry and neurology, according to Peter V. Rabins, M.D., and Constantine G. Lyketsos, M.D., of Johns Hopkins Medical Institutions at Baltimore, Maryland. The efficacy of the drug and. other drugs in the phenothiazine class demonstrated that a disease considered a "mental illness" could respond to a biologically mediated therapy, and this heralded the introduction of other neuromodulating therapies, such as levodopa for Parkinson's disease.[1] "Since their introduction, however, the phenothiazines and other antipsychotic neurologic agents have raised challenging questions about their adverse effects and toxic effects," the authors said. "Skeptics of the effectiveness of antipsychotic drugs in schizophrenia suggested that sedation rather than a direct drug action was causing patients to report fewer symptoms."

When caring for a patient with dementia, who develops psychotic symptoms or aggressive behavior, a clinician needs to evaluate other aspects of the case. First, etiologies other than dementia need to be considered. Delirium, untreated or undertreated medical illnesses, overmedication, environmental triggers, lack of engaging activities, and misinterpretation of disease symptoms are among the potential etiologies of such behaviors and symptoms. Since all have specific approaches, they should be considered when symptoms initially develop.

Second, clinicians should consider the risk/benefit ratio for each patient. For example, patients with hallucinations and delusions that are neither distressing nor placing them or others at risk or harm should not be treated with antipsychotic drugs.

Third, once antipsychotic drugs have been prescribed, careful assessment and documentation of the need for continued care is necessary.

---

1   Rabins, Peter V., M.D., and Lyketos, Constantine G., M.D. "Antipsychotic Drugs in Dementia: What Should Be Made of Risks?" JAMA 294(15): 1963-1965, 2005.

The Omnibus Budget Reconciliation Act (OBRA) of 1987 require such a reassessment in long-term care, but the need for medication continuation should be regularly reassessed and justified for all individuals, the authors continued. Given the high rates of dementia in assisted living homes, similar practices should be instituted in those settings as well.

"In their study, Schneider, et al.[1] raise an important issue that requires further research," the authors added. "Could the increased morbidity and mortality they found also occur in other groups of frail individuals exposed to this or other classes of drugs?" This hypothesis, they said, is plausible enough that immediate attention should be given to answering it. Unfortunately, the paucity of long-term data will limit the ability to study this question for many classes of drugs in the near future. International efforts are needed to improve long-term monitoring for adverse events and for research into the important questions raised by this meta-analysis.

A majority of elderly patients with dementia develop aggression, delusions, and other neuropsychiatry symptoms during their illness, reported Lon S. Schneider, M.D., and colleagues, at Keck School of Medicine, University of Southern California in Los Angeles (previously discussed).[2] "Antipsychiatric medications are commonly used to treat these behaviors, along with psychosocial and environmental interventions," Schneider said. "These drugs have been the mainstay of psychopharmacological treatment for this purpose during the last several decades, in spite of their clear overuse in the 1980s, and Federal regulations implemented in the early 1990s requiring their oversight and monitoring in nursing homes."

In the last decade, he added, the newer atypical antipsychotic drugs (risperidone, olanzapine, quetiapine, and aripiprazole) have largely replaced the older conventional or first-generation antipsychotic drugs (haloperidol and thioridazine), and have been considered preferred treatments for these behavioral disturbances associated with dementia. "Reasons for this preference include emerging clinical trials evidence, perceived relative safety advantages compared with older antipsychotic drugs, and other medications, the opinions of expert clinicians, and expectations of efficacy," Schneider added. "There is little clinical trial evidence supporting the efficacy of other classes of psychotropic medication, such as benzodiazepines, anticonvulsants, and antidepressants, for the treat-

---

1 Risk of Death with Atypical Antipsychotic Drug Treatment for Dementia: Meta-Analysis of Randomized Placebo-Controlled Trial," JAMA 294: 1934-1943, 2005

2 Schneider, Lon S., M.D., et al. "Risk of Death with Atypical Antipsychotic Drug Treatment for Dementia," JAMA 294(15): 1934-1943, 2005.

ment of aggression, psychotic symptoms, or agitation in patients with dementia."

"As a meta-analysis (a compilation of studies), our findings emphasize the need to consider certain changes in some clinical practices," Schneider continued. "Antipsychotic drugs have been dispensed fairly frequently to patients with dementia and used for long periods. The established risk for cerebrovascular adverse events together with the present observations suggest that antipsychotic drugs should be used with care in these patients."

The fact that excess deaths and cerebrovascular adverse events can be observed within 10 to 12 weeks of initiating medication, coupled with observations from individual clinical trials results that there is substantial improvement in both drug and placebo groups during the first 1 to 4 weeks of treatment, lead to the consideration that antipsychotic drugs should be prescribed and dosage adjusted with the expectation of clinical improvement within that time. If improvement is not observed, the medication should be discontinued.

A research team at the University of Texas Southwestern Medical Center in Dallas, evaluated 140 patient charts from the Center for Alzheimer's and Related Diseases at the University of Texas for the frequency of cognitive decline after exposure to anesthesia.[1] They found that 10% of the patients had evidence of acute and persistent post-operative decline in cognitive function. The type of surgery did not appear to be related to cognitive decline. The study supports other published reports which note that exposure to anesthesia may unmask, or accelerate, the symptoms of dementia in a subgroup of elderly people.

COX-2 specific inhibitors may have a role in treating and preventing Alzheimer's disease, reported John Schiezer in Medical Tribune. He quoted Patrick McGeer, M.D., of the University of British Columbia in Canada, as saying that, "what we are after in dealing with Alzheimer's is to reduce the inflammation in the brain. There is strong data that the classical NSAIDs (nonsteroidal anti-inflammatory drugs) will work in this disease, but physicians are afraid of gastrointestinal side effects."[2]

Added Preston Mason, Ph.D., of MCP Hahnemann School of Medicine in Pittsburgh, Pennsylvania, COX-2 inhibitors appear

1 Brewer, Karen K., Ph.D., et al. "Anesthesia Exposure As a Possible Risk Factor for Cognitive Decline in the Elderly," Facts and Research in Gerontology, 1996, pp. 161-171.

2 Schlezer, John. "COX-2 Inhibitors May Help Treat Alzheimer's," Medical Tribune 40(16): 2, September 23, 1999.

promising because they may slow some of the inflammatory responses that mediates the damage in Alzheimer's.

McGeer and his colleagues used various procedures to evaluate the expression of cyclooxygenase COX-1 and COX-2 in brain and peripheral organs in Alzheimer's disease patients and controls. They said that both COX-1 and COX-2 expressed in all organs tested, including the brain, heart, liver, kidney, spleen, and intestine. They reported their findings at the 9th International Congress of the International Psychogeriatric Association in Vancouver, Canada, in 1999.

Atypical antipsychotic drugs appear to increase the risk of venous thromboembolism among the elderly, according to Archives of Internal Medicine. While these episodes may be rare in clinical practice, the risk should be weighed against the effectiveness of these medications in the elderly population, the researchers said.[1]

In the study, venous thrombosis was associated with 77.6% of events and 22.4% were pulmonary embolisms. The rate of hospitalization for VTE was increased for those using atypical antipsychotic drugs, including risperidone, olanzapine, clozapine, and quetiapine fumarate. No increased incidence was found for the phenothiazines or other conventional agents.

In the Journal of Leukocyte Biology, it was reported that Alzheimer's disease may have a strong inflammatory component produced locally by brain cells which may be responsible to nonsteroidal anti-inflammatory drugs.[2]

Epidemiological data suggest that NSAIDs will reduce the risk of Alzheimer's disease by 50%. Anti-inflammatory agents cannot be expected to reverse Alzheimer's, but they should be considered in cases with mild-to-moderate symptoms or in those at genetic risk for the disease, the researchers said.

Patients with Alzheimer's disease commonly exhibit psychosis and behavioral disturbances that impair patient functioning, create caregiver distress, and lead to institutionalization, according to Archives of General Psychiatry. The study was conducted to assess the efficacy and safety of olanzapine in treating psychosis and/or agitation/aggression in Alzheimer's patients.[3]

1 Liperoti, R., et al. "Venous Thromboembolism Among Elderly Patients Treated with Atypical and Conventional Antipsychotic Agents," Archives of Internal Medicine 165: 2677-2682, 2005.

2 McGeer, P. L., and McGeer, E. G. "Inflammation of the Brain in Alzheimer's Disease: Implications for Therapy," Journal of Leukocyte Biology 65: 409-415, April 1999.

3 Street, Jamie S., et al. "Olanzapine Treatment of Psychotic and Behavioral Symptoms in Patients with Alzheimer Disease in Cursing Care Facilities: A Double-Blind, Randomized, Placebo-Controlled Trial," Archives of General Psychiatry 57: 968-976, 2000.

The double-blind, 6-week study involved 206 elderly nursing home residents with Alzheimer's disease, who exhibited psychotic and/or behavioral symptoms.

The researchers reported that low doses of the drug (5 to 10 mg/day) produced significant improvement when compared with placebo. No significant cognitive impairment was observed.

Common side effects of olanzapine (Zyprexa) include drowsiness, headache, dizziness, constipation, dry mouth, blurred vision, and runny nose, according to Prescription & Over-the-Counter Drugs. However, serious side effects, which should be reported to your doctor, include stiffness, shuffling gait, difficulty swallowing or speaking, persistent, uncontrolled chewing, lip-smacking, tongue movements, and fever, the publication added.[1]

Some Alzheimer's disease experts are suggesting hitting the disease hard and early with a "cocktail" approach combining 3 or 4 different types of medication, reported John Schlezer in Medical Tribune.[2]

Speaking at the 9th International Congress of the International Psychogeriatric Association in Vancouver, BC, Canada in 1999, George Grossberg, M.D., of St. Louis University School of Medicine in Missouri, explained that the cocktail approach involves daily treatment with a cholinesterase inhibitor, vitamin E, and either NSAID or COX-2 inhibitor. For women, estrogen replacement therapy was suggested.

Grossberg added that Alzheimer's patients can be managed on combination therapy in much the same way as HIV/AIDS patients. Doses and types of medications are tailored to the individual.

He mentioned 3 cholinesterase inhibitors — tacrine, donepezil, and rivastigmine, and, at the time of his presentation, 2 others — faeantamine and metrifonate — which were expected to be approved. "Although the cocktail approach cannot halt disease progression in either AIDS or Alzheimer's, it may moderate progression," Grossberg said. "The treatments improve quality of life and may buy people more quality time."

Added Davis Parks, M.D., who treats geriatric patients, "while all the data are certainly not in, multiple drug therapy for Alzheimer's disease is an intriguing concept."

One drug that hampers the relentless assault of late-stage Alzheimer's disease has been popular in Europe and is now available

---

1 Visalli, Gayla, project editor. Prescription & Over-the-Counter Drugs. Pleasantville, NY: The Reader's Digest Association, Inc., 1998, p. 563.

2 Schlezer, John. "Cocktail Approach Advised to Hit Alzheimer's Disease Hard," Medical Tribune 40(16): 2, September 23, 1999.

in the United States, according to Nathan Seppa in Science News. Memantine (previously mentioned) helps patients who were previously considered untreatable.[1] An early study that showed that memantine might slow late-stage Alzheimer's disease came from a 1999 report in Latvia. To corroborate that finding, Barry Reisberg, M.D., of the New York University School of Medicine, and colleagues, recruited 181 people with advanced Alzheimer's disease who lived at home with a caregiver and who retained some capacity to speak, dress themselves, and handle other daily chores. The researchers then gave memantine pills to 97 of the patients and a look-alike substance to 84 others. "After 28 weeks, the scientists found that the group getting the drug was faring significantly better than the other patients, according to 4 of 7 standard measurements of mental function," Seppa reported. "The tests gauged the patient's ability to dress, bathe, use the toilet, and participate in other common activities. Information supplied by the caregivers said that the drug-tested patients required, on average, 56 hours less assistance per month than the other patients did." Reisberg added that memantine should be complementary or even synergetic with currently prescribed drugs, since it, rather than affecting acetylcholine, inhibits the action of glutamate, a brain chemical that runs amok in Alzheimer's patients.

"Normally, glutamate binds to docking sites on neurons to initiate a signal," Seppa added. "Overstimulation of the binding sites in Alzheimer's patients kills neurons. This cell death contributes to the memory lapses and confusion seen in these patients. By occupying docking sites on the neurons, memantine prevents glutamate from binding and over stimulating the cells."

A new class of drugs is being investigated to avert aging, heart disease, diabetes, cancer, and neurodegenerative disorders.[2] By suppressing the common killers of age, the drugs, which are sirtuin activators, are designed to prolong both health and lifespan. One such drug, resveratrol, is an ingredient in red wine. (See the separate chapter.)

Initial research was done by Leonard Guarente of Massachusetts Institute of Technology in Boston, and a group of his former students, several of whom are at odds about their efficacy. "The drugs are designed to mimic the effects of caloric restriction, a low calorie but healthful diet known to make lab mice live longer and

1 Seppa, Nathan. "Progress Against Dementia: Drug Slows Alzheimer's in Severly Ill Patients," Science News, April 5, 2003, pp. 211-212.
2 Wade. Nicholas. "Aging Drugs: Hardest Test Is Still Ahead," New York Times, November 7, 2006, pp. F1, F4.

more healthily, but it is too hard for all but the most ascetic of humans to keep to it," Wade said.

At least 2 companies, Elixir Pharmaceuticals and Sirtris, are trying to develop drugs based on the potential of resveratrol, a sirtuin activator found in supplements.

The original supporters of the potential new chemical disagree about the mechanism of calorie restriction, since their research has concentrated on yeast. Both man and mice possess a gene called SIRTI, which is the counterpart to the Sir-2 gene, Wade continued. But man and mice have also evolved 6 extra SIRT genes — SIRTS 2 to 7, which seem to perform related tasks.

"The protein enzyme made by the genes are known as sirtuins, a word biologists have derived, with a simplicity likely to make etymologists wince, from Sir-2," Wade added.

A special property of the SIRT1 gene is to increase the number of mitochondria produced by neurons, and Jill Milne of Sirtris discussed this at a meeting on the molecular genetics of aging. With extra energy, brain cells may be better able to ward off neurodegenerative diseases like Alzheimer's, Wade said. The sirtuins might also improve memory, stated David Sinclair, M.D., another promoter of resveratrol. "The body's metabolism is governed by such a complex array of genetic circuits that it will be years before the role of the 7 SIRTs is fully understood," Wade concluded. "But if they really embody an ancient mechanism for fortifying the body against disease, then all that is needed is a safe drug that tricks the SIRT genes into thinking feast is famine. The theory is enticing, even if sirtuins and certainty still lie far apart."

Resveratrol is a phenolic compound in wine that may have cardioprotective benefits, according to Biotechnology Letters. It is especially present in the skin of grapes, and the authors suggest that a strain of yeast should be chosen that has alcohol-producing ability, but only slightly reduces the concentration, of resveratrol.[1]

Resveratrol, found only in red wine and peanuts, may be the agent that reduces the biological processes that are risk factors for cardiovascular disease, reported David M. Goldberg of the Banting Institute in Toronto, Canada.[2]

Resveratrol has antifungal properties, antioxidant activity, and it may increase HDL-cholesterol, the beneficial kind, according to

---

1 Vacca, Vincenzo, et al. "Wine Yeast and Resveratrol Content," Biotechnology Letters 19(6): 497-498, 1997.

2 Goldberg, David M. "More on Antioxidant Activity of Resveratrol in Red Wine," Clinical Chemistry 42(1): 113-114, 1996.

Emilio Celotti and colleagues at Universitta degli Studi di Padova in Italy.[1]

To explain the French paradox with regards to wine consumption, it has been suggested that antioxidants in wine — resveratrol, quercetin, and epicatechin — may reduce LDL-cholesterol oxidation, the bad kind, according to an article in The Lancet.[2]

The authors report that red and white wine are excellent sources of salicylic acid, and its metabolites have proven to be vasodilators and have anti-inflammatory properties. Even in white wines the total amount of these compounds per liter of wine is on the average equivalent to almost double the widely recommended daily dose of 30 mg of aspirin to maintain cardiovascular wellness, reported C. J. Muller and colleagues at California State University in Fresno. As we know, salicylic acid is a component of aspirin.

Muller goes on to say that there are synergistic effects between antioxidants and the wine's salicylic acid components. Detoxicification of ethanol (alcohol) to acetate by the liver produces reducing equivalents such as reduced nicotinamide-adenine dinucleotide (NAD). These reducing equivalents may aid in maintaining ingested antioxidants in their reduced state as well as recycling spent antioxidants, he continued.

Researchers continue to recommend NSAIDs as therapy for Alzheimer's disease patients, but many of the studies gloss over the side-effect of these anti-inflammatory drugs.

Ibuprofen, one of the most common NSAIDs, is available in numerous formulations, including Advil, Excedrin IB, Genpril, Haltran, Ibu-tab, Ibuprin, Ibuprohm, Medipren, Midol-200, Motrin, Nuprin, Pamprin IB, Rufen, Salatar, and Trendar, according to Prescription & Over-the-Counter Drugs.[3]

The drug works by interfering with the formation of prostaglandins, substances that cause inflammation and make nerves more sensitive to pain impulses.

"Do not take the drug with aspirin or any of the NSAIDs without your doctor's approval," the publication said. "Also consult your doctor if you are taking antihypertensives, steroids, anticoagulants, antibiotics, itraconazole or ketoconazole, plicamycin, penicillamine, valproic acid, phenytoin, cyclosporine, digitalis drugs,

---

1　Celotti, Emilio, et al. "Resveratrol Content of Some Wines Obtained from Dried Valpolicella Grapes — Fecioto and Amarone," Journal of Chromatography 730: 47-52, 1996.

2　Muller, C. J., and Fugelsang, K. C. "Take Two Classes of Wine and See Me in the Morning," The Lancet 343: 1428-1429, 1994.

3　Visalli, Gayla, project editor. Prescription & Over-the-Counter Drugs. Pleasantville, NY: The Reader's Digest Association, Inc., 1998, p. 406.

lithium (used during World War II as a salt substitute), methotrexate, probenecid, triamterene, or zidovudine."

Serious side effects include shortness of breath or wheezing, with or without swelling of legs or other signs of heart failure; chest pain; peptic ulcer disease with vomiting of blood; black, tarry stools; or decreasing kidney function. If you experience any of these conditions, call your doctor immediately. Other common side-effects include nausea, vomiting, heartburn, diarrhea, constipation, headache, dizziness, and sleepliness. Less common side-effects are ulcers or sores in the mouth, depression, rashes or blistering of the skin, ringing in the ears, unusual tingling or numbness of the hands and feet, seizures, and blurred vision. You may have elevated potassium levels and decreased blood counts.

About 30% of nursing home residents are on antipsychotic drugs, according to the Centers for Medicare and Medicaid Services. Most of them are given newer drugs called atypical antipsychotics.

In her print dress and coral lipstick, Mrs. F. J., who is 71, can almost pass for a staff member at Cobble Hill Health Center in Brooklyn, New York. "You have to sit and eat," she tells a fellow patient. The former manager of a local hospital, she is now a patient in the Alzheimer's unit.[1] She has been stricken with an advanced form of dementia that sometimes renders her confused, fretful, and combative. Not long ago, the staff would have given her a powerful antipsychotic drug to calm her. "Use of a new generation of antipsychotic drugs to control the behavior of dementia patients has surged in recent years," the Wall Street Journal reported, "despite the FDA's 'black box' warning labels that these drugs can increase the risk of death for elderly dementia patients."

The patient is now part of an experiment at the New York facility to wean patients off antipsychotics, Lagnado continued. The staff has figured out that when she became distraught, the best way to calm her down is to have her do what she loved to do when she was well: work. Simple tasks such as setting the table give her a renewed sense of purpose and calm.

There are few effective medicines to manage the outbursts of Alzheimer's patients who strain the resources of those trying to maintain order in nursing facilities. "Federal law strongly discourages nursing homes from physically tying down unruly patients," Lagnado continued. "But Federal health-care programs such as

---

1 Lagnado, Lucette. "Nursing Homes Struggle to Kick Drug Habit," The Wall Street Journal, December 20, 2007, pp. 1, A14.

Medicaid do pay for drugs that may help calm aggressive behavior and agitation associated with Alzheimer's."

In 2005, Medicaid spent $5.4 billion on atypical antipsychotic medicines, more than it spent on any other class of drugs, including antibiotics, AIDS drugs, or medicines to treat high blood pressure. Atypical antipsychotics are approved for schizophrenia and bipolar disorder, but in what is known as "off label" use, doctors often prescribe the drugs to elderly patients with dementia.

According to the Centers for Medicare and Medicaid Services, almost 21% of nursing-home patients who don't have a psychotic diagnosis are on antipsychotic drugs, Lagnado added. A 2005 study, published in Archives of Internal Medicine, found antipsychotics were prescribed not only for psychosis, but also for depression, confusion, memory loss, and. feelings of isolation, reported Becky Briesacher, the lead researcher. Family members can object to the use of drugs, but they risk having the facility threaten to discharge their relative on grounds that they pose a danger to themselves and others.

At Providence Rest Nursing Home, Bronx, New York, alternative procedures, such as massages and aromatherapy, are being used to calm distraught Alzheimer's patients. The facility, with 200 patients, is run by an order of nuns, and they have brought its overall reliance on antipsychotics down to 2% over the last few years, and down to zero among patients not considered psychotic.

Serena Ferguson, a physician who took care of her mother at home for years, reported that her mother would pace and wander and try to leave the apartment. It was difficult to get her to sleep, and Dr. Ferguson had to place herself by the door so that her mother wouldn't slip out. Atypical psychotics were the only way to keep her mother safe. Her mother was transferred to Cobble Hill, where she remained on the antipsychotic drug Seroquel (AstraZeneca Pharmaceuticals), but the facility decided to wean her mother off of the drug. At the time of the article, her mother had been off the drug for 11 months, and she has been getting stimulation from music and dancing. She loved to go to the Savoy Ballroom in Harlem, New York. But "not all cases work out," Lagnado said. "Some patients relapse. Others are taken off drugs and still suffer from symptoms of their brain disorder."

It is no longer news that elderly patients with Alzheimer's disease, dementia, and other mental illnesses, who are confined to hospitals and nursing homes, are overmedicated to quiet them down. The mixture of untested drugs, accompanied by ominous side effects, plus an improper diet, insure that the patients have a slim chance of recovering. Perhaps some of the geriatric wards should have a skull and crossbones posted at the door.

"The use of antipsychotic drugs to keep down the agitation, combative behavior, and outbursts of dementia patients has soared, especially in the elderly," reported Laurie Tarkan in the New York Times. "Sales of newer antipsychotics like Risperdal, Seroquel, and Zyprexa totaled $13.1 billion in 2007, up from $4 billion in 2000, according to IMS Health, a health-care information service."[1] A 2006 study of Alzheimer's patients found that for most patients, antipsychotics provided no significant improvement over placebos in treating aggression and delusions, Tarkan said.

In 2005, the Food and Drug Administration ordered that the newer drugs carry a "black box" label warning of an increased risk of death. More recently, the Agency issued a similar warning of the labels of older antipsychotics. "These antipsychotics can be overused and abused," commented Johnny Matson, M.D., of Louisiana State University. "And there is a lot of abuse going on in a lot of these places."

The first generation of antipsychotics, such as Haldol, carry a significant risk of repetitive movement disorders and sedation, Tarkan added. Second-generation antipsychotics, also called atypicals, are more commonly prescribed because the risk of movement disorders is lower. But they, too, can cause sedation, and they contribute to weight gain and diabetes.

If patients are prescribed an antipsychotic, it should be a very low dose for the shortest period necessary, explained Dillip V. Jeste, M.D., of the University of California at San Diego. Although it can take weeks or months to control behavior, the patient can often be weaned off of the drugs or kept at a very low dose.

"Some experts say another group of medications — antidementia drugs like Aricept, Exalon, and Menamda — are underused," Tarkan continued. "Research shows that 10 to 20% of Alzheimer's patients had noticeable positive responses to these drugs, and 40% more showed some cognitive improvement, even if not noticeable to an observer." Common side effects of the antipsychotic drugs include ministrokes, reparable brain hemorrhage from a mild bump on the head, hypothyroidism, malnourishment, depression, and sleep disorders, Tarkan added.

---

1 Tarkan, Laurie. "Doctors Say Medication Is Overused in Dementia," The New York Times, June 24, 2008, pp. Fl, F6.

A research team at the University of Newcastle in the United Kingdom decided to assess sudden death that has been linked to antipsychotic therapy. Their study, published in the British Journal of Psychiatry, involved psychiatric in-patients dying suddenly in 5 hospitals in the northeast of England, who were matched with surviving controls for age, gender, and mental disorder.[1] Sixty-nine case-control clusters were identified, and the probable sudden unexplained death was significantly associated with high blood pressure, heart disease, and current treatment with Thioridazine. The psychiatric drug was the main reason for the sudden unexplained death, with the likely mechanism being drug-induced arrhythmia or irregular heartbeat.

A research team from the Montreal General Hospital found that elder abuse and neglect are common among patients referred to geriatric psychiatry services, and that such facilities should have access to multidisciplinary expertise and resources to deal with abuse, and that certain situations may signal higher risk.[2]

Drug abuse by those with severe mental disorders is a significant public health problem for which there is no empirically validated treatment, according to researchers in the Archives of General Psychiatry.[3] In the study, volunteers were randomly assigned to 6 months of treatment with either the Behavioral Treatment for Substance Abuse in Severe and Persistent Mental Illness (BTSAS), or a manualized control condition, the Supportive Treatment for Addiction Recovery (STAR).

Treatment was conducted in a community-based outpatient clinic and a Veterans Affairs medical center in Baltimore, Maryland. Patients were 129 outpatients addicted to cocaine, heroin, or cannabis (marijuana), with a serious mental illness.

The researchers found that the BTSAS program was significantly more effective than STAR in the percentage of clean urine test results, survival in treatment, and attendance at the sessions. The BTSAS program also had significant effects on important community functioning variables, including hospitalization, money available for living expenses, and quality of life.

"While the BTSAS program is an efficacious treatment protocol, additional work is needed to increase the proportion of eligi-

---

1 Reiley, J. G., et al. "Thioridazine and Sudden Unexplained Death in Psychiatric In-Patients," British Journal of Psychiatry 180: 515-522, 2002.

2 Vida, Stephen, et al. "Prevalence and Correlates of Elder Abuse and Neglect in a Geriatric Psychiatry Service," Canadian Journal of Psychiatry 47: 459-467, 2002.

3 Bellack, A. S., et al. "A Randomized Clinical Trial of a New Behavioral Treatment for Drug Abase in People with Severe and Persistent Mental Illness," Archives of General Psychiatry 63: 426-432, 2006.

ble patients who are able to become engaged in treatment," the researchers added.

The trial of a drug that was expected to help Alzheimer's disease patients Fluruzan — has been halted, because it did not improve thinking ability by a statistically significant amount when compared with a placebo, reported Andrew Pollack in the July 1, 2008 issue of the New York Times.[1]

Fluruzan was similar to ibuprofen in that patients could take it in larger doses without causing gastrointestinal complaints. The drug was designed to inhibit the formation of amyloid beta 42, which is a protein called a peptide. It was developed from a larger protein called amyloid precursor protein by an enzyme called gamma secretase. Fluruzan was designed to interfere with the enzyme.

Phase 3 of the trial involved almost 1,700 patients with mild Alzheimer's disease, who were treated for 18 months with either the drug or a look-alike pill. It was designed to prevent the build-up of toxic amyloid plaques in the brain. "Such plaques are the focus of the leading theory for the cause of Alzheimer's disease, but the drug's failure may cast some new doubt on that theory, as well as on other experimental drugs designed to block amyloid plaques," Pollack said.

Meanwhile, Eli Lilly & Company is in late-stage testing of a drug that works similarly to Flurzan by inhibiting the build-up of gamma secretase. And Wyeth and Elan are in late-stage clinical trials of a drug that attempts to clear amyloid plaques from the brain in a different manner. While there were mixed results in a middle-stage study, the results were encouraging enough for the companies to move into final-stage testing, Pollack added.

Older people who are taking drugs to lower their cholesterol and reduce the risk of heart attacks, may also reduce their risk of developing Alzheimer's disease and dementia by one-half, reported Mary Haan, M.D., of the University of Michigan School of Public Health in Ann Arbor.[2]

The theory is that statins improve, help and provide some benefit in preventing dementia, Haan said.

Speaking at an Alzheimer's disease seminar in Chicago, Illinois, Aber-Claude Wischik, M.D., reported that early trials suggest that a new drug could be at least twice as effective as current medi-

1 Pollack, Andrew. "Myriad Genetics Stops Work on an Alzheimer's Drug," The New York Times, July 1, 2008, p. C4.
2 Burke, Cathy. "Surprise Alzheimer's Find," New York Post, July 29, 2008, p. 9.

cines in slowing the progression of Alzheimer's disease.[1] The drug, called Rember, slowed cognitive decline by 81%, Wischik told the conference. Rember is said to be the first drug to act on a protein, tau, that helps brain cells keep their structure and communicate with each other. As we know, in people with dementia this protein becomes tangled and results in brain cell death. Wischik added that, "this is an unprecedented result in the treatment of Alzheimer's disease. We have demonstrated for the first time that it may be possible to arrest progression of the disease by targeting the tangles which are highly correlated with the disease."

Scientists from Germany and Denmark may be able to predict new uses for existing drugs by taking a closer look at the medications' adverse effects, reported Joan Stephenson, Ph.D., in the Journal of the American Medical Association.[2] "Adverse effects are often triggered when a medication interacts with proteins other than the drug's intended target," she said. "Reasoning that chemically dissimilar drugs with similar adverse effects might sometimes act on the same target proteins, the researchers reviewed drug-package inserts of 746 marketed drugs and developed a computational method to compare 'side-effect similarities' of various drugs."

As an example, they found that donepezil, used to treat Alzheimer's disease, had adverse effects in common with the antidepressant venlafaxine, suggesting that donepezil might be of use to patients with depression.

Observational studies have suggested a reduced risk of Alzheimer's disease in those using nonsteroidal anti-inflammatory drugs. To evaluate the effects of naproxen sodium Aleve and Celecoxib on cognitive function, a research team did a randomized, double-masked chemoprevention trial using the drugs at six U.S. memory clinics.[3] Participants were men and women 70 and older with a family history of Alzheimer's disease. Of the 2,528 enrolled in the study, 2,117 had follow-up cognitive assessment. The volunteers were given 200 mg of celecoxib twice daily; 220 mg of naproxen sodium daily; or a placebo. They were then subjected to 7 tests of cognitive function and a global summary score that was measured annually. The researchers reported that the 2 drugs did

---

1 Carvel, John. "Treatment Heralds Alzheimer's Breakthrough," The Guardian, July 30, 2008, p. 16.

2 Stephenson, Joan, Ph.D. "Drugs' Adverse Effects," JAMA 300(7): 782, 2008.

3 ADAPT Research Group. "Cognitive Function Over Time in the Alzheimer's Disease Anti-Inflammatory Prevention Trial (ADAPT): Results of a Randomized, Controlled Trial," Archives of Neurology 65(7): 896-905, 2008.

not improve cognitive function, although there was weak evidence for a detrimental effect of naproxen.

The Food and Drug Administration has warned physicians that using conventional antipsychiatric drugs to treat elderly patients with dementia may increase the risk of death in these patients, according to Bridget M. Kuehn in the July 23/30, 2008 issue of the Journal of the American Medical Association.[1]

Under the new authority granted to the agency by the Food and Drug Administration Amendment Act of 2007, the FDA is insisting that manufacturers of conventional antipsychiatrics — prochlorperazine, haloperidol, loxapine, thioridazine, molindone, thiothixene, pimozide, fluphenazine, trifluoperazine, chlorpromazine, and perphenazine — to add a boxed warning to the labels notifying doctors that using conventional antipsychotics to treat behavioral problems in elderly patients with dementia is related to an increased risk of death.

Kuehn added that the FDA is also requiring manufacturers of atypical antipsychotics to revise the existing boxed warning on aripiprazole, clozapine, ziprasidone, paliperidone, risperidone, quetiapine, olanzapine, and a combination drug containing olanzapine and fluoxetine. "Antipsychotic drugs are not approved by the FDA for the treatment of patients with dementia, but these drugs are commonly used off-label to treat dementia-related psychosis in elderly patients."

A 2005 warning on atypical antipsychotics was based on an FDA meta-analysis of 17 placebo-controlled trials of olanzapine, aripiprazole, risperidone, or quetiapine in elderly patients with dementia and behavioral problems. This study found that over the 10-week trials, patients taking these drugs had a 4.5% risk of dying, while those given a placebo had a 2.6% risk of dying, according to Constantine G. Lyketsos, M.D., of the Johns Hopkins Bayview Medical Center in Baltimore, Maryland.

Kuehn went on to say that doctors treating elderly patients with dementia-related psychosis face difficult choices, since antipsychotics have been a mainstay of treatments, although demonstrating only modest effects.

"There is little evidence supporting the effectiveness of other psychotropic medications, although Lyketsos said that a recent analysis found that such drugs as selective serotonin reuptake inhibitors and anticonvulsants are not associated with an elevated mortality risk in this population (Kales, H. C., et al., Ameri-

---

1 Kuehn, Bridget M. "FDA: Antipsychotics Risky for Elderly," JAMA 300(4): 379-380, 2008.

can Journal of Psychiatry 164(10): 1568-1576, 2007)." Lyketsos added that behavioral interventions may work in some cases, but few facilities know how to implement them. "It's a huge problem because we are sort of stuck. The behavioral problems are not going away and they carry their own risks of mortality and morbidity, and we don't know how to treat them safely."

Writing in the New England Journal of Medicine, Gary W. Small, et al.[1] discussed the use of positron-emission tomography (PET) after injection of a drug FDDNP to estimate the risk of Alzheimer's disease in those with mild cognitive impairment. This report raises the question of the clinical criteria for the diagnosis of the disease, commented P. Murali Doraiswamy, M.D., of the Duke University Medical Center in Durham, North Carolina.[2] "The current criteria of the National Institute of Neurological Disorders and Stroke — Alzheimer's Disease and Related Disorder Association for diagnosing Alzheimer's disease clinically are 20 years old," Doraiswamy said.

If FDDNP-PET is validated, it poses several questions, he continued. For example, which tests are best? FDDNP-PET, Pittsburgh Compound-B PET, magnetic resonance spectroscopy, functional magnetic resonance imaging, cerebrospinal fluid biomarkers, and computerized memory tests, appear to help the diagnosis, but few studies have systematically compared these tests.

Also, how do we measure the cost-effectiveness of the markers? Is it fair to require that a marker for the diagnosis of early Alzheimer's disease improve patients' quality of life or long-term outcomes when we do not have drugs to prevent or halt the disease?

The safety of using intravenous FDDNP will be of great importance, yet there is little in the Small report that addresses questions about safety, added Gordon J. Gilbert, M.D., of St. Petersburg, Florida.[3]

For example, were there any apparent side effects? What is the fate of the brain-attached FDDNP? What effects do the drug and its metabolites have on the brain? How long does FDDNP remain attached to the targets — tau and amyloid — and how does this interaction affect their degradation or metabolism, or the integrity of the surrounding neurons and glia? And, most important, did the cognitive status of the patients and controls deteriorate or im-

---

1   Small, Gary. W., et al. "PET of Brain Amyloid and Tau in Mild Cognitive Impairment," New England Journal of Medicine 355: 2652-2663, 2006.

2   Doraiswamy, P. Murali, M.D. "PET Scanning in Mild Cognitive Impairment," New England Journal of Medicine 356(11): 1175, 2007.

3   Gilbert, Gordon J., M.D. ibid.

prove during the days, weeks, or months after injection of FDDNP? (Glia are supporting tissue.)

In response, Small, et al., of David Geffen School of Medicine at UCLA in Los Angeles, California[1], said that screening "brain checks" might be used to identify candidates for treatments that would hold brain protein deposits at bay, in order to delay the on-set of Alzheimer's disease, just as we use blood cholesterol levels to identify candidates for cholesterol-lowering drugs, in order to stave off stroke or heart disease. "Validated surrogate markers do lead to new definitions of disease, such as hypertension or hypo-thyroidism, and in the case of neurodegeneration, we may eventu-ally abandon old terminology and technology for diagnosing Al-zheimer's disease," the researchers added.

They agreed that further study will help to elucidate the effi-cacy and effectiveness of noninvasive techniques such as FDDNP-PET, but in vivo brain imaging of amyloid and tau deposits may still be useful for diagnosis and for treatment monitoring, even if these proteins are not found to cause Alzheimer's disease.

As for safety, they continued, only nanomole quantities of FDDNP are needed for detection of PET, and estimates of toxicity have confirmed the safety of the compound for these studies. "Only four people had minor adverse events during PET scanning — 2 people had minor bruising at venipuncture sites, and 2 had tran-sient headaches — and these events did not differ from those ob-served in other PET studies," the researchers said.

About 3% of the injected dose of FDDNP reaches the brain, which is similar to the percentage of the dose of many experimen-tal receptor-labeling probes used with PET, they continued.

"The short radioactive half-lives of these probes and the very low mass administered will most likely make them safe for use in humans," they said. "No effects on brain tissue in either animals or humans have been observed with any of these probes. As expected, FDDNP Injections have had no known effect on cognitive status during the days, weeks, or months after administration."

Each year, tens of millions of prescriptions are dispensed in the United States, and billions are spent for antithrombotic medica-tions (a substance that prevents blood clots) and acid-suppress-ing drugs, reported Rebecca Voelker in the August 12, 2009 issue of the Journal of the American Medical association.[2]

---

1 Small, G. W., et al., ibid. pp. 1175-1176.
2 Voelker, Rebecca. "Common Drugs Can Harm Elderly Patients," JAMA 302(6): 614-615, 2009.

While both drugs are considered safe and effective, new studies add to growing evidence that elderly patients can be at particular risk for upper gastrointestinal (GI) tract bleeding from combination antithrombotic therapy or hip fracture from prolonged use of acid suppressors, Voelker continued.

At a Digestive Disease Week meeting in June 2009 in Houston, Texas, researchers from Michael E. DeBakey VA Medical Center discussed how risky it is for elderly patients with myocardial infarction (heart attack), stroke, or peripheral vascular disease to take 2 or 3 antithrombotic drugs — aspirin, anticoagulations, or antiplatelets — as secondary cardioprophylaxis.

Neena Abraham, M.D., and colleagues, analyzed data from 78.08 patients aged 65 and older. Of the total, 40.4% received combination antithrombotic therapy, and 4% had GI bleeding. "Findings showed that those who took an anticoagulant-antiplatelet combination had a 70% increased risk of upper GI bleeding," Voelker added. "Those who received aspirin and an antiplatelet (platelets are blood constituents) were 2 and 2½ times more likely to have upper GI bleeding, while aspirin and an anticoagulant produced nearly a 3-fold increased risk." She added that those who took all 3 types of drugs had a 4-fold increase in risk, while patients who took triple therapy, the unadjusted incidence rate of upper GI bleeding was 5.3 events per 1,000 person-years.

Abraham added that the elderly often have more difficulty recovering from adverse events than do younger adults. As an example, there is a big difference between a serious, massive GI bleed, in a 75-year-old versus a 45-year-old.

Laurie Jacobs, M.D., of Albert Einstein College of Medicine of Yeshiva University in New York, said that intracranial bleeding linked with antithrombotics was what most concerned physicians. Intracranial bleeding is either a cause of death or of terrible morbidity, she added.

In a case-control study with 33,752 cases and 130,471 controls, patients who took a proton pump inhibitor (PPI) for at least 2 years had a 30% increased risk of hip fractures, according to Douglas Corley, M.D., of Kaiser Permanente in San Francisco, California. In addition, those who took a histamine-2 (H2) receptor antagonist for at least 2 years had an 18% increased risk of hip fracture. H2 is a powerful stimulant of gastric secretion, and a vasodilator that causes a fall in blood pressure. Corley estimated that about 25% of the U.S. population takes acid suppressors, at least intermittently. Some people are started on them and then kept on them.

Jane Potter, M.D., of the University of Nebraska at Omaha, added that elderly patients who take PPIs should take a supplement of calcium citrate — not calcium carbonate — because only the citrate form is absorbed when gastric acid levels are low.

A closely watched Phase III clinical trial for Dimebon, a drug for Alzheimer's diseaee, failed to show a significant effect, reported Greg Miller in the March 12, 2010 issue of Science.[1] The drug was catapulted into the limelight with a spectacularly successful trial published in The Lancet in 2008. Dimebon, an antihistamine introduced in Russia in 1983, was promoted by scientists at the Institute of Physiologically Active Compounds in Chernogolovka, Russia. In experiments, the drug improved the performance of memory-impaired rats, and a pilot study with 14 Russian Alzheimer's patients revealed encouraging results in a 2001 paper published in the Annals of the New York Academy of Sciences.

A San Francisco biotech firm, Medivation, recruited top scientists to design a larger clinical trial. "The new trial, despite a design almost identical to that of the Lancet study, yielded dramatically different results," Miller said. "It enrolled 598 patients with mild to moderate Alzheimer's. However, this time there were no significant differences between Dimebon and placebo groups." In the meantime, Medivation and Pfizer are continuing with 3 Dimebon trials for Alzheimer's disease and Huntington's disease. "I don't think the drug is dead and buried, but we need to get some clarity or good news soon," said Samuel Gandy, an Alzheimer's researcher at Mount Sinai.

An ongoing investigational intervention study utilizing naturally occurring antibodies in human blood has preserved the thinking abilities of some mild to moderate-stage Alzheimer's patients over 18 months, as well as reducing the rate of atrophy (shrinkage) of their brains.[2] An Alzheimer's disease patient's brain shrinks 3 to 4 times faster than a healthy brain because of accelerated brain cell death. This shrinkage of brain tissue causes the fluid-filled ventricles at the center of the brain to enlarge at a faster rate than a normal brain.

Ongoing trials are underway at 35 academic centers in the United States that belong to the Alzheimer's Disease Cooperative Study (ADCS). An additional 12 sites in the U.S. and Canada are being evaluated. The drug is Gammagard from Baxter Interna-

---

1   Miller, Greg. "The Puzzling Rise and Fall of a Dark-Horse Alzheimer's Drug," Science 327: 1309, March 12, 2010.

2   "Investigational Immune Intervention Slows Brain Shrinkage in Alzheimer's Disease Patients," Science Daily, April 14, 2010.

tional, Lt. Dosages range from 0.2 g/kg every 2 weeks to 0.8 g/kg monthly.

Another drug, Intravenous Immune Globulin (IVIg) has been used to treat autoimmune and immunodeficient diseases. The substance targets the amyloid beta peptide associated with Alzheimer's disease.[1]

To learn the location of a test center, and how you can participate in the study, contact NIAs Alzheimer's Disease Education and Referral (ADEAR) Center at 1-800-438-4380. The e-mail address is adearnia.nih.gov.

The brain is the most cholesterol-rich organ in the body; therefore, cholesterol is required for healthy brain function. The body requires about 2,000 mg/day of cholesterol to survive. If this amount is not obtained from the diet, the body manufactures the difference.

A research team has demonstrated that in insulin-deficient mice, there is a reduction in the regulation of cholesterol metabolism — SREBP-2 and its genes — in the hypothalamus and other areas of the brain, leading to a reduction in brain cholesterol synthesis and synaptosomal cholesterol content.[2] These changes are partly due to the direct affects of insulin to regulate these genes in neurons and glial cell, and they can be corrected by intracerebroventricular injections of insulin. This synthesis may play a significant role in the neurologic and metabolic dysfunction found in Alzheimer's disease and other disease stages.

This research may well lead to drugs that halt or slow the development of metabolic diseases such as Alzheimer's disease, Parkinson's disease, type 2 diabetes, etc. Diabetes can damage many parts of the body, which leads to a loss of vision and sensation, strokes, and heart attacks.[3]

Almost 73,000 Americans die annually from diabetes, making it a leading cause of death. Diabetes is also associated with impaired cognitive function and increased risk for dementia, including Alzheimer's disease.

---

1 "Intravenous Immune Globulin (IVIg) Study," The Gammaglobulin Alzheimer's Partnership Study, undated.
2 Suzuki, Ryo, M.D., et al. "Diabetes and Insulin in Regulating of Brain Cholesterol," Cell Metabolism 12(6): 567-579, December 1, 2010.
3 "Diabetes, the Brain, and Cognition," Brain Briefing, February 2008.

17. The Value of Red Wine

Resveratrol, one of the beneficial nutrients in red wine, is posed to become the "Nutrient of the Decade".

There is growing evidence that red wine, in spite of its alcohol content, is very beneficial to health. Research suggests that red wine can prevent platelets from sticking to arterial walls. It has been found that 2 glasses of red wine daily can significantly reduce the adherence of platelets in both human and animal studies.[1]

Furthermore, Resveratrol supplements are now on the market, and new studies are being conducted as this is written. An advantage of the supplement is that you sidestep the alcohol in wine, which can be a problem for some people.

Now, it is true that there are questions about the so-called French Paradox (in which Frenchmen eating a high-fat diet and drinking wine have the lowest incidence of heart disease of any industrialized nation, except Japan[2]). A study in the British Medical Journal threw cold water on that theory, saying that the French showed lower rates of heart disease not because of wine consumption, but because of a lag time in data collection.[3] The British researchers contend that deaths from heart disease in France reflected old data from the 1970s and not from recent studies. The numbers were taken from ratios of animal fat consumption and cholesterol intakes, the researchers said.

1 McKeown, L. A. "Red Wine Boosts Heart Health," Medical Tribune, February 10, 1994, p. 1.

2 Hurley, Joyce, and Schmidt, Stephen. "A Drink A Day?" Nutrition Action Health Letter, November 1992, pp. 5, 7.

3 "Coronary Artery Disease, French and Red Wine," British Medical Journal 196: 1471-1480, May 29, 1999.

Nonetheless, a test involving 5 men and 4 women with red and white wines and beer found that red wine had the strongest effect on platelets about twice that of white wine and beer.

It may be that red wine's protective effect comes from the way it is made. For white wine, the chunky excess — known as "must" — consisting of stems, seeds, and grape skin — is removed soon after grapes are crushed and the juice is kept for fermenting. When red wine is made, the "must" is retained during the fermenting process and removed later. It is thought that polyphenols and flavonoid are hidden in the "must."

There may be more than one mechanism, besides the HDL-raising effect of alcohol, which affects the inhibition of platelet adhesiveness. High-density lipoprotein cholesterol is the beneficial kind.

One of the best studies of dementia in the world, the Canadian Study of Health and Aging, found that drinking a glass or two of wine a day reduced the risk of Alzheimer's disease by 62% in women and 51% in all participants when men were included with the benefit, reported Disease Free.[1] "The benefit is probably due to something in the wine itself, since the protection afforded by wine was far greater than that from liquor or beer," the publication added. "Check with your doctor before increasing your alcohol intake."

The publication added that drinking any form of alcohol in moderation — up to 1 drink a day for women and 2 for men — can lower your risk of heart disease by as much as 30% by improving cholesterol ratios and helping to prevent blood clots.

"If your triglycerides are high, drink wine only in moderation or not at all," the publication said.

Researchers at the Rambam Medical Centre in Haifa, Israel, evaluated 17 people in 2 groups. One group of 8 was given 400 ml of red wine daily for 2 weeks, while a group of 9 received a similar amount of white wine.[2] Red wine consumption for 2 weeks resulted in a 20% reduction in the likelihood of the plasma (blood) to undergo lipid peroxidation as determined by thiobarfbituric acid reactive substances assay. Lipid peroxidation is an interaction of fats and oxygen, which can lead to the destruction of cells. In addition, red wine consumption reduced the propensity of LDL-cholesterol (the bad kind) to undergo lipid peroxidation as deter-

---

1 Wait, Marianne, editor. Disease Free. Pleasantville, N. Y: The Reader's Digest Association, Inc., 2009, pp. 80, 146.

2 Fuhrman, Bianca, et al. "Consumption of Red Wine with Meals Reduces the Susceptibility of Human Plasma and Low-Density Lipoprotein to Lipid Peroxidation," *American Journal of Clinical Nutrition* 61: 549-554, 1995.

mined by 46%, 72%, and 54% decrease in the amount of TBARS, lipid peroxides in conjugated dienes in LDL, respectively. TBARS stands for thiobarbituric acid substances.

Dietary consumption of white wine for 2 weeks resulted in a 34% increase in plasma propensity to undergo lipid peroxidation. There was also a 41% increase in the propensity of LDL to undergo lipid peroxidation. The antioxidant effect of dietary red wine on plasma lipid peroxidation was not secondary to the changes in plasma vitamin E or beta-carotene, but could be related to the elevation of polyphenol concentrations in the blood.

As reported in Clinica Chimica Acta, 24 men, between the ages of 26 and 45, were evaluated after the consumption of red wine, white wine, commercial grape juice, and the same grape juice enriched with trans-resveratrol.[1] The research team said that the trans-resveratrol can be absorbed from grape juice in biologically active quantities, and in amounts that are likely to cause reductions in the risk of hardening of the arteries.

Red wine's antiatherosclerotic activity may be due to its ability to reduce platelet aggregation and thromboxane production, the antioxidant effect of red wine phenolics, and the red wine polyphenols, which include resveratrol, which can reduce lipoprotein synthesis. Thromboxanes are a group of compounds related to the prostaglandins.

As reported in the European Journal of Clinical Investigation, 22 type 2 diabetics (55.1 years of age, duration of disease of 9.2 years) were studied during fasting consumption of 300 ml of red wine, or during a meal accompanied with or without red wine.[2] Plasma glucose, insulin, triglycerides, and LDL oxidation significantly increased, while total plasma radical-trapping parameter significantly decreased during the meal test, the researchers said.

The study suggests that consumption of a moderate amount of red wine during meals may help prevent cardiovascular disease in diabetics. Elderly people with type 2 diabetes have an 8.8 percent increase risk of developing dementia, including Alzheimer's disease.

Epidemiologic studies have suggested that several forms of alcohol may reduce the risk for mortality from cardiovascular dis-

1 Pace-Asciak, Cecil R., et al. "Wines and Grape Juice as Modulators of Platelet Aggregation in Healthy Human Subjects," Clinica Chimica Acta 246: 183-192, 1996.

2 Ceriello, A., et al. "Red Wine Protects Diabetic Patients from Meal-Induced Oxidative Stress and Thrombosis Activation: A Pleasant Approach to the Prevention of Cardiovascular Disease in Diabetics," European Journal of Clinical Investigation 31(4): 322-328, 2001.

ease.[1] The alcohol components of red wine may reduce thrombosis (blood clot), fibrinogen levels, and collagen-induced platelet aggregation, all of which reduce cardiovascular disease, the researchers said.

Red wine appears to have a greater protective effect than beer, which is said to have a greater protective effect than distilled spirits. While it was not discussed in this article, it is well known that there is a risk factor between heart disease and Alzheimer's disease.

Resveratrol, found in peanuts and red wine, may be the agent that reduces the biological processes that are risk factors for cardiovascular disease, reported Clinical Chemistry.[2]

In an earlier article in the same publication, Andrew Day and David Stansbie of the British Royal Infirmary in the United Kingdom, evaluated 5 men who consumed 250 ml of port wine on 1 occasion, and 250 ml of water containing the equivalent amount of alcohol (40 grams) on another occasion.[3] The research team found a 23% increase in serum urate concentrations 30 minutes after the ingestion of the wine. There was a significant correlation between the increase in serum antioxidant capacity and the increased serum urate concentrations. (Urate is a salt of uric acid.)

The researchers reported that their data suggest that approximately 73% of the acute increase in serum total antioxidant capacity after the ingestion of port wine may be attributable to an increase in serum urate concentrations.

The beneficial antioxidant effect of red wine may not only be due to polypnenolics, but also due to the increase in urate, which may, in part, explain the French Paradox. An antioxidant is a substance that prevents free-radical or oxidative damage. Free radicals are highly unstable molecules, characterized by an unpaired electron, which can bind to and destroy cellular compounds.

About 300-500 mg of an extract of red wine grape fermentation (ANOX) is equal to the daily dose of red wine polyphenols that appear to be protective against cardiovascular disease, reported the Journal of International Medical Research.[4]

---

1 Wollin, S. D., and Jones, P. J. H. "Alcohol, Red Wine and Cardiovascular Disease," Journal of Nutrition 131: 1401-1404, 2001.

2 Goldberg, David M., M.D. "More on Antioxidant Activity of Resveratrol in Red Wine," Clinical Chemistry 42(1): 113-114, 1996.

3 Day, Andrew, and Stansbie, David. "Cardioprotective Effect of Red Wine May Be Modulated by Urate," Clinical Chemistry 41(9): 1319-1320, 1995.

4 Halpern, M. J., et al. "Red-Wine Polyphenols and Inhibition of Platelet Aggregation: Possible Mechanisms, and Potential Use in Health Promotion and Disease Prevention" Journal of International Medical Research 26: 171-180, 1998.

There may be a synergistic effect of these red wine polyphenols and vitamin C, due to their vasorelaxation activity and their possible role in preventing over-cross linking of connective tissues.

The polyphenols and flavonoids found in red wine-derived extract may have beneficial effects in a variety of chronic diseases due to their ability to scavenge free radicals, prevent lipid peroxidation, protect LDL-cholesterol from oxidation, inhibit the hydrolytic and oxidative enzymes, and by their anti-inflammatory actions, the research team explained.

They may also have the ability to reduce platelet activity/thrombotic tendencies. It has been estimated that if every adult in North America consumed 2 glasses of wine daily, cardiovascular disease, which accounts for 50% of all deaths in the population, would be cut by 40%, and $40 billion could be saved annually, the researchers said.

As reported in Atherosclerosis, 7 male volunteers consumed 375 ml of red wine (30 grams of alcohol) daily for 2 weeks after abstaining from alcoholic beverages, grape juices, and tea for 1 week.[1] A significant shortening of lag-time was found in vivo regarding LDL oxidation after 2 weeks of red wine consumption.

The researchers said that the study confirms a strong antioxidant effect of red wine in vitro, which should not be attributed to alcohol but to other components like polyphenols. Experts say that doctors rarely ask older patients how much and how often they drink, and not knowing the answers to these questions can result in misdiagnosis, medical complications, and life-threatening accidents, reported the New York Times.[2] "Doctors may also fail to recognize the symptoms of alcohol abuse, a problem that is expected to become increasingly common as baby boomers, who have been found to drink more than previous generations, reach age 65 and beyond."

Even at lower levels of consumption, alcohol can be problematic for older people, added Frederick C. Blow, M.D. Because of an increased sensitivity to alcohol and decreased tolerance as one ages, lower amounts of alcohol can have a bitter effect. Older people get into trouble with doses of alcohol that wouldn't be a problem with a younger person, he said. Immoderate consumption of alcohol — more than 3 drinks a day — can be hazardous for people of all ages, but it is especially so for the elderly, who reach higher levels of

---

1 Van Golde, P. H. M., et al. "The Role of Alcohol in the Anti Low-Density Lipoprotein Oxidation Activity in Red Wine," Atherosclerosis 147: 365-370, 1999.

2 Brody, Jane E. "Query for Aging Patients: How Much Do You Drink?" New York Times, December 16, 2008, p. D7.

blood alcohol faster and maintain them longer than younger people. "Potential hazards include an increased risk of falls and vehicular accidents, a decline in short-term memory, a worsening of existing health problems, and interactions with other medications that may diminish the effectiveness of some drugs and increase the toxic effects of others," Blow continued.

Alcohol abuse and alcoholism in aging adults is a silent epidemic, said Maria Pontes Ferreira, who with M. K. Suzy Weems, co wrote an article in the October 2008 issue of the Journal of the American Dietetic Association.

Added Madeline A. Naegle, M.D., of the New York College of Nursing, many older people pursue drinking patterns established earlier in life, and may not realize that continuing to drink the same amount of alcohol as they did when they were younger may place them at risk for health problems. Naegle suggested diet and exercise as a way to reduce cardiac risk; trying alternate relaxation methods like meditation, yoga, and exercise, and, for those who drink cutting down on the amount of alcohol or by mixing it with water, taking an hour to finish one drink, and. alternating alcohol with nonalcoholic drinks.

Speaking on "60 Minutes," David Sinclair said that he believed a new resveratrol product his colleagues were testing contained 250 mg of the nutrient.[1] "Until human tests are completed, we believe that most people can start with 250 to 500 mg/day of the supplement." He added that his scientists say that most people can take 100 mg if it is micronized (pulverized) and used by those under 35, but that those who are older need a higher dosage.

Patients with dementia or Alzheimer's disease have large amounts of plaques that are found outside neurons or nerve cells within the brain, according to P. Marambaud, et al., in the Journal of Biological Chemistry.[2, 3] In an in vitro study, trans-resveratrol secreted beta-amyloid peptides, which are responsible for the build-up of plaques in the brain. Resveratrol is useful in stimulating the break-down of beta-amyloid peptides, the researchers said.

In a study involving laboratory animals, who were given resveratrol for 45 days, there was a 45% reduction in plaques in the medial cortex, 89% in the stratum, and 90% in the hypothalamus.

1 Sinclair, David. "60 Minutes," October 5, 2008.
2 Marambaud, P., et al. "Resveratrol Promotes Clearance of Alzheimer's Disease Amyloid-Beta Peptides," Journal of Biochemical Chemistry 280(45): 37377-37382, 2005.
3 Karuppagounder, S. S., et al. "Dietary Supplementation with Resveratrol Reduces Plaque Pathology in a Transgenic Model of Alzheimer's Disease," Neurochemical International 54(2): 111-118, 2009.

This suggests that resveratrol may delay the onset of various neurodegenerative diseases.

Researchers at Queen Charlotte's and Chelsea Hospital in London, England fractionated (broke into portions) a red wine known high in vitro 5-hydroxytryptamine (HT)-releasing potency. The 5-HT-releasing potency was mainly associated with the phenolic flavonoid fraction, including red anthocyanins (red pigments).[1]

When 14 other red wines were assessed for their in-vitro platelet, 5-HT-releasing potency, there was no significant correlation with the red color. Flavonoids, other than the anthocyanins, must be involved in 5-HT-releasing potency, the researchers added.

Phenolic fractions of red wine may have clinical effects other than on those with low-density lipoprotein (LDL), the researchers added.

Red blood cells preincubated with micromolar (one millionth of a mole) amounts of wine extract, and challenged with hydrogen peroxide, showed an inhibition of the oxidative changes by incubating the red blood cells with oak barrel-aged red wine extract containing 5.3 micromolar galic acid equivalent of phenolic compounds, according to the Journal of Nutritional Biochemistry.[2]

The protective effect was reduced when red blood cells were incubated with wines containing lower amounts of polyphenols.

Resveratrol and quercetin, known antioxidants in red wine, showed lower antioxidant properties compared with the specific red oak-barrel aged red wine extracts, which suggests that the interaction between the components of the red wine may provide the antioxidant effect compared with single components.

The researchers added that it appears that the nonalcoholic components of red wine, specifically the polyphenols, have proven antioxidant properties.

In an Italian study reported in the European Journal of Clinical Nutrition, volunteers drank 3 different beverages of red wine, which provided 30 grams of alcohol per day; 30 grams of alcohol diluted in 320 ml of clear fruit juice, or 320 ml of de-alcoholized red wine over 2 meals.[3] The alcohol by itself or from the red wine resulted in similar decreases in platelet aggregation (sticking together), and fibrinogen levels. The beneficial effects of red wine on ho-

1   Pattichis, K., et al. "Phenolic Substances in Red Wine and Release of Platelet 5-Hydroxytryptamine," The Lancet 341: 1104, April 24, 1993.

2   Tedesco, I., et al. "Antioxidant Effect of Red Wine Polyphenols in Red Blood Cells," Journal of Nutritional Biochemistry 11: 114-119, February 2000.

3   Pellegrini, N., et al. "Effects of Moderate Consumption of Red Wine on Platelet Aggregation and Haemostatis Variables in Healthy Volunteers," European Journal of Clinical Nutrition 50: 209-213, 1996.

meostasis (balance) appeared to be due to the alcohol and not to some nonalcoholic fraction in the red wine.

De-alcoholized red wine contains polyphenolic compounds capable of synergizing with vitamin E, and long-term moderate consumption can decrease hardening of the arteries in apolipoprotein E gene-deficient mice, reported Roland Stocker and Ruth A. O'Halloran of the University of South Wales in Sydney, Australia, and colleagues at other facilities.[1] Wines contain abundant quantities of polyphenolic compounds that are not necessarily present in other alcoholic beverages. They chose de-alcoholized red wine because it has antioxidant activities similar to those of red wine, and because it inhibits in vivo lipid peroxidation, whereas alcohol increases that process and may, therefore, contribute to fatty deposits in the arteries.

The beneficial effect of moderate wine intake on the risk of all-cause mortality in those with high blood pressure has been observed in France and Great Britain, according to Serge C. Renaud, et al., of Hopital Emile in Limeil-Brevannes, and colleagues elsewhere in France.[2] [3] [4] "These findings may have important implications for hypertensive-middle-aged and elderly patients who are already moderate wine drinkers," the researchers said. "This habit may lower these patient's risk of death, especially that from all causes, which has not improved, even with recent antihypertensive drugs." They added that, concordant with that hypothesis are results suggesting a specific effect on wine drinking on protection from ischemic stroke in aged subjects.

In a population-based study involving 5,033 stroke-free men and women, researchers at the University of Tromso in Norway, reported that light-to-moderate consumption of red wine may be associated with improved cognitive function.[5] The patients were assessed during the 7-year study, which involved cognitive func-

1   Stocker, Roland, and O'Halloran, Ruth A. "De-alcoholized Red Wine Decreases Atherosclerosis in Apolipoprotein E Gene-Deficient Mice Independently of Inhibition of Lipid Peroxidation in the Artery Wall," American Journal of Clinical Nutrition 79: 123-130, 2004.

2   Renaud, Serge C., et al. "Moderate Wine Drinkers Have Lower Hypertension-Related Mortality: A Prospective Cohort Study in French Men," American Journal of Clinical Nutrition 80: 621-625, 2004.

3   Palmer, A. J., et al. "Alcohol Intake and Cardiovascular Mortality in Hypertensive Patients: Report from the Department of Health Hypertension Care Computing Project," Hypertension 12: 957-964, 1995.

4   Djousse, L., et al. "Alcohol Consumption and Risk of Ischemic Stroke: The Framingham Study," Stroke 33: 907-912, 2002.

5   Arntzen, K. A., et al. "Moderate Wine Consumption Is Associated with Better Cognitive Test Results: A 7-Year Follow-Up of 5,033 Subjects in the Tromso Study," Acta Neurologica Scandinavia Supplement 190: 23-29, 2010.

tion, verbal memory tests, etc. The researchers reported an independent association between moderate wine consumption and a better performance on all cognitive tests.

18. Don't Smoke!

It was probably Bette Davis and the other Hollywood divas who enticed women around the world to light up, because it was oh so glamorous and chic. Who can forget Miss Davis, cigarette in hand, strolling onto a porch and proclaiming, "What a dump!"

But wait. The Marlboro Man came along and convinced us that smoking is oh so masculine and macho, even though he died an agonizing death from tobacco use.

And then the cigarette companies converted generations of children to the weed because it was oh so sophisticated.

So which is it? The lowly cigarette can't possibly be all of those things.

In the meantime, cigarette smokers continue to battle emphysema, lung cancer, COPD, throat cancer, and other life-threatening diseases, while their sidestream smoke endangers all of those around them.

Like the Energizer bunny, the cigarette just keeps on going.

Smoking and Alzheimer's Disease

Heavy smoking in midlife is associated with the development of Alzheimer's disease, according to researchers at Kaiser Permanente Division of Research in Oakland, California, and colleagues in Finland.[1] The research team followed 21,123 men and women from midlife on for 23 years. The volunteers participated in a survey be-

---

1   Rusanen, Minna, M.D., et al. "Heavy Smoking in Midlife and Long-Term Risk of Alzheimer's Disease and Vascular Dementia," Archives of Internal Medicine 171(4): 333-339, 2011

tween 1978 and 1985. Diagnosis of dementia, Alzheimer's disease, and vascular dementia were collected from January 1, 1994 to July 31, 2008. During that time, 5,367, or 25.4%, were diagnosed with dementia. Compared with non-smokers, those who smoked over 2 packs a day had more than a 157% increased risk of Alzheimer's disease, and a 172% increased risk of vascular dementia during the 23 years of follow-up.

Vascular dementia is the second most common form of dementia after Alzheimer's disease. It is a group of dementia syndromes caused by conditions affecting the blood supply to the brain. "This study shows that the brain is not immune to the long-term consequences of heavy smoking," commented Rachel A. Whittaker, Ph.D., of the California facility, the lead researcher. Added co-author, Minna Rusanen, M.D., of the University of Eastern Finland and Kuopio University Hospital in Finland, "While we don't know for sure, we think the mechanism between smoking and AD and vascular dementia are complex, including possible deleterious effects to brain blood vessels and brain cells."

In a meta-analysis — a compilation of studies — of 43 studies examining the relationship between smoking and Alzheimer's disease, a research team concluded that smoking is definitely a significant risk factor for Alzheimer's disease, according to the Journal of Alzheimer's Disease.[1]

Those who quit smoking by age 50 had a no higher risk for developing the disease. Those who smoked less than half a pack of cigarettes a day were not at a higher risk for developing dementia.

Note that 11 of the 43 studies had authors with tobacco industry ties. Not surprisingly, they were not all that concerned about the consequences of smoking.

EVOLVING ATTITUDES TOWARD SMOKING

Believed to have medicinal properties, tobacco was introduced into Europe and the rest of the world, where it became the chief commodity that British colonists exchanged for European manufactured goods, reported Merriam-Webster's Collegiate Encyclopedia.[2] Native to South America, Mexico, and the West Indies, tobacco (Nicotina tabacum) has been used for smoking, chewing,

---

1 Cataldo, J. K., et al. "Cigarette Smoking Is a Risk Factor for Alzheimer's Disease: An Analysis Controlling for Tobacco Industry Affiliation," Journal of Alzheimer's Disease 19(2): 465-480, January 2010.

2 Stevens, Mark A., editor. Merriam-Webster's Collegiate Encyclopedia. Springfield, MA: Merriam-Webster's, Inc., 2000, p. 1623.

and snuffing. When Columbus reached the Americas, he found natives smoking tobacco as well as using it in religious ceremonies.

The Aztecs and other New World people smoked tobacco in hollow reeds, canes, or wrapped in leaves, but it was in pipes and cigars that the Europeans first smoked tobacco. Early in the 16th century, beggars in Seville, Spain, began picking up discarded cigar butts and wrapping them in scraps of paper to smoke, creating the first European cigarettes.[1]

About 5.4 million people in the world die prematurely from tobacco-related causes, such as cancer, annually, reported Betsy McKay in Wall Street Journal. In 2030, the World Health Organization (WHO) predicts that number to increase to some 8.3 million annual deaths.[2] About 80% of those deaths will come from low and middle-income nations, which are least equipped to deal with the financial, health, and social consequences of tobacco-related illness. Over half of the world's smokers live in 15 such countries, including China, India, Indonesia, Russia, and Bangladesh. "While Philip Morris International and other international tobacco giants deny that they are targeting new smokers, or seeking to expand in areas with minimal regulation, they are moving to build sales in countries where populations are growing," McKay said.

In those countries, people are joining the middle class, and smoking is viewed as a sign of upward mobility. At the same time, tobacco companies are developing and promoting new products, such as shorter cigarettes, to attract new customers, and to adapt to tobacco restrictions that are already in place, McKay continued.

On February 7, 2008, Margaret Chan, director-general of the WHO, and New York City's Mayor Michael R. Bloomberg, unveiled a report to offer suggestions for combating smoking around the world. The Bloomberg Philanthropies helped the UN agency to fund the report. He had pledged $125 million towards a global anti-smoking campaign. Smoking is entrenched in many emerging economies, McKay added. For example, in Bulgaria, 52% of health professionals — potential role models for healthy living — smoke, according to the Tobacco Atlas, which is published by the American Cancer Society.

"Young people with rising incomes and women, whose smoking rates have historically been low, are especially at risk," McKay continued. "Health experts note that tobacco marketers are employing tactics similar to those in the United States as far back as

---

1 ibid, p. 346.
2 McKay, Betsy. "Where There's Smoke: Emerging World," The Wall Street Journal, February 7, 2008, pp. B1, B2.

the 1920s, when, for instance, women marching for equality were urged to display cigarettes as 'torches of freedom.'"

Writing in the January 9/16, 2008 issue of the Journal of the American Medical Association, Mike Mitka reported that a Senate Committee hearing explored the accuracy of the Federal Trade Commission's tar and nicotine cigarette rating system, and the marketing claims of cigarette companies based on those findings.[1] At the hearing, Senator Frank R. Lautenberg (D., N. J.), who chaired the session, said that he had uncovered a lengthy history of false and deceptive cigarette ratings and marketing practices. "It is now clear that the tobacco industry has been aware of the inaccuracy of these findings for more than 3 decades," Lautenberg said.

Mitka explained that at issue is the method used by the Federal Trade Commission to determine tar and nicotine levels in each brand. Cigarettes that contain comparatively lower levels of tar and nicotine are marketed as "light" or "low-tar." "But smokers of these products often inhale more tar and nicotine than they would with conventional cigarettes by taking longer and deeper puffs, and smoking more to compensate for the lower nicotine levels," Mitka said.

If trends continue, an estimated 8 million deaths from smoking will be recorded by 2030, and the eventual toll from tobacco products could be 1 billion deaths in this century, or 10 times the 100 million smoking-related deaths that were recorded in the 20th century. Bill Marsh reported in the New York Times[2] that the World Health Organization, an arm of the United Nations, tracked the vigor of tobacco controls worldwide, and found them especially weak in poor nations. "One reason," he continued, "is that many governments are in the tobacco business, and rely on it for revenue. A case in point is the state-owned China National Tobacco Corporation."

More than 100 additives in cigarettes have pharmacological actions that camouflage the odor of cigarette tobacco smoke, and thus enhance or maintain nicotine delivery.[3] Some of the additives contain chemicals that can make it easier for cigarette smoke to penetrate the lungs, perhaps increasing the addictiveness of cigarettes. Other cigarettes have properties that may mask symptoms, such as an anesthetizing effect that makes it easier for smokers to avoid coughing.

1   Mitka, Mike. "Cigarette Ratings Questioned," JAMA 299(2): 163, 2008.
2   Marsh, Bill. "A Growing Cloud Over the Planet," The New York Times, February 24, 2008, p. 4.
3   Hampton, Tracy, Ph.D. "Cigarette Additives," JAMA 298(10): 1152, 2007.

Cigarette manufacturers have about 1,000 different tobacco flavorings to choose from to make a unique taste for their products.[1] Included in the list of cigarette additives are fragrant and flavoring extracts of anise, cinnamon, molasses, dandelion roots and walnut hulls, juices from apples, raisins, figs and plums, black currant buds, peppery capsicum oleoresin, clover tops, nutmeg powder, vanilla, vinegar, smoke flavor, tea leaves, orange blossom water and oils of basil, bay leaves, caraway, carrots, dill seeds, ginger, lavender, lemon, lime, pepper, Scotch pine, oak chips and patchouli, butter, chocolate, coffee, cognac oil, cocoa, honey, rum, sherry, yeast, and others.

Tobacco smoke contains over 4,000 chemicals, many of which are free radicals, that is, highly reactive compounds that damage cells and initiate a cascade of dangerous health problems.[2]

Antioxidant nutrients, including vitamin A, beta-carotene, vitamin C, and vitamin E help to neutralize these damaging reactions caused by exposure to tobacco smoke, but, unfortunately, antioxidant defenses are overwhelmed by the amount of free radicals in the tobacco.

While progress against smoking has been impressive, tobacco use remains an enormous health threat, as 45 million U.S. adults continue to smoke.[3] "Given that more than 70% of these smokers visit a health care facility each year, clinicians are ideally situated to increase the rate of tobacco cessation among these smokers, and reduce the risk of tobacco-caused disease." The promise of the clinical visit is enhanced because, as shown in the 2008 guideline update, numerous effective tobacco dependence treatments exist — treatments that significantly increase the likelihood of tobacco users both making quit attempts and successfully quitting.

REASONS TO STOP SMOKING

Your health starts improving the minute you quit smoking, according to the New York City Department of Health and Mental Hygiene.[4]

- In 20 minutes your heart rate and blood pressure fall.
- In 24 hours your risk of heart attack drops.

1   Raloff, Janet. "What's In a Cigarette? Tobacco Companies Blend Hundreds of Additives into Their Products," Science News, May 21, 1994, pp. 330-331.

2   Garrison, Robert H., Jr., R.Ph., and Somer, Elizabeth, R.D. The Nutrition Desk Reference. New Canaan, CT: Keats Publishing, Inc., 1995, p. 341.

3   Fiore, Michael C, M.D., MPH, and Jaen, Carlos Roberto, M.D., Ph.D. "A Clinical Blueprint to Accelerate the Elimination of Tobacco Use," JAMA 299(17): 2083-2085, 2008.

4   "Still Smoking? Cigarettes Are Eating You Alive." Health Bulletin, New York City Department of Health and Mental Hygiene. Health Bulletin 5(12), 2008.

- In 2 days your ability to taste and smell improves.
- In 2-3 weeks your lung function improves, your circulation is better, and walking is easier.
- In 1 year your risk of heart disease is cut in half.

In five years:
- Your risk of cancer of the mouth, throat, and esophagus drops by half.
- Your risk of stroke and heart disease begins to equal that of non-smokers (in 5–15 years).
- In 10 years your risk of dying of lung cancer is about the same as that of non-smokers.

How to Stop Smoking

Seven smoking cessation medications are now approved by the Food and Drug Administration for treating tobacco use and dependence. These include 2 non-nicotine medications — bupropion and varenicline — and 5 nicotine replacement medications — gum, patch, nasal spray, inhaler, and lozenge.

All of these medications have been found to be effective, and combinations of these drugs have also been found to be useful. Fiore and Jaen note, "Half of all U.S. smokers alive today — over 20 million — will die prematurely from a disease directly caused by their tobacco use if they are unable to quit, making treatment of tobacco dependence a chief medical and public health challenge." They go on to say that the 2008 guideline update serves as a benchmark of the progress made and the challenges that remain to eliminate tobacco dependence from society. Thus, the update should reassure clinicians, policy makers, funding agencies, and the public that tobacco use is amenable for both scientific analysis and clinical interventions. "This history of remarkable progress in treating tobacco dependence should encourage renewed efforts by clinicians, policy makers, and researchers to help the 43 million U.S. individuals who continue to smoke," they concluded. "Adherence to the recommendations in the 2008 U.S. Public Health Service guidelines, which were published May 7, 2008, will provide such help, ensuring that every smoker who visits a U.S. health-care setting can receive effective treatment for their tobacco dependence."

When you smoke, toxic chemicals from tobacco enter your bloodstream, and some of these chemicals send signals to your heart to beat harder and faster, explains Sharon Parmet, MS. Smoking also causes blood vessels to constrict, that is, become narrower, forcing blood to travel through a smaller space. Both of these effects contribute to high blood pressure.[1] "Smoking also lowers high-density lipoprotein cholesterol, the beneficial kind, in your body and increases the likelihood of plaques (fatty deposits), which collect on the inside of blood vessels, a condition called atherosclerosis (hardening of the arteries)" Parmet said. "Smoking also increases the risk of thrombosis (blood clots blocking a blood vessel). Over time, these effects increase the risk of having a myocardial infarction (heart attack)."

Smoking can also increase the risk of having a stroke (sudden blockage of blood circulation to the brain). A stroke is often caused by a blood clot lodging in the blood vessels supplying the brain with blood and oxygen. When this happens, brain cells begin to die. "This can cause permanent brain damage or even death," Parmet continues. "Women who smoke and use oral contraceptives — birth control pills — are at a much higher risk of developing heart disease or having a stroke than are women taking oral contraceptives who do not smoke."

Tobacco use remains the leading preventable causes of death in the United States, and globally about 5 million premature deaths were attributable to smoking in 2000, according to Stacey A. Kenfield, Sc.D., of the Harvard School of Public Health in Boston, Massachusetts, and colleagues at various facilities in Massachusetts and Missouri.[2] Their study involved an evaluation of 104,519 women participants in the Nurses' Health Study with a follow-up from 1980 to 2004. During that time, 12,483 deaths occurred in the cohort: 4,485 among never-smokers, 3,602 among current smokers, and 4,396 among past smokers.

"Our findings indicate that 64% of deaths in current smokers and 29% of deaths among past smokers are attributable to smoking, the research team said. "Quitting reduces the excess mortality rates for all major causes of death we examined. Most of the excess risk of vascular mortality due to smoking may be eliminated rapidly upon cessation, and within 20 years for lung diseases, in which the damaging effects of smoking are greatest."

They added that early-age at initiations associated with an increased mortality risk, so implementing and maintaining school tobacco prevention programs, in addition to enforcing youth access laws, are key preventive strategies. In addition, effectively

---

1 Parmet, Sharon, M.S. "Smoking and the Heart," JAMA 299(17): 2112, 2008.
2 Kenfield, Stacey A., Sc.D., et al. "Smoking and Smoking Cessation in Relation to Mortality in Women," JAMA 299(17): 2037-2047, 2008.

communicating risks to smokers and helping them quit success-fully should be an integral part of public health programs.

Quitting smoking, even with pharmacological and behavioral assistance, is extremely difficult, according to Robert C, Klesges, Ph.D., and colleagues at the University of Tennessee Health Science Center in Memphis, and colleagues at other locations. Patients currently cannot and probably never will simply be able to "take a pill" that will make them stop smoking, so smokers must want to stop smoking and must be willing to work hard to achieve the goal of smoking abstinence.[1]

"While much research needs to be conducted to establish the effectiveness of varenicline, stop smoking researchers and clinicians, as well as smokers wanting to quit smoking, now have another product available that appears to help increase the probability of smoking cessation," the research team said.

They reviewed 3 studies reported in the Journal of the American Medical Association on the efficacy of the nicotine acetylcholine receptor partial agonist varenicline for achieving smoking cessation.

In the trial by D. E. Jorenby, et al.[2], the drug showed significantly better long-term (at 52 weeks) cessation rates with use of varenicline when compared with bupropion.

The trial by D. Gonzales, et al.[3], revealed a trend in the same direction. The trial by S. Tonstad, et al.[4] reported that extended use of varenicline significantly reduced relapse at nearly 1-year follow-up among those who could successfully quit smoking while using the drug, based on continuous abstinence during weeks 11 to 12 of therapy.

Most drugs, whether they are swallowed or injected, enter the venous side of the bloodstream first, explained Jim Thornton in the June 2008 issue of Men's Health. This means that the drug must circulate back to the right side of your heart, travel to your lungs, then return to the left side of your heart, which finally pumps the drug to your brain.[5]

1 Klesges, Robert C., Ph.D., et al. "Varenicline for Smoking Cessation: Definite Promise, But No Panacea," JAMA 296(1): 94-95, 2006.

2 Jorenby, D. E., et al. "Efficacy of Varenicline, An Alpha-4-Beta-2 Nicotine Acetylcholine Receptor Partial Agonist vs Placebo or Sustained-Release Bupropion for Smoking Cessation: A Randomized Controlled Trial," ibid, pp. 56-63.

3 Gonzales, D., et al. "Varenicline, an Alpha-4-Beta-2 Nicotinic Acetylcholine Receptor Parial Agonist vs Sustained-Release Bupropion and Placebo for Smoking Cessation: A Randomized, Controlled Trial," ibid, pp. 47-55.

4 Tonstad, S., et al. "Effect of Maintenance Therapy with Varenicline on Smoking Cessation: A Randomized Controlled Trial," ibid, pp. 64-71.

5 Thornton, Jim. "Why Are Men Still Smoking?" Men's Health, June 2008, pp. 142ff.

Smoking shortens this trip considerably, since you send nicotine directly into your lungs, bypassing the venous system. Nicotine goes straight to the left side of your heart and out to your brain, reaching it within a few heartbeats. "Because of their small size, nicotine molecules can cross the blood-brain barrier and cell membranes alike with relative ease," Thornton added. "Nevertheless, Philip Morris invested huge amounts of money to find an additive that would produce an even quicker hit. The result: ammonia."

Thornton quoted an article in the Journal of the American Medical Association in 1998, which revealed the real reason for the addition of ammonia: It's the most effective way to freebase nicotine.

"Freebasing is a specific chemical process designed to remove hydrogen ions from the outside of molecules — nicotine or cocaine — and by stripping off these ions, the drug becomes streamlined, allowing it to cross cell membranes even faster," he continued.

Smoking and obesity are leading causes of illness and death worldwide, and the co-occurrences of overweight and smoking have substantial consequences for health, according to Arnaud Chiolero and colleagues at Centre Hospitalier Universitaire Vaudois and the University of Lausanne in Switzerland.[1]

They reviewed the famous Framingham Study which showed that the life expectancy of obese smokers was 13 years less than of normal-weight nonsmokers. In the study, one-third to one-half of obese smokers had died between the ages of 40 and 70, while only about 10% of normal weight nonsmokers died.

"Smoking's effect on body weight could lead to weight loss by increasing the metabolic rate, decreasing metabolic efficiency, or decreasing caloric absorption (reduction in appetite), all of which are associated with tobacco use," the researchers reported in the April 2008 issue of the American Journal of Clinical Nutrition. "The metabolic effect of smoking could explain the lower body weight found in smokers."

They added that smoking a single cigarette has been shown to induce a 3% rise in energy expenditure (EE) within 30 minutes. Smoking 4 cigarettes, each of which contains 0.8 mg of nicotine, increased resting EE by 3.3% for 3 hours. In regular smokers whose metabolism was assessed in a metabolic ward, smoking 24 cigarettes in 1 day increased the total EE from 2,230 kcal/day to 2,445, and stimulation of the sympathetic nervous system activity could be involved.

---

1 Chiolero, Arnaud, et al. "Consequences of Smoking for Body Weight, Body Fat Distribution, and Insulin Resistance," American Journal of Clinical Nutrition 87: 801-809, 2008.

The effect of smoking on EE was weaker among obese people, and it also depended on the degree of physical activity and fitness, the researchers added. After 30 days of stopping smoking, the resting metabolic rate in female quitters was shown to be 16% than it had been when they were smoking, and an increase in body weight was attributable to a decrease in resting metabolic rate and an increase in caloric intake. Smokers may be at a higher risk of hyperthyroidism than are nonsmokers, which could also increase metabolic rate.

Physicians have long recognized that a disproportionate number of people with mental illness smoke, according to Bridget M. Kuehn in the Journal of the American Medical Association. She quoted K. Lesser, et al., as saying that about 41% of all those who have had a mental illness in the past month smoke, compared with 22.5% of those who have never had a mental illness. Further, studies show that those with mental illnesses are less likely to stop smoking.[1]

Apparently those with schizophrenia, ADHD, or other mental illnesses may experience more positive effects from smoking than those without such disorders, and those benefits may make them more vulnerable to initiating smoking and make them less likely to quit, Kuehn said.

"The results of several studies suggest that nicotine remediates some of the cognitive deficits associated with certain mental illnesses, including Alzheimer's disease, ADHD, and schizophrenia," she added.

If we can understand the relationship between nicotine intake and Alzheimer's disease, we may have a greater understanding of the pathogenesis of the disease, reported R. C. A. Pearson, M.D., of Sheffield University in the United Kingdom. It has been theorized that causative agents of Alzheimer's may enter the brain through the nose and spread from neuron to neuron along the neuroanatomical pathway, beginning in the olfactory area of the medial temporal lobes, he reported in the British Medical Journal.[2]

Pearson added that this evidence is supported by the distribution of the pathology and also by early deficits of smell that occur in some people.

It is believed that smoking may damage the olfactory mucosa, thereby rendering this means of entry less permeable to such

---

1 Kuehn, Bridget M. "Link Between Smoking and Mental Illness May Lead to Treatments," JAMA 295(5): 483-484, 2006.
2 Pearson, R. C. A., et al. "Nicotine Intake in Alzheimer's Disease," British Medical Journal, August 10, 1991, p. 361.

agents, he added. Researchers have suggested that anemia occurred 2 years before cognitive decline in a patient with Alzheimer's, which was associated with mutation in the beta-amyloid precursor protein gene.

There is a negative association between smoking and the risk and age of Alzheimer's, and Pearson and colleagues state that the investigation of the mechanism by which smoking exerts a protective effect against the disease may give considerable information to the pathogenesis of Alzheimer's, and it should focus on the role of the olfactory system.

In studying 6,870 people, 55 years of age or older, during a follow-up of 2.1 years, 146 cases of dementia were reported, according to The Lancet. Of these, 105 were diagnosed with Alzheimer's disease.[1] Compared with never-smokers, smokers had an increased rate of dementia and Alzheimer's disease, and smoking was regarded as a strong risk factor for Alzheimer's disease in those without the Apo-E gene, but it had no effect on those with this gene.

The U.S. Public Mental Health System must address the issue of tobacco use in psychiatric hospitals, reported Jill M. Williams, M.D., of University of Medicine and Dentistry of New Jersey-Robert Wood Johnson Medical School in New Brunswick. Programs that treat behavioral health-problems such as depression and schizophrenia are the only remaining sector of health care where they fail to systematically help patients quit smoking, she reported in the February 8, 2008 issue of the Journal of the American Medical Association.[2]

"As mental health systems move toward addressing tobacco use, advocates can provide an important role in demanding increased access to tobacco dependence treatment and increasing staff education on the evidence-based treatments," she continued. "Only then can more people with mental illness successfully overcome nicotine addiction and strive toward full mental health recovery." Patients with serious mental illness die, on average, at least 25 years earlier than the general population. Heart disease is the leading cause of death among those with serious mental illnesses, resulting in more deaths than from injuries or obesity-related diseases such as diabetes.

"A survey of 222 state-operated psychiatric facilities in the United States found that the majority of hospitals had begun the pro-

1 Ott, A., et al. "Smoking and Risk of Dementia and Alzheimer's Disease in a Population-Based Cohort Study: The Rotterdam Study," The Lancet 351: 1840-1843, June 20, 1998.
2 Williams, Jill M., M.D. "Eliminating Tobacco Use in Mental Health Facilities," JAMA 299(5): 571-573, 2008.

cess of becoming tobacco-free facilities or were planning to do so," Williams said.

Facilities that had undergone these changes indicated improved patient health, cleaner indoor environments, and hospital grounds, increases in staff satisfaction, and more time to provide treatment. These findings are consistent with national trends calling for a transformation of U.S. mental health care to be more oriented toward wellness and recovery. Smoking is an accepted part of the culture of care in some psychiatric hospitals in which staff — often those who smoke themselves — take patients outdoors to smoking shelters several times during the day. These smoke breaks — often 1 per 8-hour staff shift — can serve both as fillers of time and as a reward for patients who have been cooperative.

"Much time is spent in the bartering and control of tobacco products between staff and patients, and this can be the source of conflicts and incident reports," Williams continued. "Not surprisingly, studies of psychiatric hospitals becoming tobacco-free report fewer behavioral problems and less violence after policies take effect."

There is evidence that those who have mental illness smoke at higher rates, consume more tobacco products, and have greater difficulty in quitting smoking. This is especially true of those with the most severe forms of mental illnesses, who often are disabled from their illness. While nicotine may provide temporary benefit, this benefit should not be a rationale for continued smoking, she said. "Patients with mental illnesses deserve the same protection from tobacco exposure that benefits the rest of the public," she concluded.

As more communities have banned smoking, cigarette manufacturers have been increasing nicotine in their products, making it more difficult for people to quit, reported Carol Potera in the May 2007 issue of the American Journal of Nursing. According to the Harvard School of Public Health in Boston, Massachusetts, from 1998 to 2005, nicotine content rose 11.3% in all types of cigarettes, even for those branded light or ultra light.[1] "The researchers analyzed 1997 to 2005 data on the smoke yield of nicotine that cigarette makers submitted to the Massachusetts Department of Public Health, and the nicotine content of the Camel, Doral, GPC, Cool, Marlboro, Newport, and Salem brands increased significantly, whereas that of Basic and Winston did not," Potera said.

---

1 Potera, Carol, "Tobacco Companies Increased Nicotine in Cigarettes," American Journal of Nursing 107(5): 22, May 2007.

Added Gregory Connolly, director of Harvard's Tobacco Control Research Program, "Our analysis shows that the companies have been subtly increasing the drug nicotine year by year, without any warning to consumers."

ADDICTION AND WAYS TO QUIT

Today, seven forms of medication have been shown to improve the chances of smoking cessation, and toll-free telephone quit lines exist in every state (1-800QUITNOW), and there are more exsmokers than current smokers.[1] "A risk of the marginalization of smoking is that it further isolates the group of people with the highest rates of smoking — those with mental illness, problems with substance abuse, or both. These people are already stigmatized by their underlying psychiatric condition. Somehow we must find a way to integrate the twin goals of reducing smoking and integrating people with mental illness into mainstream society." However, tobacco remains our nation's No. 1 health problem. Over 400,000 people die every year from smoking, and 20 times that number struggle with severe smoking-related disabilities. If the United States is to improve its current dismal performance in health status as compared to other countries, it must do better in reducing tobacco use.

Like other addicting substances, nicotine produces pleasurable effects that prompt smokers to keep up the habit and, ultimately, lose control over smoking, often even when dire consequences like a heart attack, cancer, or emphysema result, explained Jane E. Brody in the New York Times.[2] "Among the addiction-maintaining effects of nicotine are arousal, relaxation, improved mood, reduced anxiety, and stress, better concentration and faster reaction time." However, when deprived, smokers report withdrawal symptoms that include irritability, depression, restlessness, anxiety, difficulty concentrating, increased hunger, insomnia, a craving for tobacco, difficulty getting along with others, and a feeling that life lacks pleasures.

She went on to say that these effects have a biological connection. Nicotine crosses the blood-brain barrier, where it binds to nicotine-specific receptors in the brain. This results in the release of a number of neurotransmitters, primarily dopamine. She quoted Neal L. Benowitz, M.D., of the University of California at San Fran-

---

1 Schroeder, Steven, M.D. "Stranded in the Periphery — The Increasing Marginalization of Smokers," New England Journal of Medicine 358(12): 2284-2286, 2008.
2 Brody, Jane E. "Trying to Break Nicotine's Grip," The New York Times, May 20, 2008, p. F7.

cisco, as saying that, "this signals a pleasurable experience and is critical to the reinforcing effect of nicotine and other drugs that are abused."

Brody added that repeated exposure to nicotine increases the receptors and induce tolerance to and dependence on nicotine. Smokers typically take in the amount of nicotine needed to bind to the receptors.

Nicotine-specific receptors in the brain promote the release of various neurotransmitters, including:

- Acetylcholine, which produces arousal and cognitive enhancement.
- Beta-endorphin, which reduces anxiety and tension.
- Dopamine, which creates pleasure and appetite suppression.
- Glutamate, which enhances learning and memory enhancement.
- Norepinephrine, which stimulates arousal and appetite suppression.
- Serotonin, which affects mood and appetite suppression.

Smokeless tobacco users have a higher urinary level of a potent carcinogen than cigarette smokers do, according to the American Journal of Nursing in November 2007.[1]

Levels of carcinogen — 4-methylnitrosamino)-3-pyridyl)-1-butan — one of the metabolites, are higher in smokeless tobacco users even after adjusting for demographic variables and creatine levels.

The researchers, who originally reported their study in the August 2007 issue of Cancer, Epidemiology, Biomarkers, and Prevention, said that smokeless tobacco products should not be promoted as safer alternatives to smoking because they still carry substantial risks for cancer.

Topiramate (Topamax) had previously been shown to be an effective treatment for alcohol dependence, and researchers reported in Archives of Internal Medicine that they wanted to find out if cigarette smoking, alcohol-dependent volunteers from an earlier study also improved cigarette smoking outcomes.[2] In the study, involving 94 cigarette-smoking, alcohol-dependent people, 45 were assigned to receive the drug, and 49 received a placebo. The treatment group was given from 25 to 300 mg/day of the drug for 12 weeks. Topiramate, at up to 300 mg/day, showed potential as a safe

---

1 "In the News," American Journal of Nursing 107(11): 22, November 2007.
2 Johnson, B. A., et al. "Use of Oral Topiamate to Promote Smoking Abstinence Among Alcohol-Dependent Smokers: A Randomized Controlled Trial," Archives of Internal Medicine 165: 1600-1605, 2005.

and promising medication for the treatment of cigarette smoking in alcohol-dependent people.

Originally designed as an anticonvulsant, the just-named drug may cause intense pain in the kidney, suggesting kidney stones, according to Prescription and Over-the-Counter Drugs.[1] Common side effects include drowsiness, fatigue, dizziness, anxiety, strange eye movements, tingling sensations, speech problems, depression, mood changes, memory impairment, weight loss, and tremor.

African-American smokers are mere likely to experience tobacco-related illness and death than European American smokers, and menthol cigarette smoking may contribute to these disparities, according to an article in Archives of Internal Medicine.[2] The research team measured cumulative exposure to menthol and nonmenthol cigarettes and smoking cessation behavior from 1985 to 2000, coronary calcification, and 10-year change in pulmonary function in both races. They found that 89% of the African-Americans preferred menthol cigarettes, compared with 29% of the whites. After adjusting for ethnicity, demographics, and social factors, it was also reported that nonsignificant trends in menthol smokers toward lower cessation, and recent quit attempts, and a significant increase in the risk of relapse.

Menthol and nonmenthol cigarettes seem to be equally harmful per cigarette smoked in terms of hardening of the arteries and pulmonary function decline, however, menthol cigarettes may be harder to quit smoking, the researchers added.

It takes only two questions to assess a patient's nicotine dependence, reported Lynne Lamberg in the September 15, 2004 issue of the Journal of the American Medical Association. Those are: how soon after you wake up do you smoke your first cigarette? How many cigarettes do you smoke per day?[3]

"Smoking at least 20 cigarettes a day or within 30 minutes of arising indicates high nicotine dependence," Lamberg said. "Smoking at least 10 cigarettes a day or smoking within 60 minutes of arising suggests moderate nicotine dependence." She quoted Jonathan Foulds, Ph.D., as saying that primary care physicians can double a patient of quitting smoking with brief counseling and phar-

1 Visalli, Gayla, project editor. Prescription and Over-the-Counter Drugs. Pleasantville, NY: The Reader's Digest Association, Inc., 1998, p. 719.

2 Fletcher, M. J., et al. "Menthol Cigarettes, Smoking Cessation, Atherosclerosis, and Pulmonary Function: The Coronary Artery Risk Development in Young Adults (CARDIA Study)," Archives of Internal Medicine 166: 1915-1922, 2006.

3 Lamberg, Lynne. "Patients Need More Help to Quit Smoking: Counseling and Pharmacotherapy Double Success Rate," JAMA 292(11)286, 2004.

macological therapies. However, the higher a person's dependence on nicotine, the more difficult withdrawal is likely to be.

Withdrawal symptoms include a dysphoric or depressed mood, insomnia, irritability, anxiety, difficulty concentrating, restlessness, and a decreased heart rate. And those who stop smoking usually gain on average 6 pounds. This fear of gaining weight prompts some smokers from trying to quit. Foulds added that while withdrawal symptoms usually subside within a month, 50% of smokers still report cravings 6 months later, but their mood usually improves.

A patient entering the New Jersey facilities dependence withdrawal program has made on average 9 unsuccessful attempts to quit. About 45% of the participants report that they wake at night to smoke. "Patients with such high nicotine dependence rarely succeed in quitting without psychological support and medications," Foulds continued. "Those who live with or work with other smokers, especially those with high current stress and comorbid psychiatric disorders, have a harder time quitting than those who do not."

A research team at Osaka University in Japan reported in the Journal of Occupational and Environmental Medicine that cigarette smoking is highly associated with development of high-frequency hearing impairment in the Japanese male office workers who were investigated.[1] As the number of pack-years of exposure increased, the risk for high-frequency hearing loss increased in a dose-dependent manner, however, the risk for low-frequency hearing impairment did not.

People at risk of a heart attack should avoid smoke-filled rooms, since researchers have found that lab animals were far less likely to survive a heart attack if they had regularly breathed secondhand smoke during the previous week, reported Janet Raloff in Science News.[2] She quoted Paul F. McDonagh of the University of Arizona Health Sciences Center in Tucson, that he and his colleagues had found that blood platelets in the smoke-exposed animals attached themselves to white blood cells more frequently than did those in the control animals. Platelets play a role in clotting, and the white cells participate in inflammation.

---

1 Nakanishi, Noriyuki, et al. "Cigarette Smoking and Risk for Hearing Impairment: A Longitudinal Study in Japanese Male Office Workers," Journal of Occupational and Environmental Medicine 42: 1045-1049, 2000.
2 Raloff, Janet. "Cigarette Smoke Worsens Heart Attacks," Science News 159(16): 248, April 21, 2001.

The excessive linking of these 2 types of cells may have made the blood form more fatal clots, McDonagh added. In addition, immune cells activated by exposure to smoke in the lungs may have triggered the systemic release of chemical messengers — cytokines — that somehow aggravated the heart attacks.

In a double-blind, placebo-controlled trial, a vitamin cocktail containing 272 mg of vitamin C, 31 mg of vitamin E, and 400 mcg of folic acid was given to 37 smokers and 38 nonsmokers. The population was selected for a low intake of fruit and vegetables, who were recruited in the San Francisco Bay area, reported Jens Lykkesfeldt of the University of California at Berkeley, and colleagues at other facilities in California, Denmark, and Switzerland.[1] Following 3 months of supplementation, vitamin C was efficiently repleted in the smokers. Blood levels of the other vitamins increased in both supplemented groups.

The high oxidant content of smoke explains the low antioxidant status and increased oxidative stress and damage that is consistently observed in smokers, the researchers reported. Thus, it has been suggested that smokers would benefit from increasing their dietary intake of antioxidants. "Dietary guidelines recommend 5 to 9 servings a day of fruits and vegetables," the researchers continued. "Recent studies indicate that only a relatively small portion of the American population routinely has an intake in the recommended range. Like smoking, a low daily intake of fruit and vegetables has been associated with an increased risk of developing chronic diseases."

Smokers have been found to have poorer diets than nonsmokers, the researchers continued. Of the major plasma antioxidants, vitamin C is the only one apparently depleted by smoking, therefore, a supplement may be warranted. Nineteen healthy smokers were put on a low vitamin C diet of less than 30 mg/day for 2 weeks, and then they were given either a placebo or 1,000 mg/day of the vitamin for 2 weeks at the University of Texas-Southwestern Medical Center in Dallas.[2]

The vitamin C group had a significant reduction in LDL-oxidative susceptibility, reported Jialal Iswarlal and colleagues. There was no increased signs of iron body stores in the vitamin C group.

1 Lykkesfeldt, Jens, et al. "Ascorbate Is Depleted by Smoking and Repleted by Moderate Supplementation: A Study of Male Smokers and Nonsmokers with Matched Dietary Antioxidant Intakes," *American Journal of Clinical Nutrition* 71: 530-536, 2000.
2 Iswarlal, Jialal, et al. "Effect of Ascorbate Supplementation on Low-Density Lipoprotein Oxidation in Smokers," *Atherosclerosis* 119: 139-150, 1996.

As reported in the International Journal of Epidemiology, men who smoked over 20 cigarettes a day had significantly lower beta-carotene (provitamin A) and vitamin C intakes than men who never smoked, due to an almost 60% lower intake of fruit.[1] "Our results indicate that male heavy smokers and to a lesser extent female moderate and heavy smokers have a lower dietary antioxidant intake with respect to vitamin C and beta-carotene, but not vitamin E, and that heavy smoking men seem to use supplements relatively infrequently." Since smokers have increased oxidative stress compared to nonsmokers, it is generally assumed that they require a higher intake of antioxidants.

In 50 fasted male smokers, compared with 50 age-matched controls who had never smoked, ranging in age from 50 to 59, lower vitamin A and vitamin C concentrations were found in smokers than in those who never smoked, reported the European Journal of Clinical Nutrition.[2] The cause is unknown, but smokers may benefit from increased carotenoid (vitamin A) and vitamin C, the research team added.

A research team at the University of Nevada at Reno evaluated the effect of environmental tobacco smoke in exposed antioxidant supplemented and nonsupplemented participants, reported Cancer Epidemiology, Biomarkers and Prevention. They found a marker of oxidative DNA damage was 63% greater in the exposed group compared with the nonexposed volunteers.[3]

With a 60-day supply of over-the-counter antioxidants, including 3,000 mcg of beta-carotene, 60 mg of vitamin C, 30 IU of vitamin E, 40 mg of zinc, 40 mcg of selenium, and 2 mg of copper, there was a 62% decrease in the marker for oxidative damage after supplementation. Lipid peroxidation levels were also reduced, as were antioxidant enzyme activities. (Lipid peroxidation is an interaction of fats and oxygen, which can lead to the destruction of cells.) The researchers added that environmental tobacco smoke in the workplace increases oxidative stress and antioxidant supplementation may provide some protection.

As reported in the British Medical Journal, 100 Finnish volunteers were assigned to a quit-smoking group, while 82 others con-

1 Zondervan, E. T., et al. "Do Dietary Supplementary Intakes of Antioxidants Differ with Smoking Status?" International Journal of Epidemiology 25: 70-79, 1996.

2 Rose, M. A., et al, "Plasma Concentrations of Carotenoids and Antioxidant Vitamins in Scottish Males: Influences of Smoking," European Journal of Clinical Nutrition 49: 861-865, 1995.

3 Howard, D. J., et al. "Oxidative Stress Increased by Environmental Tobacco Smoke in the Workplace Is Mitigated by Antioxidant Supplementation," Cancer Epidemiology, Biomarkers and Prevention 7: 981-988, November 1998.

tinued to smoke for 4 weeks. When given vitamin C, blood levels of the vitamin increased by an average of 23.3% in those who quit, and 9.8% in those who continued to smoke.[1] Even within 4 weeks of smoking- cessation, there is a remarkable recovery of vitamin C levels, and this effect is probably related to the physiology of smoking rather than dietary change, the researchers said.

Vitamin E appears to be one factor that is important in the protection against reactive oxygen species, according to K. M. Brown, M.D., of Rowett Research Institute in Aberdeen, United Kingdom, and colleagues.[2] In the study, 50 nonsmokers and 50 smokers of greater than 15 cigarettes per day for at least 10 years, were divided into 4 treatment groups. For 10 weeks, each volunteer took 1 capsule of either a 250 mg supplement of vitamin E as dl-alpha-tocopherol acetate, or a placebo containing hydrogenated coconut oil with little vitamin E.

It was found that vitamin E increased erythrocyte catalase in both smokers and nonsmokers, and erythrocyte glutathione peroxidase and glutathione reductase activities in nonsmokers. Brown added that vitamin E supplements resulted in a fall in erythrocyte superoxide dismutase activity, and total glutathione concentrations. In both smokers and nonsmokers, there was a significant decrease in the susceptibility of erythrocytes to peroxidation. Glutathione peroxidase works with vitamin E to convert harmful oxidized fats into less harmful substances.

As reports of suicide and other serious psychiatric problems among patients taking the smoking cessation drug varenicline continue to surface, the Food and Drug Administration is requiring a boxed warning on the drug's label to alert physicians and patients to these risks, reported Bridget M. Kuehn in the Journal of the American Medical Association.[3]

The net labeling will prominently warm of the risk of behavioral changes, depression, hostility, aggression, suicidal thoughts, and suicide in those taking the drug. The revised labeling includes a more prominent warning about the risks of vehicle crashes while taking the medication.

A similar warning is being added to the label of bupropion, an antidepressant and smoking cessation therapy that already carries

1 Lykkesfeldt, Jens., et al. "Vitamin C Levels in Former Smokers," British Medical Journal 313(7049): 91, 1996.

2 Collins. Karen, M.S., R.D. "Is Weight Gain Unavoidable When Someone Quits Smoking?" Nutrition Wise, American Institute for Cancer Research, Washington, D. C, June 2, 2008.

3 Kuehn, Bridget M. "Varenicline Gets Stronger Warnings About Psychiatric Problems, Vehicle Crashes," JAMA 302(8): 834, 2009.

a warning about suicidality in those treated with the drug for depression. "An FDA analysis, released in early 2009, of varenicline adverse events submitted to the agency between May 2006 and November 2007, documented 19 suicides and 18 reports of suicidal attempts, including 13 suicide attempts," Kuehn said. However, in a press briefing in July 2009, Curtis Rosenbaugh, M.D., of the FDA, said that based on accounts the agency now has reports of 98 suicides and 188 suicide attempts. The analysis also covered bupropion events between 1997 and 2007, and found 10 suicides and 19 suicidal behaviors, while the current estimated counts were 14 suicides and 17 suicide attempts. Rosenbaugh reported that varenicline and bupropion have shown effectiveness as cessation aids, and if physicians choose to prescribe them, they are advised to monitor their patients for behavioral changes to prevent serious psychiatric outcomes.

Robert J. Temple, M.D., also of the FDA, said that during nicotine withdrawal, some people experience symptoms such as depression, anxiety, and irritability that are similar to those reported in patients taking varenicline and bupropion. However, he added, some reports have occurred in those who were still using nicotine, and in many reports the symptoms stopped after the drugs were discontinued, suggesting the drugs are triggering the symptoms.

The FDA is recommending that the manufacturers conduct additional randomized controlled trials, Kuehn continued. Unlike previous studies, these trials will include people with preexisting mental health issues, who make up a disproportionate number of smokers.

COMMON MEDICATIONS TO HELP STOP SMOKING[1]

Nicotine patch (NicoDerm). Releases nicotine into the skin, thereby easing smoking withdrawal. May cause skin irritation, dizziness, racing heartbeat, sleep problems, headache, nausea, and muscle aches.

Nicotine gum (Nicorette). Releases nicotine into the body when chewed. To avoid stomach upset, chew a few times to break it down, then park it in your teeth. Don't continue to chew the gum; don't chew more than 24 pieces of gum daily and don't use for more than 3 months.

Nicotine lozenge (Commit). Releases nicotine into the body as the lozenge dissolves in the mouth. May cause sore teeth or gums,

---

1 This list is from Kane, Tracy, M.Ed. Albert Einstein Health Care Network, Philadelphia, PA. Reprinted in "Smoking Cessation," *Nursing* 37(5): 58, 2007.

indigestion, and throat irritation. Don't use over 20 lozenges a day; don't use more than 3 months.

Nicotine nasal spray (Nicorette Nasal Spray). Releases nicotine through membranes in the nose. May cause nose and throat irritation. Don't use over 40 doses daily.

Nicotine inhaler (Nicotrol Inhaler). Delivers nicotine as you inhale. Delivers nicotine equal to 2 cigarettes. May cause mouth and throat irritation and coughing. Don't use more than 16 cartridges daily, and don't use over 3 months.

Non-nicotine pill (Zyban, bupropion hydrochloride). Reduces symptoms of nicotine withdrawal. May cause insomnia, dry mouth, and dizziness. Nonnicotine Pill (Chantix, varenicline). Reduces pleasure of smoking, and eases withdrawal symptoms. May cause nausea, headache, vomiting, gas, insomnia, abnormal dreams, and a change in taste perception. (See earlier comment on varenicline.)

WEIGHT CONTROL

Although modest weight gain is not unusual when someone quits smoking, it is not universal, according to Karen Collins, M.S., R.D. There is increased calorie consumption as people begin to eat when they otherwise would have smoked.[1]

These extra calories, combined with a return to a normal metabolic rate — nicotine may elevate the metabolism, helping smokers turn calories more quickly — can lead to excess pounds. "Exercise is one of the most effective ways to avoid weight gain after you quit smoking," she said. "Two to three 10 to 15 minute blocks of activity can burn enough calories to compensate for a drop in metabolic rate. In addition, by reducing stress and improving mood, regular exercise can decrease emotion-based eating."

She added that many people find that snacking on small amounts of food several times a day is helpful as well. Eating more frequently can help people avoid rapid drops in blood sugar, which can stimulate cravings. The key is to choose balanced snacks, not just sweets or chips.

If you want to lose weight to avoid obesity, diabetes, heart disease, etc., the following tips have long been known:

1. Throw the diet books in the trash.

---

1 Collins. Karen, M.S., R.D. "Is Weight Gain Unavoidable When Someone Quits Smoking?" Nutrition Wise, American Institute for Cancer Research, Washington, D. C., June 2, 2008.

2. Eliminate all sugar. True, the body/brain crave glucose/sugar, but the body is equally adept at converting meat, cheese, etc. into glucose.

3. Eat 5 small meals daily. The largest meal of the day should be a nutritious breakfast, and the smallest meal should be at night. Have a nutritious mid-morning snack and a healthful mid-afternoon snack.

4. Exercise. Walking is the best, since you don't need any expensive gear. Put on your old clothes and shoes and head out of the house or apartment. Swimming is probably next on the list. Running is fine, but avoid jogging, in which your body is pounding the pavement and possibly doing other damage.

APPENDIX 1. WHEN IT'S TIME FOR A NURSING HOME

There often comes a time when the family has to relinquish home care because of inability to manage problematic patient behavior, or because they lack the resources to provide 24-hour a day care, and must seek institutionalized care.

Ann C. Hurley, RN, and Ladislav Volicer, M.D., discussed this in the November 13, 2002 issue of the Journal of the American Medical Association.[1] They added that C. E. Smith, et al., reported in Neurology in 2001 that during 3,600 person-years of surveillance, 203 (40%) of 512 AD patients were placed in nursing homes.[2]

Also, in a study of 5,788 community-residing elders with AD and their caregivers, K. Yaffe, et al., found that both patient and caregiver characteristics independently predicted nursing home placement.[3] Patient predictors include living alone, being white, having cognitive and functional impairment, and having behavioral problems.

"Caregiving costs are enormous," Hurley and Volicer note. "Family caregiving can distress caregivers, causing intense physical, emotional, and functional burden, yet families provide unpaid care for Alzheimer's disease valued at $65 billion annually, of the at least $100 billion spent by all sectors of U.S. society." They say that annual pre-patient costs of informal care are estimated to range

1 Hurley, Ann C, RN, and Volicer, Ladislav, M.D. "Alzheimer Disease. 'It's Okay, Mama, If You Want to Go, It's Okay,'" JAMA 288(18): 2324-2331, 2002.

2 Smith, G. E., et al. "Prospective Analysis of Risk Factors for Nursing Home Placement of Dementia Patients," Neurology 57: 1467-1473, 2001.

3 Yaffe, K., et al. "Patient and Caregiver Characteristics and Nursing Home Placement in Patients with Dementia," JAMA 287(22): 2090-2097, 2002.

from \$10,140 to \$34,517. Medical expenses for those with AD are 70% higher than for other beneficiaries. "Because nursing home admissions for those with AD are almost twice as long as for the average beneficiary, when Medicaid pays for long-term care, the cost is almost \$7,700 more for those with AD."

Deciding to place a patient in a nursing home carries dual concerns of finding an appropriate facility and managing the guilt of giving up primary caregiver responsibilities, the authors continued. The family selects the nursing home, and the physician can help the family in this process by providing a list of questions to ask when visiting potential nursing homes.

"After transferring the patient, family caregivers should have emotional support to help them cope with their own sense of 'failing' the patient," Hurley and Volicer said. "Physicians and other health care professionals should be willing to help family members deal with their guilt, depression, and grief. At this juncture, symptoms of grieving seem to cycle around two losses: admitting a loved one to long-term care and needing to make an advanced care plan for the end of life."

It takes a team of nurses working 3 shifts a day, 7 days a week to do what caregivers have been doing. The physician should also reiterate that no matter how fine the nursing home care is, the disease still progresses relentlessly, the patient's condition will continue to worsen, and the patient will ultimately die, either from the consequences of AD or from some other disease.

Following are some of the issues to consider when selecting a nursing home. This report was supported by Brigham and Women's Hospital, in Boston, the U.S. Department of Veterans Affairs, the United States Public Health Service, the Perspective of Care at the Close of Life, and a grant from the Robert Wood Johnson Foundation.

1. Safe Physical Environment
   Is the unit locked?
   Are there protected and outdoor wandering paths?
   How is elopement prevented?
   How are falls prevented?
   Are physical or chemical restraints ever used?
   What types of assistive devices were used?

2. Dementia Health
   How often does a physician or nurse practitioner routinely visit each resident?
   What memory enhancing medications are typically used?

What cognitively enhancing activities are used?

3. Overall Health

What is the range of drugs and treatment for other medical conditions that are available without being transferred?

How are chronic preexisting and other new problems assessed and managed?

What are the procedures if acute care is needed?

Where is terminal care provided?

Is hospice available on the unit?

4. Knowledgeable and Available Staff

What kind of staff training programs are there?

How often are they provided?

What percentage of staff attend?

What percentage of nursing assistants are certified?

What percentage of nursing assistants are certified in dementia care?

What special consultants are available?

How many hours of direct nursing care does each resident receive each 24-hour segment?

How many full-time equivalent registered nurses are there per resident?

5. Quality-of-Life Issues

What programs are there to maintain physical functioning (toileting, feeding assistance, ambulation)?

What is the pain management program?

How much time in each 24-hour period do residents stand outside their bedrooms?

What are the ongoing activities and daily events?

6. Support Services

What types of family support groups are there and how frequently do they meet?

What family education programs are provided?

7. Interdisciplinary Team Approach

How are individual residents' care-plans developed, evaluated, revised, and shared with the family?

How frequently does the team evaluate each resident's care plan?

Is there a system to include family input?

APPENDIX 2. INCIDENCE OF ALZHEIMER'S DISEASE BY STATE

State	Year 2000	Year 2010	% Change
Alabama	84,000	91,000	8
Alaska	3,400	5,000	47
Arizona	78,000	97,000	24
Arkansas	56,000	60,000	7
California	440,000	480,000	9
Colorado	49,000	72,000	47
Connecticut	68,000	70,000	3
Delaware	12,000	14,000	17
D. C.	10,000	9,100	-9
Florida	360,000	450,000	25
Georgia	110,000	120,000	9
Hawaii	23,000	27,000	17
Idaho	19,000	26,000	37
Illinois	210,000	210,000	0
Indiana	100,000	120,000	20
Iowa	65,000	69,000	6
Kansas	50,000	53,000	6
Kentucky	74,000	80,000	8
Louisiana	73,000	83,000	14
Maine	25,000	25,000	0
Maryland	78,000	86,000	10

Massachusetts	120,000	120,000	0
Michigan	170,000	180,000	6
Minnesota	88,000	94,000	7
Mississippi	51,000	53,000	4
Missouri	110,000	110,000	0
Montana	16,000	21,000	31
Nebraska	33,000	37,000	12
Nevada	21,000	29,000	38
New Hampshire	19,000	22,000	16
New Jersey	150,000	150,000	0
Few Mexico	27,000	31,000	31
New York	330,000	320,000	-3
North Carolina	130,000	170,000	31
North Dakota	16,000	18,000	13
Ohio	200,000	230,000	15
Oklahoma	62,000	74,000	19
Oregon	57,000	76,000	33
Pennsylvania	280,000	280,000	0
Rhode Island	24,000	24,000	0
South Carolina	67,000	80,000	19
South Dakota	17,000	19,000	12
Tennessee	100,000	120,000	20
Texas	270,000	340,000	26
Utah	22,000	32,000	45
Vermont	10,000	11,000	10
Virginia	100,000	130,000	30
Washington	83,000	110,000	33
West Virginia	40,000	44,000	10
Wisconsin	100,000	110,000	10
Wyoming	7,000	10,000	43

Source: "Alzheimer's Disease Facts and Figures", Alzheimer's Association, Chicago, Illinois, 2008. Also, Herbert, L. E., et al. "State-Specific Projections through 2025 of Alzheimer Disease Prevalence." Neurology 62:1645, 2004.

APPENDIX 3. ALZHEIMER'S ASSOCIATIONS AROUND THE WORLD

These listings are provided courtesy of Alzheimer's Disease International, London, England (infoalz.co.uk). Listed associations are members of the Alzheimer's Disease International, except those marked with an asterisk (*). Regional groups for Europe and Latin America are listed at the end.

Albania*

Albanian Alzheimer Society
Rr. Themistokli Germenji
Pall 10, Tirana, Albania
Tel/Fax: +355 4223 3289
Email: fleurapsy@yahoo.co.uk

Argentina

Asociacion de Lucha contra el Mal de Alzheimer
Lacarra No 78
1407 Capital Federal, Buenos Aires, Argentina
Tel/Fax: +54 11 4671 1187
Email: info@alma-alzheimer.org.ar
Web: www.alma-aizheimer.org.ar

Armenia

Alzheimer's Disease Armenian Association
Prof Michail Aghajanov Ph.D

Head of the Biochemistry Dept.
Yerevan State Medical University
2 Koriun Str
Yerevan 375025 Armenia
Tel: + 3741 582 412
Fax: + 3741 589 219
Email: michail.aghajanov@meduni.am

Aruba

Fundacion Alzheimer Aruba (FAA)
Avenida Milo Croes 29, Suite C
Oranjestad, Aruba
Tel: +297 582 1684
Fax: +297 584 8416
Email: alzheimeraruba@gmail.com
Web: www.alzheimer-aruba.org

Australia

Alzheimer's Australia
P.O. Box 4019
Hawker ACT 2614 Australia
Tel: +612 6254 4233
Helpline: 1800 100 500
Fax: +612 6278 7225
Web: www.alzheimers.org.au

Austria

Alzheimer Angehorige Austria
Reisnerstrasse 41
1030 Vienna, Austria
Tel/Fax: +43 1 713 6208
Email: alzheimeraustria@aon.at
Web: www.alzheimer-selbsthilfe.at

Bahrain*

Alzheimer Support Group
Dr Adel Al-Offi
Psychiatric Hospital
P.O.Box 5128
Kingdom Of Bahrain
Tel: +973 17 279 326

Bangladesh

Alzheimer Society of Bangladesh
Hall Para
PO: Thakurgaon-5100
Thakurgaon Sader
Bangladesh
Tel: +88 0172 049 8197
Email: alzbangladesh@yahoo.com

Barbados

Barbados Alzheimer's Association Inc

Room #3 Bethesda
Black Rock
St Michael
Barbados
Tel: +1 246 438 7111
Fax: +1 246 427 4256
Email: barbadosalzheimersassociation@caribsurf.com

Belgium

Ligue Nationale Alzheimer Liga
Rue Brogniezstraat, 46
B-1070
Brussel – Bruxelles – Brussels
Helpline: (within Belgium) 0800 15 225
Email: info@alzheimer-belgium.be
Web: www.alzheimer-belgium.be

Bermuda

Alzheimer's Family Support Group

P.O. Box DV114
Devonshire DVBX
Bermuda
Tel: +441 238 2168 (pm)
Fax: +441 234 1765
Email: JulieKay@ibl.bm

Bolivia *

Asociación Boliviana de Alzheimer y Otras Demencias
Casilla No. 9302
La Paz
Bolivia
Tel: +591 2249 4143
Email: elvio904@gmail.com

Brazil

FEBRAZ - Federacao Brasileira de Associacaoes de Alzheimer
CF 542214 e o endereco
Rua Frei Caneca, 915
conjunto 2, Sao Paolo, Brazil
01307-003
Tel/Fax: +55 11 3237 0385
Helpline: 0 800 55 1906
Email: abraz@abraz.org.br

Bulgaria

Compassion Alzheimer Bulgaria
Tzanko Djustabanov 30, fl.3
9000 Varna
Bulgaria
Tel: +359 52 505 873
Fax: +359 52 505 873
Email: compassion.alz@abv.bg

Canada

Alzheimer Society of Canada
20 Eglinton Avenue, W., Suite 1600
Toronto, Ontario M4R 1K8
Canada
Tel: 416 488 8772
Helpline: 800 616 8816
Fax: 416 488 3778
Email: info@alzheimer.ca
Web: www.alzheimer.ca

Chile

Corporación Alzheimer Chile
Desiderio Lemus 0143

(alt 1400 Av. Peru)
Recoleta
Santiago, Chile
Tel: +562 7321 532
Fax: +1 562 777 7431
Email: alzchile@adsl.tie.ci
Web: www.corporacionalzheimer.ci

China

Alzheimer's Disease Chinese

Department of Neurology
First Hospital Peking University
Beijing 100034
PR China
Tel: +8610 6521 2012
Helpline: +973 39425525
Email: alzbahrain@gmail.com

Colombia

Asociacion Colombiana de Alzheimer y Desordenes Relacionados
Calle 69 A No. 10-16
Sante Fe de Bogota D.C.
Colombia
Tel/Fax: +57 1 521 9401
Email: alzheimercolombia@hotmail.com

Costa Rica

Asociación Costarricense de Alzheimer y otras Demencias Asociadas

991-2070, Sabanilla de Montes de Oca
San Jose 11502 2070
Costa Rica
Tel: +905 285 3919
Email: ascada.alzcr@gmail.com
Web: ascadacr.wordpress.com

Croatia

Alzheimer Disease Societies Croatia
Vlaska 24a
HR-10000 Zagreb
Croatia

Tel/Fax: +385 1560 1500
Email: alzheimer@alzheimer.hr
Web: www.alzheimer.hr

Cuba

Sección Cubana de la Enfermedad de Alzheimer

Policlinico Docente Playa
Proyecto Alzheimer, Avenida 68 # 29B y 29F
Playa Ciudad de la Habana, CP. 11400
Cuba
Tel: +537 220 974
Fax: +537 336 857
Email: mguerra@infomed.sld.cu
Web: www.scual.sld.cu

Curacao

Stichting Alzheimer Curacao
Roodeweg 111
Willemstad
Curacao
Tel: +5 999 462 3900
Fax: +5 999 462 8554
Email: info@alzheimercuracao.org

Cyprus

Pancyprian Association of Alzheimer's Disease

31A Stadiou
6020 Larnaca
Cyprus
Tel: +357 24 627 104
Fax: +357 24 627 106
Email: alzhcyprus@cytanet.com.cy

Czech Republic

Ceská alzheimerovská spolecnost

Centre of Gerontology
Simunkova 1600
18200 Praha 8
Czech Republic

Tel: +420 286 883 676
Fax: +420 286 882 788
Email: martina.matlova@gerontocentrum.cz
Web: www.alzheimer.cz

Denmark

Alzheimerforeningen
Sankt Lukas Vej 6, 1
DK 2900 Hellerup
Denmark
Tel: +45 39 40 04 88
Fax: +45 39 61 66 69
Email: post@alzheimer.dk
Web: www.alzheimer.dk

Dominican Republic

Asociacion Dominicana de Alzheimer
Apartado Postal # 3321
Santo Domingo
Republica Dominicana
Tel: +1 809 544 1711
Fax: +1 809 544 1731
Email: asocalzheimer@codetel.net.do

Ecuador*

Fundacion Alzheimer Ecuador
Centra Medico Pasteur
Ave. Eloy Alfaro e Italia
2do Piso. Consultorio 204
Quito
Ecuador
Tel: +593 2 2521 660
Fax: +8610 6521 2386
Email: wyhbdyy@gmail.com

Egypt

Egyptian Alzheimer Group
c/o Professor A Ashour
233 26 July Street
Giza 12411
Cairo
Egypt

Tel: +202 334 70 133
Fax: +202 330 23 270
Email: ashour200835@yahoo.com

El Salvador

Asociacion de Familiares Alzheimer de El Salvador
Sara Zaldivar,
Colonia Costa Rica, Avenida Irazu
San Salvador
El Salvador
Tel: +503 2237 0787
Email: jrlopezcontreras@yahoo.com

Ethiopia*

Ye Ethiopia Alzhiemers Beshitegnoch Mahber
P. O. Box 28657/1000
Addis Ababa
Ethiopia
Tel: +251 91 113 8547
Email: ninates2002@yahoo.com

Finland

Alzheimer Society of Finland
Luotsikatu 4E
00160 Helsinki
Finland
Tel: +358 9 6226 2010
Fax: +358 9 6226 2020
Email: susann.morck@muistiliitto.fi
Web: www.muistiliitto.fi

France

Association France Alzheimer
21 Boulevard Montmartre
75002 Paris
France
Tel: +33 1 42 97 52 41
Fax: +33 1 42 96 04 70
Email: contact@francealzheimer.org
Web: www.francealzheimer.org

Germany

Deutsche Alzheimer Gesellschaft
Friedrichstr 236
10969 Berlin
Germany
Tel: +49 30 315 057 33
Helpline: 01803 171 017
Fax: +49 30 315 057 35
Email: deutsche.alzheimer.ges@t-online.de
Web: www.deutsche-alzheimer.de

Gibraltar*

The Gibraltar Alzheimer's and Dementia Support Group

P.O. Box 1196
Gibraltar
Tel: +350 2007 1049
Email: adsupportgroup@hotmail.com

Greece

Greek Association of AD and Related Disorders
Petrou Sindika 13
Thessaloniki
Hellas
Greece
Tel/Fax: +30 2310 810 411
Helpline: +30 2310 909 000
Email: info@alzheimer-hellas.gr
Web: www.alzheimer-hellas.gr

Guatemala

Asociación ERMITA, Alzheimer de Guatemala
10a. Calle 11-63
Zona 1, Ave. 1-48 Zona 1
Apto B, P O Box 2978
01901 Guatemala
Tel: +502 2 320 324
Fax: +502 2 381 122
Email, alzguate@quetzal.net

Honduras

Asociación Hondureña de Alzheimer

Apartado Postal 5005
Tegucigalpa Honduras, C.A.
Tel: +504 239 4512
Fax: +504 232 4580
Email: alzheimerhn@ashalz.org
Web: www.ashalz.org

Hong Kong SAR

Hong Kong Alzheimer's Disease Association

G/F, Wang Yip House
Wang Tau Hom Estate
Kowloon, Hong Kong SAR
China
Tel: +852 23 381 120
Carer Hotline: +852 23 382 277
Fax: +852 23 38 0772
Email: headoffice@hkada.org.hk
Web: www.hkada.org.hk

Hungary

Hungarian Alzheimer Society
Csaba u. 7A
H-1022
Budapest 1122 Hungary
Tel: +36 1 214 1022
Fax: +36 1 214 1022
Email: ehimmer@axelero.hu

Iceland*

FAAS
Austurbum 31
104 Reyjkjavik
Iceland
Tel: +354 533 1088
Fax: +354 533 1086
Email: faas@alzheimer.is
Web: www.alzheimer.is

India

Alzheimer's & Related Disorders Society of India

Guruvayoor Road
PO Box 53
Kunnamkulam
Kerala 680 503
India
Tel: +91 4885 223 801
Fax: +91 4885 224 817
Email: ardsinationaloffice@gmail.com *or* alzheimr@md2.vsnl.net.in
Web: www.alzheimer.org.in

Iran

Iran Alzheimer Association
Shahrak Ekbatan
North Sattari Exit
Next to Bassij Building
Tehran 13969
Iran
Tel: +98 21 4651 122
Fax: +98 21 4651 122
Email: info@alzheimer.ir
Web: www.alzheimer.ir

Ireland

Alzheimer Society of Ireland
National Office
Temple Road
Blackrock, Co. Dublin
Ireland
Tel: +353 1 284 6616
Helpline: +353 1 800 341 341
Fax: +353 1 284 6030
Email: info@alzheimer.ie
Web: www.alzheimer.ie

Israel

Alzheimer's Association of Israel

P O Box 8261
Ramat Gan

Israel 52181
Tel: +972 3 578 7660
Fax: +972 3 578 7661
Email: a-a-i@zahav.net.il
Web: www.alz-il.net

Italy

Federazione Alzheimer Italia
Via Tommaso Marino 7
20121 Milano
Italy
Tel: +39 02 809 767
Fax: +39 02 875 781
Email: alzit@tin.it
Web: www.alzheimer.it

Jamaica

Alzheimer's Jamaica

52 Duke Street
Kingston
Jamaica
Tel: +1 876 927 8967
Fax: +1 876 927 6155
Email: alzheimerja@cwjamaica.com

Japan

Alzheimer's Association Japan

c/o Kyoto Social Welfare Hall
Horikawa-Marutamachi, Kamigyo-Ku
Kyoto
Japan 602-8143
Tel: +81 75 811 8195
Fax: +81 75 811 8188
Email: office@alzheimer.or.jp
Web: www.alzheimer.or.jp

Jordan*

Jordanian Alzheimer Association
Faculty of Medicine
University of Jordan

P.O. Box 13490
Amman 11942
Jordan
Tel: +96 279 659 6390 or +96 265 355 000
Fax: +96 265 356 746
Email: e.alkhateeb@ju.edu.jo

Kenya*

Alzheimer's Association of Kenya

University of Nairobi
AIC Building, Flat No. 4
Ralph Bunche Road
P.O. Box 48423-00100
Nairobi
Kenya
Tel: +254 0202 716 315
Fax: +254 0202 717 168
Email: dmndetei@uonbi.ac.ke

Lebanon

Alzheimer's Association Lebanon

Tabet Bldg., 4th floor
Monot Street – Achrafieh
Lebanon
Tel: +961 3 245 606
Email:d.mansour@aizlebanon.org
Web: www.alzlebanon.org

Luxembourg*

Association Luxembourg Alzheimer
BP 5021
L-1050
Luxembourg
Tel: +352 42 16 76 1
Fax: +352 42 16 76 30
Helpline: +352 26 432 432
Email: info@alzheimer.lu
Web: www.alzheimer.lu

Macau SAR

Macau Alzheimer's Disease Association

9/F, Macau Landmark
555 Avenida da Amizade
Macau SAR
China
Fax: +853 8295 6225 or +853 2878 2233
Fax: +853 2836 5204 or +853 2878 1218
Email: info@mada.org.mo
Web: www.mada.org.mo

Macedonia

Association of Alzheimer Disease - Skopje Macedonia
UI. 50 Divizija br 34
Ordinacija Pasoski
1000 Skopje
Macedonia
Tel: +389 7576 1025 or +389 2317 9805
Email: makalzheimer@yahoo.com

Madagascar*

Madagascar Alzheimer Association
Masoandro Mody
Lot VK 70 Bis A
Fenomanana Mahazoarivo
BP 3081 - 101 Antananarivo
Madagascar
Tel: +26 120 226 1202
Email: contact@madagascar-alzheimer.org
Web: www.madagascar-alzheimer.org

Malaysia

Alzheimer's Disease Foundation Malaysia

No. 6 Lorong 11/8E, Sec. 11
46200 Petaling Jaya
Selangor Darul Ehsan
Malaysia
Tel: +603 7956 2008 or +603 7958 3008
Fax: +603 7960 8482
Email: adfmsec@streamyx.com

Web: www.adfm.org.my

Malta

Malta Dementia Society
Room 135
Department of Pharmacy
University of Malta
Msida
Malta
Email: info@maltadementiasociety.org.mt
Web: www.maitadementiasociety.org.mt

Mauritius

Foundation Mauritius Alzheimer
42/302 Stevenson Ave
Quatre Bornes
Mauritius
Tel: +230 467 6564
Helpline +230 800 1111
Fax: +230 466 4604
Email: assocalzheimer@intnet.mu
Web: http://mauritiusalzheimer.intnet.mu

Mexico

Federación Mexicana de Alzheimer

Av. Manrique 540
Colinas de San Gerardo
Tampico, Tamaulipas 89367
Mexico
Tel: +52 81 8333 6713 or +52 81 8347 4072
Helpline: 01 800 00 33362
Email: alzheimerfedma@yahoo.com
Web: http:/fedma.org.mx/

Namibia*

Elizabeth Swart (support groups)
Tel/Fax: + 264 61 227 023
Email: jtpot@mweb.com.na

Nepal*

Alzheimer's Association Nepal

P.O. Box 4795
20200 Kathmandu
Nepal
Tel: +977 1557 0361 or +977 1557 4380
Fax: +977 1 446 3029
Email: alz.nepal@gmail.com

Netherlands

Alzheimer Nederland
Post Bus 183
3980 CD BUNNIK
The Netherlands
Tel: +31 30 659 6900
Helpline: 030 656 7511
Fax: +31 30 659 6901
Email: info@alzheimer-nederland.nl
Web: www.alzheimer-nederland.nl

New Zealand

Alzheimers New Zealand
Level 3, Adelphi Finance House
15 Courtenay Place
PO Box 3643
Wellington
New Zealand
Tel: +64 4 381 2362
Helpline: 0800 004 001
Fax: +64 4 381 2365
Email: nationaloffice@alzheimers.org.nz
Web: www.alzheimers.org.nz

Nigeria

Alzheimer's Disease Association of Nigeria

c/o Dept. of Psychiatry
Nnamdi Azikiwe University Teaching Hospital
Nnewi
Anambra State
Nigeria

Tel: +234 46 463 663
Fax: +234 46 462 496
Email: alzheimernigeria@yahoo.com

Norway*

Nasjonalforeningen Demensforbundet
Oscarsgt 36 A, Postboks
7139 Majorstua
N 0307 Oslo
Norway
Tel: +47 23 12 00 00
Helpline: +47 815 33 032
Fax: +47 23 12 00 01
Email: post@nasjonalforeningen.no
Web: www.nasjonalforeningen.no

Pakistan

Alzheimer's *Pakistan*

146/1 Shadman Jail Road
Lahore 54000
Pakistan
Tel: +92 42 759 6589
Fax: +92 42 757 3911
Email: info@alz.org.pk
Web: www.alz.org.pk

Panama

AFA PADEA
Via Fernandez de Cordoba
Edificio Julimar, Primer Piso, Oficina #3
Apartado Postal 6-6839
El Dorado. Panama
Email: afapadea@gmail.com

Peru

Asociacion Peruana de Enfermedad de Alzheimer y Otras Demencias
Calle Inquisicion No 135, 2do piso
Esquina Av. Caminos del Inca
Santiago de Surco
Lima 33
Peru

Tel: +511 279 2331
Email: alzheimer2109@gmail.com
Web: www.alzheimerperu.org

Philippines

Alzheimer's Disease Association of the Philippines
St Luke's Medical Center
Medical Arts Bldg, Rm 410
E Rodriguez Sr Avenue, Quezon City
Philippines
Tel/fax: +632 723 1039
Email: adap@alzphilippines.com
Web: www.alzphilippines.com

Poland

Polish Alzheimer's Association
ul. Hoza 54/1
00-682 Warszawa
Poland
Tel/Fax: + 48 22 622 11 22
Email: alzheimer_pl@hotmail.com
Web: www.alzheimer.pl

Portugal*

Associacāo Portuguesa de Familiares e Amigos de Doentes de
   Alzheimer
Avenida de Ceuta Norte
Lote 1 - Lojas 1 e 2 - Quinta do Loureiro
1350-410 Lisboa
Portugal
Tel: +351 21 361 0460
Fax: +351 21 361 0469
Email: geral@alzheimerportugal.org
Web: www.alzheimerportugal.org

Puerto Rico

Asociación de Alzheimer y Desórdenes Relacionados de Puerto Rico
Apartado 362026
San Juan

Puerto Rico 00936-2026
Tel: +1 787 727 4151
Fax: +1 787 727 4890
Email: alzheimerpr@alzheimerpr.org
Web: www.alzheimerpr.org

Romania

Romanian Alzheimer Society
52 Austrului Street
2nd District 024074 Bucharest
Romania
Tel: +402 1 334 8940
Fax. +402 1 334 8940
Email: contact@alz.ro
Web: www.alz.ro

Russia*

Association for Support of Alzheimer's Disease Victims

34 Kashirskoye shosse
115522 Moscow
Russia
Tel: +7 095 324 9615
Fax: +7 095 114 4925
Email: sigavrilova@yandex.ru
Web: www.alzrus.org

Saint Martin*

Sint Maarten Alzheimer Foundation
St Petersroad 65
St Peters
Sint Maarten
Tel: + 599 520 0777
Email: alzheimersxm@gmail.com

Scotland

Alzheimer Scotland - Action on Dementia
22 Drumsheugh Gardens
Edinburgh
EH3 7RN
Scotland
Tel: +44 131 243 1453

Helpline: 0808 808 3000
Fax: +44 131 243 1450
Email: alzheimer@alzscot.org
Web: www.alzscot.org

Serbia*

Alzheimer Society of Serbia and Montenegro
Dr Subotica 6
Institute of Neurology
Belgrade 11000
Serbia
Tel: +381 11 361 4122
Fax: +381 11 684 577
Email: dpavlovic@drenik.net

Singapore

Alzheimer's Disease Association

Blk 157 Lorong 1 Toa Payoh
#01-1195
Singapore 310157
Tel: +65 6353 8734
Fax: +65 6353 8518
Email: adahq@alz.org.sg
Web: www.alz.org.sg

Slovak Republic

Slovak Alzheimer's Society

Mlynarovicova 21
851 03 Bratislava
Slovak Republic
Tel: +421 7 594 13 353
Fax: +421 7 547 74 276
Email: nilunova@savba.sk
Web: www.alzheimer.sk

South Africa

Alzheimer's South Africa

10 Boskruin Business Park
Bosbok Road

Randpark Ridge ext 58
2169
South Africa
Tel: +27 11 792 2511/8387
Fax: +27 11 792 7135
Helpline: 0860 102 681 (Mornings from 09h00)
Email: info@alzheimers.org.za
Web: www.alzheimers.org.za

South Korea

Alzheimer's Association, Korea

#52, Machon 2-Dong
Songpa-ku
Seoul 138-122
South Korea
Tel: +82 2 431 9963
Helpline: +82 2 431 9993
Fax: +82 2 431 9964
Email: afcde01@unitel.co.kr
Web: www.alzza.or.kr

Spain

Confederación Española de Familiares de Enfermos de
    Alzheimer
C/ Pedro Miguel Alcatarena n° 3
31014 Pamplona (Navarra)
Spain
Tel: +34 902 174 517
Fax: +34 948 265 739
Email: ceafa@ceafa.es
Web: www.ceafa.es

Sri Lanka

Lanka Alzheimer's Foundation

19 Havelock Road
Colombo 5
Sri Lanka
Tel: +94 1 583 488
Fax: +94 1 732 745
Email: alzheimers@alzlanka.org

Web: www.alzlanka.org

Suriname*

Surinam Alzheimer Society (SAS)
Lallk Rookhweg 91
Paramaribo
Suriname
Tel: +00 597 490261
Tel/Fax: +00 597 431261
Fax: +94 1 732 745
Email: H.vanDis@uva.nl

Sweden

Alzheimerföreningen i Sverige
Karl XII gatan 1
221 00 Lund, Sweden
Tel: +46 46 14 73 18
Fax: +46 46 18 89 76
Email: info@alzheimerforeningen.se
Web: www.alzheimerforeningen.se

Switzerland

Association Alzheimer Suisse
8 Rue des Pêcheurs
CH-1400 Yverdon-les-Bains
Switzerland
Tel: +41 24 426 2000
Fax: +41 24 426 2167
Email: alz@bluewin.ch
Web: www.alz.ch

Syria

Syrian Alzheimer and Memory Diseases Society
PO Box 14189
Damascus
Syria
Tel: +963 94 74 1955
Fax: +963 11 54 21893
Email: afodafro@scs-net.org

TADA Chinese Taipei

TADA

10F-1, No. 206, Sec. 2
Nanchang Road
100
Taipei
Taiwan
Tel: +886 2 23 149 690
Fax: +886 2 23 147 508
Email: tada.tada@msa.hinet.net
Web: www.tada2002.org.tw

Thailand

Alzheimer's and Related Disorders Association of Thailand

114 Pinakorn 4
Boramratchachunee Road
Talingchan
Bangkok 10170
Thailand
Tel: +66 2 880 8542/7539
Fax: +66 2 880 7244
Web: www.azthai.org

Trinidad and Tobago

Alzheimer's Association of Trinidad and Tobago

c/o Soroptimist International Port of Spain
15 Nepaul Street
St James, Port of Spain
Republic of Trinidad and Tobago
Tel: +1 868 622 6134
Fax: +1 868 627 6731
Email: nebinniss@gmail.com

Tunisia*

Association Alzheimer Tunisie
BP N°116
Cité Elkhadra
1003 Tunis
Tunisia

Tel: +216 98 613 976
Fax: +216 98 704 592
Email: alzheimer.tunisie@gmail.com
Web: www.alzheimertunisie.com

Turkey

Turkish Alzheimer Association
Halaskargazi Cad. No: 115 Da: 4 Harbiye
Istanbul
Turkey
Tel: +90 212 224 41 89
Helpline: 0800 211 8024
Fax: +90 212 296 05 79
Email: alzdernek@alzheimerdernegi.org.tr
Web: www.alzheimerdernegi.org.tr

Ukraine*

The Association for the Problems of Alzheimer's Disease

Institute of Gerontology
67 Vyshgorodskaya Street
04114 Kiev
Ukraine
Tel: +380 44 431 0526
Fax: +380 44 432 9956
Email: admin@geront.kiev.ua

United Kingdom (except Scotland)

Alzheimer's Society

Devon House
58 St Katharine's Way
London
E1W 1JX
United Kingdom
Tel: +44 20 7423 3500
Helpline: 0845 300 0336
Fax: +44 20 7423 3501
Email: enquiries@alzheimers.org.uk
Web: www.alzheimers.org.uk

United States of America

Alzheimer's Association

225 N Michigan Avenue
Suite 1700
Chicago, Illinois 60601
United States of America
Tel: +1 312 335 8700
Helpline: 0800 272 3900
Fax: +1 312 335 1110
Email: info@alz.org
Web: www.alz.org

Uruguay

Asociación Uruguaya de Alzheimer y Similares

Magallanes 1320
11200 Montevideo
Uruguay
Tel: +598 2 400 8797
Fax: +598 2 400 8797
Email: audasur@gmail.com
Web: http://audas.wordpress.com

Venezuela

Fundación Alzheimer de Venezuela

Calle El Limon, Qta Mi Muñe, El Cafetal
Caracas
Venezuela
Tel: +58 212 414 6129
Fax: +58 212 9859 183
Email: alzven@gmail.com
Web: www.alzheimer.org.ve

Zimbabwe

Zimbabwe Alzheimer's and Related Disorders Association

PO Box CH 832
Chisipite
Harare

Zimbabwe
Tel: +263 4 860 166
Fax: +263 4 704 487
Email: zarda@zol.co.zw

Regional groups

Europe

Alzheimer Europe
145 route de Thionville
L-2611
Luxembourg
Tel: +352 29 79 70
Fax: +352 29 79 72
Email: info@alzheimer-europe.org
Web: www.alzheimer-europe.org

Latin America

Alzheimer Iberoamerica
C/ Pedro Alcatarena n° 3 Bajo
31014 Pamplona (Navarra)
Spain
Tel: +34 902 174 517
Fax: +34 948 265 739
Email: ceafa@ceafa.es
Web: http://www.alzheimeriberoamerica.org/